705

GW00601798

Applied Neurophysiology

With particular reference to anaesthesia

J.A. Simpson MD, FRCP, FRCP (Ed), FRCP (Glas), FRS (Ed)
Professor of Neurology, University of Glasgow
and Institute of Neurological Sciences, Glasgow

W. Fitch PhD, MB ChB, FFARCS
Reader in Anaesthesia, University of Glasgow
and Royal Infirmary, Glasgow

WRIGHT
London · Boston · Singapore ·
Sydney · Toronto · Wellington

John Wright
is an imprint of Butterworth Scientific

First published 1988

© Butterworth & Co. (Publishers) Ltd., 1988

British Library Cataloguing in Publication Data

Simpson, J.A.
  Applied neurophysiology: with particular
  reference to anaesthesia.
  1. Neurophysiology
  I. Title I. Fitch, W.
  612'.8   QP 361

ISBN 0 7236 0707 9

Typeset by Activity Limited, Salisbury, Wiltshire
Printed and bound in Great Britain at the University Press, Cambridge

Preface

This book has not been entitled 'Clinical Neurophysiology' as that term has been adopted for the diagnostic specialties of electroencephalography, electromyography and related investigative procedures in neurology. No more is this a systematic textbook of vertebrate neurophysiology for neuroscientists. We were asked to write a book for anaesthetists primarily, to promote understanding of the structure and function of the human nervous system. For that reason we have presented concepts rather than critical discussions of experimental work. To give detailed references to original work would have required a different kind of book: we have instead recommended further reading where such information can be obtained.

We anticipated that the trainee practical anaesthetist would need to understand the neural mechanisms for consciousness and awareness, respiration, pain, muscle tone and the autonomic control of the cardiovascular system but that cellular physiology could be summarized as being readily available in other texts. It soon became apparent, however, that a selective approach had serious limitations. Although these topics are given special prominence, it was evident that a comprehensive though less detailed coverage was necessary for understanding of these important areas, and that the conventional arrangement of sensory and motor 'systems' etc. was detrimental to understanding the roles of the diencephalon and cerebral cortex.

The material has been organized to stress the distributed nature of functional systems and their integration, and attention is drawn to anatomical structures or important functional concepts by free use of italic type since their use in context usually makes it unnecessary to give formal definitions. In the main, the anatomical nomenclature and connections described are from *Human Neuroanatomy* by M. B. Carpenter. Unfortunately the elegant but simplified drawings of anatomical connections in other publications omit the important connections of the mid-brain and diencephalon and are often more relevant to laboratory animals than to man. Most of the illustrations in the present text attempt to show distributed systems more accurately. Unfortunately there is no substitute for a knowledge of the anatomy of the human nervous system but the already complicated drawings would be impossible to follow if they were burdened with lettering. As an alternative, the reader is 'talked through' the illustration by means of an extended legend, but at a second reading it is recommended that a good anatomical atlas should be compared.

Anaesthesiology is now probably the largest hospital specialty in collaboration with specialists in intensive care, ophthalmology, orthopaedics and many others. Certain chapters, such as those on vision, control of gaze, hearing and locomotion, are intended for such specialists but they have also been included to introduce concepts on brain stem automatisms and cortical function necessary to understand respiration and conscious awareness. It is hoped that the additional coverage of these chapters may interest other clinicians, psychologists, speech pathologists and even neurologists in training. The final section on the autonomic nervous system continues with an account of the regulation of the cerebral circulation. In view of the importance of this for the practising anaesthetist, we have provided quantitative data and references to original studies which were not thought necessary in other sections.

J.A.S.
W.F.

Acknowledgements

Acknowledgement is made to the following authors, publishers and journals for permission to reproduce illustrations.

Fig. 1.3   P. Seaman, 1972: *Pharmacol. Rev.* **24**, 583–655.

Fig. 2.3   J. del Castillo, 1960: *Res. Publ. Assoc. Res. Nerv. Ment. Dis.* **38**, 90–143.

Fig. 4.2   L. Bindman, O. Lippold, 1981: *The Neurophysiology of the Cerebral Cortex.* London, Edward Arnold.

Fig. 9.2   I. A. Boyd, 1985: In M. Swash and C. Kennard, ed., *Scientific Basis of Clinical Neurology.* Edinburgh, Churchill Livingstone.

Fig. 10.1   R. L. Gregory, 1966: *Eye and Brain: the Psychology of Seeing.* London, Weidenfeld and Nicolson.

Fig. 16.1   R. Cooper, J. W. Osselton, J. C. Shaw, 1980: *EEG Technology*, 3rd ed. London, Butterworths.

Fig. 16.2   L. G. Kiloh, A. J. McComas, J. W. Osselton, A. R. M. Upton, 1981: *Clinical Electroencephalography*, 4th ed. London, Butterworths.

Fig. 16.3   Dr Anne P. McGeorge, Department of Clinical Neurophysiology, Institute of Neurological Sciences, Glasgow.

Fig. 19.5   J. A. Simpson, 1969: In R. N. Herrington, ed., *Current Problems in Neuropsychiatry, Schizophrenia, Epilepsy, the Temporal Lobe. Br. J. Psychiat.* Special Publication No. 4.

Fig. 20.3   F. Plum, J. B. Posner, 1966: *The Diagnosis of Stupor and Coma.* Philadelphia, Davis.

Fig. 24.2   R. E. Burke, V. R. Edgerton, 1975: In J. H. Wilmore and J. F. Keogh, ed., *Exercise and Sport Sciences Review*, vol. 3. New York, Academic Press.

Fig. 25.3/4   F. Knowles, 1974: In R. Bellairs and E. G. Gray, ed., *Essays on the Nervous System.* Oxford, Oxford University Press.

Fig. 26.1/2   G. Ross, 1979: *Essentials of Human Physiology.* Chicago, Year Book.

Fig. 26.7b   K. H. Jakobs, G. Schultz, 1982: *J. Cardiovasc. Pharmacol.* **4**, S63–S67 (adapted).

Fig. 26.14 and *Table* 26.4   R. Bannister, 1983: *Autonomic Failure. A Textbook of Clinical Disorders of the Autonomic Nervous System.* London, Oxford University Press.

Table 26.3   W. S. Nimmo, 1984: *Br. J. Anaesth.* **56**, 29–36 (adapted).

Fig. 27.2   A. M. Harper, J. McCulloch, 1985: In M. Swash and C. Kennard, ed., *Scientific Basis of Clinical Neurology.* Edinburgh, Churchill Livingstone.

Fig. 27.5   A. M. Harper, H. I. Glass, 1965: *J. Neurol. Neurosurg. Psychiatry* **28**, 449–52.

Fig. 27.6   D. G. McDowall, 1966: In J. P. Payne and D. W. Hill, ed., *Oxygen Measurements in Blood and Tissues.* London, Churchill.

Fig. 28.4   B. Jennett, G. Teasdale, 1981: *Management of Head Injuries.* Philadelphia, Davis.

Fig. 28.5   W. Fitch, D. G. McDowall, 1969: *Int. Anesthesiol. Clin.* **7**, 639–62.

Contents

PART 1 Cellular Organization of the Nervous System

Chapter 1
The excitable cell

The resting potential

Every living cell has a potential difference across its membrane due to the fact that charged particles are separated by a semi-permeable membrane which prevents the charged particles (ions) from redistributing themselves randomly. The special feature of the so-called 'excitable cells' (nerve, muscle) is that the permeability can be changed by processes which either increase (hyperpolarize) or decrease (depolarize) the potential difference.

The membrane is a double layer of phospholipid molecules with specialized protein molecules inserted into it, some of which are structured to form channels which allow passage of water and ions (*Fig. 1.1*). There are at least two types of *ion channels* which differ in channel diameter, so restricting the ion species which each will pass (in fact the ion and its shell of water). Thus, one type allows ready passage of potassium and chloride ions. The other will pass, less readily, sodium ions and the similarly dimensioned lithium ions. The channels also have a selectivity filter for certain ion species, apparently because of energy barriers which remove the shell of water molecules around the ions. In the sodium channel the sodium ions bind to fixed negatively charged sites (probably oxygen atoms) which force them into single file. Similar constraints probably exist in the potassium channel. Thus the resting membrane has little permeability to ions. There are some molecules which are capable of inactivating the passage of ions by blocking the channels. Tetrodotoxin (from the puffer fish and other poisonous animals) is a complex molecule which can bind to the outward-facing molecule of the sodium chan-nels and so block passage of sodium ions. Similarly, tetraethylammonium ion applied internally blocks potassium conductance.

In addition to these specialized channels, there is an *active pumping mechanism* which transports sodium ions out of the cell and potassium ions into it. The structural basis for the pump is unknown but the action of certain poisons indicates that its carrier molecules are driven by energy derived from metabolic processes within the cell, probably from energy-rich ATP hydrolysed by Na-K-ATPase. The important part of this process is the removal of sodium from the cell cytoplasm as this permits the intracellular substance to have a sodium concentration only about 10 per cent of that of the extracellular fluid since the pump extrudes sodium at a rate that exactly balances the net passive inward membrane current. However, the membrane is slightly leaky to cations even when the channels are 'closed', although it is impermeable to anions other than Cl^- (eg glutamic and aspartic ions) and the imbalance of positive charges produced by the pump sets up an electric potential across the membrane (the *resting potential*). Potassium ions, which pass more readily than sodium, are retained within the cell in higher concentration than in the external fluid and chloride ions are extruded until the combined electrochemical gradient for potassium and chloride ions is about zero, while the imbalance of sodium ions makes the interior of the cell at a negative potential relative to the exterior.

The increased permeability to K^+ ions on depolarizing the membrane is vastly greater than the opposite effect of a hyperpolarizing current. This phenomenon is termed *delayed rectification*. Muscle membrane has an additional *anomalous rectification* in the opposite

1

2

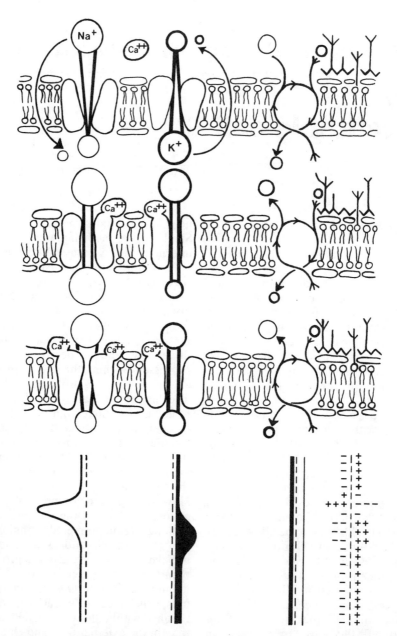

Fig. 1.1. Schematic diagram of the outer membrane of an excitable cell (extracellular space above, cytoplasm below). The structural protein bounding layers are separated by a double layer of orientated lipids. The outer surface has a glycoprotein 'backbone' into which are set a 'fuzz' of polysaccharides, glycoproteins and glycolipids (*right*) with fixed anions. The membrane is leaky (*upper*) but a metabolically driven pump extrudes Na^+ and introduces a smaller number of K^+ ions into the cell. The difference in charge is seen as a resting potential across the membrane (positive outside with respect to the cytoplasm). This sets up a gradient of both potential and cation concentrations across the membrane. This is abolished and temporarily reversed when an electric current activates the opening gates of specific channels allowing Na^+ ions to rush in and K^+ to emerge more slowly. Calcium ions (Ca^{++}) are necessary to open the gates. The sodium channel is soon closed by a voltage- and calcium-dependent inactivation gate but passive flux of K^+ continues until the balance is restored. Specific channels for transfer of calcium are not shown in the diagram which illustrates three states — resting (*upper*), activated (*middle*) and inactivated (*lower*).

Beneath each channel and the Na–K–ATPase pump are illustrated the fluxes of Na^+ and K^+ due to each. Intracellular shifts are to the left of the dashed line, extracellular extrusions to the right. The net charge distribution across the membrane is shown bottom right. This illustrates the change from resting to action potential (depolarization) with after-hyperpolarization which is slowly abolished by the sodium pump.

direction. Membrane permeability decreases during the outward flow of potassium current and increases with inward flow. Depolarizing drugs cause sufficient loss of potassium from muscles to raise the level of plasma potassium. In patients with severe burns or with extensive injuries to soft tissues, administration of succinylcholine may raise the potassium efflux to levels which may cause cardiac arrest. There is a similar risk in its administration to patients with widespread denervation (polyneuritis) or myotonic dystrophy.

The total body potassium is obviously significant for the excitable cell, but for its polarization and ability to produce action potentials, the external sodium level is more important than the level of potassium — a fact commonly overlooked in clinical medicine. Muscle is much more vulnerable than nerve to low potassium levels. Anomalous rectification seems to indicate a valve-like mechanism to resist a net outflow of potassium ions from the muscle cell, probably in the sarcoplasmic reticulum.

So long as the sodium–potassium pump operates, the intracellular cytoplasm is rich in potassium and organic anions but poor in sodium and chloride compared to the external fluid. This is a potentially unstable situation with *ion diffusion gradients* across the membrane. If the metabolic pump fails, there is a slow but continuous inward movement of Na^+ ions and compensatory loss of K^+ ions so that both concentration gradients gradually disappear. This is a comparatively slow process as the permeability to sodium is so low. It takes many hours for the resting potential to drop significantly and during this time action potentials can still be generated. The electrochemical gradients are the motive force; but eventually the gradients are dissipated. This demonstrates the importance of the metabolic process for 're-charging the battery', but also indicates that the ion shifts across the membrane are too slow to account for the action potential which is the hallmark of excitable cells, differentiating them from other cells which share the above mechanisms for polarizing the cell by electrochemical gradients.

The action potential

The time courses of passive diffusion of ions into and out of the cell described so far are insufficient to account for the generation of an action potential. If the membrane of an excitable cell is depolarized beyond a critical level (by passing an electric current through it, or by increasing the extracellular concentration of potassium) it develops a high permeability to Na^+ ions which then pass into the cell until the sodium equilibrium potential is reached. The influx of positive charges reverses the potential across the membrane. Activation of a sodium carrier has been postulated but it now seems that an adequate explanation is a voltage-regulated adjustment of a 'gate' mechanism at the external opening of the *sodium channels* (*Fig.* 1.2). At the normal resting potential, the channel appears to be occluded at its external opening by charged particles. When the membrane is depolarized (internal potential more positive) these gating particles are believed to change configuration by a series of steps to an 'open' position which allows sodium ions to pass freely through the channel. Passage of these positive ions into the cell further depolarizes it and therefore opens the gate still wider and the permeability increases explosively. The increase in conductance of sodium (with passage of sodium ions into the cell) is regenerative because of this gate effect, which is the characteristic feature of excitable cells. So far as nerve is concerned, the channel remains open for a very short time (about 1 ms) during which about 100 sodium ions pass through. Then the gate appears to be inactivated, even though the membrane remains depolarized. The method of *inactivation* of the gate is not clear, probably a further configurational change. Whatever it is, the gate is refractory to further opening for a short period.

Ion channels are believed to be protein polymers floating in the lipid membrane of the cell, with subunits of the complex arranged to form an obstructed pore through the membrane. Appropriate ions or an applied voltage alter the architecture of the channel and this *conformational change* opens or closes the channel to allow passage of ions, atoms or molecules if they are sufficiently small, appropriately charged and have a concentration gradient across the cell membrane. The conformational change may be induced by specific chemical substances (hormones or neurotransmitters) attached to receptor sites. The

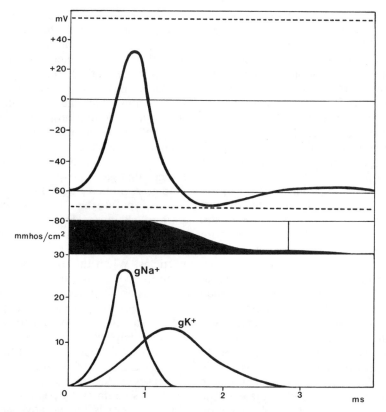

Fig. 1.2. *Upper*: Typical action potential recorded intracellularly. The dotted lines represent the sodium (*upper*) and potassium (*lower*) equilibrium potentials. The resting potential is −60 mV. *Lower*: The ionic conductances for sodium (g Na$^+$) and potassium (g K$^+$) across the cell membrane which generate the current responsible for the action potential. Between the graphs is an index of threshold to a second stimulus. During the first part of the action potential the membrane is completely unresponsive to a second stimulus (absolutely refractory). This is followed by a relatively refractory period. Under certain environmental conditions, a period of supernormality may follow the absolutely refractory period. Cyclical alternation of supernormality and subnormality leading to autorhythmicity occurs with low extracellular Ca^{++}.

architecture of each polymer is critical and may be distorted by changes in the fluidity of the lipid membrane in which it floats. Many lipid-soluble substances alter the fluidity and increase the rotational mobility of the protein structures, distort their architecture and permit increased passive diffusion of ions between the structures. Substances that do this act as local anaesthetics (*Fig.* 1.3).

Although the evidence is less satisfactory, it is likely that a similar voltage-dependent gate is opened at the internal end of the *potassium channel*. Depolarization of the membrane opens this a little later than the sodium channel and about ten times more slowly. Furthermore, the number of potassium channels per unit area of surface membrane is only about 10

per cent of the sodium channels (for nerve axon). For these reasons, the potassium conduction following depolarization is much slower than the sodium. Indeed it does not reach its peak until the sodium conductance has almost stopped, but it then continues for about three times the duration of the sodium conductance. While each gate is open the appropriate ion is transferred through its channel according to the concentration gradient, ie sodium passes rapidly into the cell and potassium flows out more slowly.

The sodium flux goes on until the sodium equilibrium potential is reached. As this takes place before significant K$^+$ loss has occurred, there is now a surplus of positive charges within the cell and the potential across the

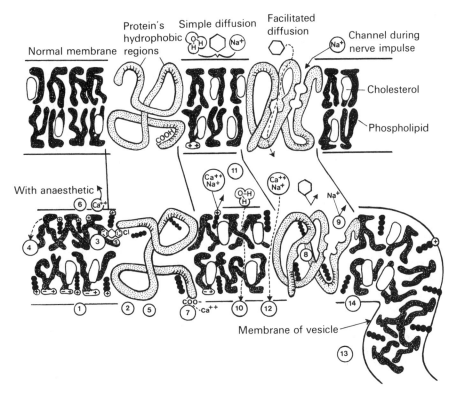

Fig. 1.3. Diagram of cell membrane showing some effects of drug occupation of membrane by anaesthetic agent. The lower diagram indicates: 1, drug occupation of membrane at low concentrations; 2, expansion of membrane with pressure alteration at higher concentrations; 3, increased rotational mobility of membrane units ('fluidization'); 4, decreased translocation of membrane lipids; 5, membrane enzymes activated or inhibited; 6, displacement of Ca^{++} by amine anaesthetics or; 7, increased membrane Ca^{++} by neutral anaesthetics; 8, diffusion of glucose and choline decreased; 9, ion exchange decreased during nerve impulse; 10, increased passive diffusion of water and urea; 11, decreased passive diffusion of ions by anaesthetic amines, or; 12, increased passive diffusion of ions by neutral anaesthetics; 13, increased exocytosis (neurosecretion); 14, dissociation of lipid-protein complexes at high anaesthetic concentrations.

membrane is reversed. Inactivation of the sodium channel while the potassium outflow is still increasing rapidly restores the potential to its resting value, but the potassium conductance continues beyond this stage so that the cell becomes hyperpolarized (*positive after potential*) until the resting state is restored by passive diffusion of potassium and active extrusion of sodium by the sodium pump. The relative proportion of potassium to sodium channels varies between tissues and species. The node of Ranvier of the mammalian myelinated nerve fibre is now believed to have many sodium but few potassium channels.

The other important cation is *calcium*. Although it plays a vitally important role in most physiological processes, the mechanisms involved are not well understood. At the excitable cell membrane, Ca^{2+} and (possibly Mg^{2+}) enters the cell by at least two channels. One of these is probably the Na^+ channel as Ca^{2+} entry is linked with Na^+. It occurs at the time of peak inward Na^+ current of the action potential and is blocked by tetrodotoxin. It is suggested that sodium–calcium exchange occurs and this channel is *voltage-dependent*. There is also at least one 'late' calcium channel (sometimes called the *slow channel*) which is not voltage-dependent and which may act as a second K^+ channel. These channels are still somewhat speculative and may not be represented in all excitable membranes. Evidence for their existence is mainly in invertebrate axons and in cardiac and smooth muscle, but they have been provisionally identified in the soma-dendritic area of vertebrate motoneurones and autonomic neurones with α-adrenoceptors and it seems likely that they will also be found in axons, which show accommodation properties (*see below*). In muscle (striated and cardiac) the calcium channels are mainly in the transverse tubular system and sarcoplasmic reticulum.

The sodium–calcium linkage promotes outward diffusion of sodium from the cell and the 'late' calcium channel increases K^+ conductance, both processes tending to restore the membrane potential after depolarization and indeed temporarily to hyperpolarize the membrane immediately after the action potential. These 'stabilizing' effects will be discussed after the action potential proper. Further important actions of calcium ions, including the release of neurotransmitters at nerve terminals, will be discussed in the appropriate section (p. 24). The calcium flux does not contribute materially to the action potential except in special experimental circumstances. Modulation of voltage-sensitive Ca^{2+} channels is a probable mechanism for the known effects of certain neurotransmitters and neuropeptides (p. 36) on the duration of neuronal action potentials. Despite the considerable amount of calcium entering the nerve cell, the concentration of calcium ions in axoplasm is low as most is sequestered in mitochondria and endoplasmic reticulum and some is bound to protein (calmodulin). Calcium in axoplasm is required for axoplasmic transport. In muscle fibre it binds reversibly with specific sites on myofibrils, causing them to contract.

In summary, the rapid change of potential (the 'action potential') is due to opening of voltage-dependent channels with different time courses, and the role of the energy-dependent pump mechanism is to restore the resting potential. The amplitude and time course of the action potential depends on the ionic gradients and channel sizes and hence the action potential is an 'all or none' response to adequate ('threshold') depolarization of the membrane. Calcium plays an important role in restoration of the membrane potential.

PROPAGATION OF ACTION POTENTIAL

The facility with which ions cross the membrane determines its electrical resistance. Flow of charge through a resistance constitutes electrical current but this can only take place when a circuit is completed. Ionic charge is drawn from an adjacent region of the excitable cell and the circuit is completed through the neighbouring membrane, most readily at those parts where current can easily flow across it — ie at the next potassium channels. This, of course, depolarizes the adjacent membrane setting up an action potential there, and so the action potential is propagated in all directions away from the initial site of depolarization (*Fig.* 1.4). What happens next depends on the structure of the excitable cell and differs for nerve cell soma, axon, dendrites or muscle. Further differences between these cells, the effective stimulus for depolarization, will depend on peculiarities of membrane structure, including the presence of specialized receptor sites which, like the ionic channels considered so far, are specialized protein molecules traversing the lipid membrane.

Chemical substances with affinity for each of these sites may depolarize the cell or block evocation of an action potential (and hence block conduction of the impulse). It will be convenient to postpone discussion of drugs

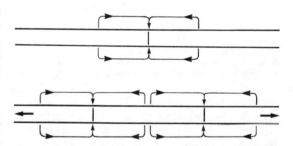

Fig. 1.4. *Orthodromic and antidromic propagation of a nerve impulse.* An area of depolarization of nerve membrane (*upper*) acts as a sink for current to flow into from neighbouring polarized membrane on each side. This creates depolarized areas which act as further current sinks and this change propagates in both directions (*lower*). The direction for normal transmission is termed 'dromic' and the other direction (e.g. towards the soma of a motoneurone) is 'antidromic'. An orthodromically conducted action potential spreads into collateral or terminal branches of an axon but an antidromic impulse starting in a branch tends to block at the confluence (T-junction effect). Action potentials will not spread retrogradely across a synapse, which conducts only in one direction, usually by release of a transmitter chemical by the pre-synaptic neurone which binds to receptors on the dendrites or soma of the post-synaptic neurone(s).

with affinity for receptors to the chapters on synapses and neuromuscular junction. Those that depolarize or block by action on the ion channels or the 'electrogenic' pump affect all excitable tissues to a greater or lesser degree. *Local anaesthetics* are believed to act by blocking activation of both sodium and potassium conductances; possibly ion channels are blocked only in the open state. The rate of rise, overshoot and rate of fall of the action potential are decreased and eventually depolarization is blocked. There are quantitative differences between nerve and muscle — the action being mainly on sodium conductance in nerve and on potassium conductance in muscle. The effects are transient.

A more complete block is produced by some naturally occurring toxins. *Tetrodotoxin* from the puffer fish (and certain other aquatic animals) has already been mentioned. Another is *saxitoxin*, a paralytic poison of equally high toxicity elaborated by a species of marine plankton (*Gonyaulax*) which may be so numerous in certain conditions as to cause a 'red tide'. Shellfish feeding in these waters concentrate the toxin and are highly poisonous. These biotoxins have a complex organic molecule. At one end of it there are one (tetrodotoxin) or two (saxitoxin) positively charged guanidium groups which can enter the sodium channel, but the main part of the molecule cannot do so and effectively plugs the sodium channel. (The effect is very specific and the affinity very high. Modern measurements of the number and distribution of sodium channels on an excitable membrane depend on the counting of isotopically labelled molecules of one of these paralytic poisons fixed to the surface of the cell.) A related molecule, guanidine hydrochloride, has its main effect on the cell membrane of cholinergic nerve terminals where it facilitates the release of acetylcholine (p. 19).

Anions

The most important anions within the cell are the comparatively large organic ions (eg glutamate, aspartate and organic phosphates), too large to move freely across the membrane and hence not contributing to the action potential but playing a role in the resting potential of the cell. On the other hand, the cell membrane is so freely permeable in both directions to chloride ions that their movements play no more than a negligible role during the action potential, the net flux being very small. Chloride shift out of the cell plays a greater part in the repolarization of the membrane. When the external sodium concentration is lowered (passively followed by the internal sodium) the action potential takes longer to subside to normal (*see* negative after potential, p. 4). During this time the membrane is more readily depolarized by a further stimulus and repetitive firing may occur, especially if external potassium is also low. A similar membrane hyperexcitability occurs if there is reduction in the permeability of the resting membrane to chloride. It appears that this abnormality is the cause of the membrane hyperexcitability of human myotonia congenita and that of goats with hereditary myotonia. The chloride permeability of cell membrane is also reduced by monocarboxylic aromatic acids and by certain sterols such as 20,25-diazocholesterol. Potassium and chloride conductances of mammalian muscle are both reduced by denervation. This reduces the critical membrane depolarization required to produce an action potential and reduces the repolarization electrolyte shifts, causing fibrillation potentials. No doubt similar spontaneous activity is generated in dying neurones.

Myotonic activity is reduced by procainamide, phenytoin or quinine as well as by reducing extracellular potassium.

Membrane stabilizers

The action of local anaesthetics such as procaine in blocking activation of the gate of the sodium channel (p. 3) has been described as 'membrane stabilization'. Phenytoin has a highly complex action, including stimulation of the sodium pump (driving Na^+ out of and K^+ into the cell) and increasing the availability of high-energy phosphates. The effects of quinine and quinidine are grossly similar to those of the local anaesthetics but their actions have not been identified at the molecular level. Cardiac glycosides (like ouabain) and aglycones (like strophanthidin) act specifically to inhibit Na^+

and K^+ transport. It is possible that this action is on the sodium–potassium pump ATPase which is sensitive to cardiac glycosides. This enzyme is also inhibited by calcium ions but only when applied intracellularly.

The role of *calcium* as a membrane stabilizer is still controversial. One theory is that it occupies and neutralizes negative charges of adjacent molecules in the membrane. The external calcium ion concentration alters the dependence of the membrane permeability channels on the membrane potential, as described above. Decreasing the external calcium ion concentration facilitates depolarization and increasing it facilitates hyperpolarization. During the action potential there is an increased influx of calcium. Since almost all of the intracellular calcium is bound, a large influx during the action potential could cause a significant change in the amount of 'free' Ca^{2+} within the cell. It could be speculated that it might play a role in activating the K^+ channel gate. It has additional important actions in muscle cells.

It is perhaps misleading to use the vague term 'membrane stabilization' to cover all of the effects described in this section. They are certainly not identical. Procaine, for instance, reduces the maximum Na^+ and K^+ permeability without any great effect on the rate processes, whereas Ca^{2+} ions located on the cell surface reduce excitability by altering dependence of the rate processes on the membrane potential without affecting maximum Na^+ and K^+ permeabilities. To put it another way, high calcium ion concentration on the surface of the membrane opposes the increase in potassium conductance associated with small depolarizations and hence the explosive self-regenerative action potential mechanism is less likely to follow. Conversely, with low calcium at the cell surface the action potential mechanism is evoked by quite small depolarizations of the membrane — ie it is more excitable. Since at the time the action potential is prolonged and the negative after potential (p. 4) may still be significant after inactivation of the Na^+ channel gate has subsided, the slightly depolarized membrane again swings into the action potential phase, and so on repetitively. The normal process, termed *accommodation* (p. 10), is defective.

This 'oscillation' of the membrane means that a single stimulus is followed by a train of action potentials and, if the calcium level at the cell surface is sufficiently low, by 'spontaneous' trains of action potentials. These are the basis of the sensory and motor phenomena of *hypocalcaemic tetany*. The same mechanism is invoked if the calcium ions are competitively displaced by certain other divalent cations, as in hypermagnesaemic tetany. The effect is most obvious on nerve axons. Muscle is also affected (eg the prolonged Q–T segment of the ECG), but the clinical manifestations of tetany are due to repetitive firing of peripheral nerve fibres. Latent tetany can be identified by measuring the time constant of accommodation (p. 10). Further lowering of the extracellular calcium is accompanied by failure to produce action potentials.

ANOXIA OF EXCITABLE CELLS

A similar decrease of accommodation, membrane instability and repetitive firing of action potentials going on to failure is caused by anoxia of excitable cells. This is the basis of paraesthesia or tetanic cramp when a sphygmomanometer cuff is applied, preceding loss of excitability and of conduction. Similar spontaneous phenomena are associated with hypoxia of the central nervous system. The sodium–potassium pump ATPase mechanism is oxygen-dependent. Its failure is preceded by an inability to restore membrane potential by extrusion of sodium ions. The effects of low calcium and hypoxia are so similar as to suggest a common site of action. They are additive in the Trousseau sphygmomanometer test used to diagnose latent tetany. The calcium effects are ionic, so there is no paradox in the fact that tetany may be provoked by hyperventilation, in which the respiratory alkalosis causes reduced ionization of extracellular calcium.

So far as we know, the sodium–potassium pump is the only 'electrogenic' mechanism that is oxygen-dependent. Calcium is also required for the resynthesis of ATP. There are other metabolic pumps which exchange cationic species across the membrane (no net gain in charge) and so are 'non-electrogenic'. They also require oxygen and calcium but their malfunction is not recognizable as excitability changes.

There is an optimal level for extracellular calcium. Above this level, the accommodation of excitable tissues becomes so great that it becomes increasingly difficult to depolarize them. In human disease *hypercalcaemic states* cause hypotonia, muscular weakness, loss of reflexes and drowsiness. Calcium is less well tolerated after pretreatment with narcotics and rapid injection intravenously may cause falls in blood pressure and pulse rate. The action of cardiac glycosides on heart muscle is potentiated.

CALCIUM ANTAGONISTS

A number of substances block the entry of calcium into cells with slow calcium channels. In mammals these are mainly cardiac and smooth muscle cells and their effect is similar to that of reducing extracellular calcium — prolongation of the action potential and negative inotropic effect on heart muscle, and decrease of smooth muscle tone. These actions have some use in the treatment of angina pectoris, hypertension and supraventricular tachycardia. Examples are nifedipine, verapamil, lidoflazine and perhexiline. In therapeutic doses they have no significant effect on nerve membrane or skeletal muscle. Dantrolene sodium reduces the intracellular calcium in skeletal muscle, probably by an action on the membrane of the transverse tubules and possibly the triad junctions, so inhibiting the inward movement of 'triggering calcium', which would normally release 'activator calcium' from the sarcoplasmic reticulum. This is a large flux of calcium ions which diffuse to the adjacent myofibrils and bind to the troponin situated on the actin filament, a combination which is considered to cause a conformational change of the actin filament resulting in exposure of active sites on the actin molecule at which a reaction with cross bridges of myosin filaments occurs, leading to muscle contraction by a ratchet mechanism. This intracellular calcium flux is an essential part of the link between action potential and contraction of the muscle fibre (*excitation–contraction coupling*). The active sites are probably ADP molecules. The energy source for muscle

contraction is ATP which is believed to combine with the head of each myosin cross bridge which then tilts and draws the actin filament which shortens the muscle fibre. The energy is provided by hydrolysis of the ATP (to ADP and phosphate ion) and so the head of the bridge returns to its normal position until further ATP is supplied (by creatine phosphokinase acting on ADP plus creatine phosphate) to initiate another cycle. The triggering calcium is reabsorbed into the sarcoplasmic fluid by an energy-dependent calcium pump in the walls of the longitudinal tubules and this ends the muscle contraction.

Failure of the reabsorption mechanism would cause persistent contraction of muscle fibre without further action potentials. This is termed *contracture*. It may be caused by potassium or caffeine and possibly by some anaesthetics (notably halothane), especially if there is a genetic defect of the sarcoplasmic regulation of calcium in muscle as in the rare muscular disease associated with malignant hyperpyrexia in man and pig. The hypermetabolism associated with the contracture causes oxygen desaturation despite increased oxygen uptake, respiratory acidosis followed by severe metabolic acidosis (as the hypoxic muscle changes to anaerobic metabolism) and leakage of creatine phosphokinase, potassium and myoglobin from the muscle cell into the bloodstream. The hypermetabolism rapidly raises body temperature to a dangerous level. The train of events can be arrested by inhibiting trigger calcium inflow into the skeletal muscle cell with dantrolene sodium, resulting in a decreased release of activator calcium in the terminal cisternae. Oral dantrolene may be of some prophylactic value before anaesthesia in known cases but treatment requires intravenous administration (10 mg/kg). There is a slight calcium-antagonist effect on smooth muscle (vascular and intestinal) but apparently only weak inotropic effect on heart muscle and no detectable effect on nervous tissues.

The train of events leading to contracture may be initiated by anything causing depolarization of muscle. This includes potassium, inhalational anaesthetics and depolarizing myoneural blocking drugs such as succinylcholine.

Membrane constants

The discussion on permeability of cell membranes to charged ions passing through narrow channels or exchanged by a metabolic pump has indicated that the membrane has 'resistance' in the electrical sense so that the basic laws of electricity flowing through chains of resistances may be applied. Additionally, the more extensive bilipid non-conducting part of the membrane has layers of ions on each side, ie space charges separated by an insulator. It therefore also has the properties of a condenser (capacitor). Since it has both capacity and resistance in parallel, any small potential change across the membrane (depolarization or hyperpolarization) will tend to decay exponentially to the normal resting potential. The time to decay to 1/e of the initial value is the electric *time constant* of the membrane.

The membrane resistance separating the central conducting core of the cell from the external conducting medium also gives it the properties of a cable, especially with elongated cell (fibres). If a steady potential change is produced at one transverse zone of the fibre (nerve or muscle) there is a distribution of current along its length. Steady current cannot easily pass through the membrane capacity so the through membrane current (and hence the membrane potential) will drop with increasing distance from the applied voltage. It decays exponentially according to a formula which contains a factor termed the *length constant*. The time constant and length constant of nerve and muscle fibre are such that they make inefficient cable conductors. The excitable cell tends to 'ignore' a continuous stimulus but responds maximally to an abrupt one. Less 'powerful' (eg lower voltage) stimuli have to be applied for a longer time to allow depolarization to reach the critical value (*threshold*). For this reason there is a *strength–duration curve* related to the membrane time constant, and the curve changes in degenerating neurones. Because there is a threshold for activation of the self-regenerative Na^+ conductance, even a stimulus current of infinite duration has a finite minimum strength (*rheobase*) which excites at the end of a finite maximum *utilization time*. For transmission of a signal over long distances some 'signal boosters' are required — the nodes of Ranvier and synapses at which the signal strength is renewed.

Refractoriness and accommodation

The voltage change which activates sodium and potassium conductances across the excitable membrane rapidly terminates the self-regenerative process by inactivating the sodium current, while potassium efflux continues (resulting in after-hyperpolarization). Both processes make the cell refractory to an immediately following depolarizing stimulus. During the sodium channel inactivation there is a *completely refractory period*, followed by a *relatively refractory period* of hyperpolarization.

Sodium inactivation occurs during the passage of an electric current, even if this is insufficient to cause the channel activation response. Thus a brief subthreshold stimulus increases excitability and lowers the threshold to a further stimulus following shortly, but a prolonged subthreshold stimulus raises the threshold to a following brief stimulus because the sodium channel inactivation and potassium efflux are dominant. In old terminology, the excitable cell is said to 'accommodate' to the passage of current through its membrane, regardless of whether it activates the sodium channel or not. If a stimulating current increases (linearly or exponentially) over a brief period but not instantaneously, there is a relation between the slope of current rise and its final exciting strength. There is a minimal current gradient. Currents rising at less than this critical rate will never excite. The rising threshold proportional to rate of rise of current is specified by a *time constant of accommodation*. Note that it is not the same as adaptation (p. 57) or habituation (p. 165). There is a limit to accommodation. It breaks down at a certain current level at which the excitable cell responds repetitively as long as the current is applied.

A consequence of accommodation is that — at threshold intensity — a constant current stimulates at the cathode when the circuit is completed ('*make*' excitation) but no repetitive firing occurs while current flows. When the current is stopped suddenly, a '*break*' excitation occurs at the anode. However, if there is no accommodation, repetitive excitation occurs at the cathode as long as current continues to flow. When the external Ca^{2+} concentration is reduced or the excitable cell is made hypoxic, the accommodation is reduced and the breakdown of accommodation occurs at a lower level. Slowly rising stimuli excite at a threshold level little above that for instantaneously rising stimuli. At extreme, with accommodation abolished (as in peripheral nerve in severe tetany) the fibre continues to fire iteratively so long as the stimulus continues, or it even fires spontaneously. The rate of firing depends on the duration of refractoriness following each action potential. These factors of excitability, accommodation and recovery phenomena are fundamental to an understanding of the production of trains of action potentials ('spikes') by long-acting depolarizing stimuli, such as transmitter action at synapses or any other 'generator potential' as at sensory transducers.

Excitability, refractoriness and accommodation are not uniform throughout the cell. A typical *nerve cell* consists of a nucleated cell body (*soma*), with afferent fibres (*dendrites*) and an *axon hillock* leading into a more or less elongated axon which commonly branches at its distal end, each branch ending in a specialized knob-like structure containing vesicles of transmitter substance. The excitability factors just described vary considerably. The nerve cell dendrite–soma–axon hillock part is more excitable than the axon and terminal and its accommodation breaks down readily. Even the axon has a gradient of excitability and accommodation, with excitability and conduction velocity decreasing and accommodation increasing from proximal to distal. Finally, at the *nerve terminal* there is a specialized role for Ca^{2+} with respect to release of transmitter substance when the terminal is depolarized. Thus, spontaneous discharges are more likely to start in the proximal part of the neurone and to fire repetitively. Indeed, special inhibitory controls, such as the *Renshaw loop* (p. 244), are required to limit this tendency. When a neurone becomes metabolically deranged, this form of excitability tends to spread distally along the axon (a possible mechanism for the production of fasciculation in muscle). Long nerve fibres accommodate better than short

ones, and motor neurones better than sensory neurones or muscle fibres. Clearly these regional variations must be correlated with the ultrastructure of the cell membrane, possibly the distribution of ion channels. For instance, in a myelinated nerve fibre the sodium channels are numerous at the nodes of Ranvier and relatively sparse in internodal segments.

Conduction velocity

We have already seen that regarded as a conductor of electricity, even a nerve fibre is a poor cable because its membrane is leaky and it has a space factor which makes the potential across the membrane drop in a rather short distance from the activated area. However, if there are ion channels within a suitable distance, the flow of current in the local circuits through adjacent membrane is sufficient to activate the voltage-dependent sodium channels and so induce the self-regenerative mechanism which starts off the action potential at full amplitude. The analogy of a spark passing along a line of gunpowder particles is a better analogy than an electric cable. The rate of conduction is, similarly, rather slow (about 10–15 m/s) and dependent on the diameter of the fibre (velocity is approximately proportional to fibre diameter). This is the situation in unmyelinated nerve fibres. Rapid conduction in unmyelinated fibres is only possible if the fibre diameter is very large (as in the giant axon of the squid).

In myelinated nerves the *myelin sheath* (*Fig. 2.1*) provides further insulation and local circuits can only be completed through the 'bare' *nodes of Ranvier* separating the myelin segments. Each segment is laid down by a single cell (the Schwann cells in peripheral nerve, the oligodendrocytes in the central nervous system). These nodes concentrate the electrical current density and, as just described, direct it to areas of membrane with high concentration of sodium channels. The next action potential is therefore generated at the next node (*Fig. 1.5*). The action potential jumps from node to node (*saltatory conduction*) (*Fig. 1.5*). This considerably increases the conduction velocity without requiring uneconomically large diameter axons. The fastest motor and sensory fibres in human peripheral

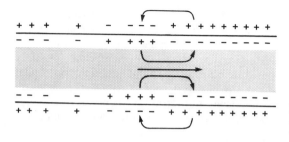

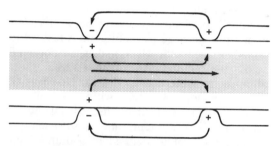

Fig. 1.5. Propagation of nerve impulse in a non-myelinated and myelinated nerve fibre (*lower*). The conduction velocity is increased in the myelinated fibre by saltatory conduction from one node of Ranvier to the next. A stimulus applied at a point on the fibre will propagate both ways (orthodromic and antidromic) but must then continue in that direction as it vacates a zone with inactivated sodium channels (absolutely refractory). Similarly, if two stimuli are applied at separate zones they will each evoke an action potential. These will eventually meet at a refractory zone and will not continue beyond it (occlusion).

nerve conduct at 50–85 m/s. The velocity depends mainly on (i) fibre diameter and (ii) internodal distance, and these factors are not constant throughout the length of a nerve. Conduction velocity is slower distally. Disease processes that decrease fibre diameter or, more importantly, decrease the internodal distance, will decrease the velocity of conduction.

Activation and inactivation of the ion channels vary with the ambient temperature. Raising the temperature increases conduction velocity until a temperature is reached at which impulse block occurs (about 46°C). Conversely, lowering the temperature slows conduction velocity but it also increases excitability and lowers accommodation (probably the mechanism for the tetany-like rigidity of muscle in hypothermia). These temperature effects are important in measuring conduction velocity of

nerves for diagnostic purposes, and are also responsible for the clinical deterioration caused by overheating patients with multiple sclerosis. The initial beneficial effect on conduction velocity of raising the temperature is due to a more rapid increase of outward potassium current during the generation of the action potential, but inward sodium current at the node is also decreased and this ultimately blocks conduction.

Anaesthetics, general and local

A definition of an anaesthetic is 'a drug that directly blocks the membrane action potential without appreciably affecting the resting potential'. Many lipid-soluble substances conform to the definition and the potency of an anaesthetic is directly proportional to its oil/water partition coefficient (Meyer–Overton rule). The anaesthetic drugs electrically stabilize the membranes of excitable cells, partly by changing the fluidity of the membrane; it swells, becomes more fluid and its components are disordered, with modification of its enzyme activities. Membrane-bound Ca^{2+} may be increased or displaced and the transmembrane ionic fluxes may be increased or decreased according to the anaesthetic species. Neutral anaesthetics increase the passive fluxes of ions, amine anaesthetics decrease them. In some instances the effect is greatest in small fibres such as the pre-synaptic region so that transmission block occurs there additionally. Furthermore, certain drugs selectively block specific receptors. These factors, plus local morphological characteristics, cause regional or local predilection to blocking by some drugs.

Compound action potential

If all nerve fibres were identical, stimulation of a bundle of fibres would cause a summed action potential with amplitude proportional to the number of fibres stimulated, but with rise time and fall time, and conduction velocity identical with the action potential of one of the fibres. In practice, the fibres differ at least in diameter, internodal distance and myelin thickness. For these reasons alone the compound action potential is not a simple multiple of any single fibre potential and its components propagate at different rates along the bundle of fibres, so increasing the discrepancy in recordings made at a distance (*Fig.* 1.6). The problem of interpretation is increased by the fact that neither of the recording electrodes can be intracellular for all fibres. Extracellular recording must be carried out with the fibres in an electrolytic medium (tissue fluid or an organ bath). Interpretation of differences of potential between two points in a conducting medium requires understanding of the properties of a *volume conductor*. In practice all biological potential measurements made in intact man have this limitation. Furthermore, measurement involves potential *difference* and this implies two electrodes. One of these can be made relatively 'indifferent' by siting it suffi-

ciently far from the 'active' electrode (so called monopolar recording) or by placing it at a permanently depolarized area (injured cells). A discussion of the principles of volume conduction would be out of place in this book, but any reader intending to make a detailed study of action potentials must study this subject and in reading original papers it is essential to identify the type of recording used. For didactic presentation it is simplest to describe the compound nerve action potential as recorded monophasically (as nearly as possible 'monopolar').

The compound action potential recorded very near the site of stimulation has a single 'spike' with a hump on its falling phase. If the recording is made progressively further from the source, the 'spike' decreases in amplitude and the hump separates off into a separate wave, increasingly separated in time as conduction distance increases. Clearly the second wave is formed by action potentials from fibres conducting more slowly than those contributing to the initial 'spike'. With appropriate amplification and conduction distance it becomes clear that the 'compound action potential' is the algebraic summation of unit action potentials which differ in threshold, amplitude, duration and velocity of conduction (*Fig.* 1.6). These differences reflect the differences in diameter, myelination and internodal distances of the fibres and so it is possible to characterize the fibre type by the place where its action potential appears in the compound potential. There have been several nomenclature systems (requiring care in reading earlier literature). Unfortunately there is no universally agreed terminology related to fibre diameter and conduction velocity. The following terms in common usage depend on the type of nerve studied and so this must also be identified by the reader.

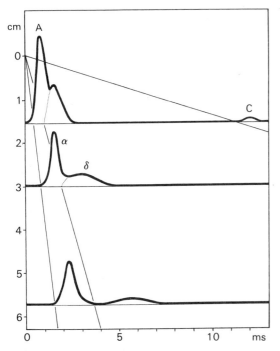

Fig. 1.6. Compound action potential of sural nerve. Diagram to illustrate dispersal with increasing distance from stimulating cathode. (In fact, C fibre potential would be at 30 ms or later in the top trace.) Progressive asynchrony, dependent on differing conduction velocities of fibre groups, causes each peak to widen and drop in amplitude. The diagrams are based on monopolar recording of a moist nerve in air. Each wave would be triphasic if recorded in a volume conductor. The compound wave is the summed potential at the site of the recording electrode. *In vivo*, the A_δ and later peaks can be identified by computer averaging of numerous responses.

An estimate of fibre diameter may be obtained by dividing the conduction velocity by a factor of 6 (large myelinated fibres) or 4·5 (small myelinated fibres), bearing in mind that the nerve fibre is not a true cylinder but has longitudinal grooves. The different conversion factors make it difficult to determine the spectrum of fibre diameters from a compound action potential. Conduction velocities shown in *Table* 1.1 are mainly derived from cat and

Table 1.1

Category	Group		Fibre type	Conduction velocity (m/s)	Function
Cutaneous afferent	Aα	II	Myelinated	20–100	Mechanoreceptors
Joint afferent	Aδ	III	Myelinated	4–30	Mechanoreceptors, cold, first pain
Visceral afferent	C	IV	Unmyelinated	2·5	Warm, second pain, post-ganglionic autonomic
Muscle afferent	A	Ia	Myelinated	50–125	From spindle primary
		Ib	Myelinated	50–120	From Golgi tendon organ
		II	Myelinated	24–71	From Golgi tendon organ
		II	Myelinated	20–70	Spindle secondary
		IV	Unmyelinated	2·5	Muscle nociceptors
		III	Unmyelinated	5–40	Muscle nociceptors
		IV	Unmyelinated	2·5	Muscle nociceptors
Efferent	Aα	I	Myelinated	41–120	Skeletomotor
	Aβ	II	Myelinated	50–85	Skeletofusimotor
	Aγ	III	Myelinated	10–40	Fusimotor
	B	III	Myelinated	3–15	Preganglionic autonomic

The efferent fibres are classified α–γ according to Leksell, muscle afferents I–IV according to Lloyd and other afferents (A–C) according to Erlanger and Gasser (their original A$_β$ and $_γ$ groups, based on analysis of the compound action potential, were shown to be recording artefacts). Modern classification based on receptor of origin has not yet established a unified system of nomenclature but approximate equivalents are shown.

primate studies but are probably representative for human nerves.

The different types of nerve fibres have some important consequences for the anaesthetist as they have differing susceptibility to anoxia and to local anaesthetics. Conductivity of sensory fibres is blocked in the following order by compression with sphygmomanometer cuff B, Aα, Aδ (ie preganglionic autonomic, then large followed by progressively smaller myelinated somatic fibres). Similar sized motor fibres are blocked at the same time as afferent fibres (skeletomotor before fusimotor). Note the relative resistance of unmyelinated C fibres, important in conduction of pain impulses. (The literature on this should be consulted as various accounts of order of susceptibility are inconsistent.) With local anaesthetics the small myelinated sensory and (gamma) motor fibres fail first, followed by large myelinated fibres, as with compression block, but the order of unmyelinated C fibre blockade appears to depend on anatomical factors such as whether the nerve is sheathed (peripheral nerve) or unsheathed (posterior roots) and this factor confuses interpretation of many experimental studies on excised nerve. The susceptibility to cold block appears to be substantially the same as to cuff compression and local anaesthetics. (Note: the situation is rather different with tourniquet compression which damages the Schwann cell–myelin sheaths in the paranodal zones.)

Interaction between nerve cells and satellite cells

There is experimental evidence that glial cells are not necessary for production of action potentials by neurones but it has been suggested that they act as a buffering mechanism to limit local concentrations of K^+ outside nerve membranes producing action potentials and at the same time they accumulate potassium which would otherwise diffuse away from the nerve cell. This is a controversial subject. The glial cells, especially astroglia, probably regulate the extracellular fluid of the central nervous system to a constitution typified by cerebrospinal fluid rather than blood plasma. The blood–brain barrier formed by capillary endothelial cells (Chapter 27) buffers the nerve cells and glia from changes in the chemistry of the blood involving large molecules, but small molecules can penetrate the CNS rapidly from the blood. Nevertheless the CSF varies little in its pH, P_{CO_2} and HCO_3 and this regulation may be effected by glial cells. This is an active metabolic regulatory process rather than a barrier function.

There is also controversy regarding the suggestion, based on ultramicroscopic evidence of small vesicles in some glial cells, that they mediate exchange between the nerve cells and intercellular space by pumping material from one surface of the glial cell to the other. It is also suggested that glial cells prepare substrates for the nerve cells, acting as energy donors to them.

There is little doubt that astrocytes are not merely structural scaffolding for the central nervous system. Microglia are the histiocytes of the central nervous system, constituting a non-haemic source for macrophages and for production of antibodies. The main satellite cells are the oligodendrocytes in the CNS and the Schwann cells in the peripheral nervous system. These are intimately wrapped around all axons. Around the larger axons they wrap multiple layers of myelin, one satellite cell to each node. The insulating effect and contribution to saltatory conduction of the nerve impulse have been described above. Small fibres without myelin coverage are also infolded into oligodendrocytes or Schwann cells, often several nerve fibres to one satellite cell. The thickness of the myelin sheath is not proportional to the diameter of the axon and the ratio varies from one nerve to another. In statements about the relation between diameter and conduction velocity of myelinated nerve fibres the diameter refers to total diameter (including myelin).

Further reading

Boyd I.A. and Davey M.R. *Composition of Peripheral Nerves*. Edinburgh: Livingstone, 1968.

Hodgkin A.L. *The Conduction of the Nervous Impulse*. Liverpool: Liverpool University Press, 1964.

Hodgkin A.L. and Huxley A.F. A quantitative description of membrane current and its application to conduction and excitation in nerve. *J. Physiol.* 1952; **17**:500–44.

Hille B. Ionic channels in excitable membranes: current problems and biophysical approaches. *Biophys. J.* 1978; **22**:283–94.

Hubbard J.I., Llinas R. and Quastel D.M.J. *Electrophysiological Analysis of Synaptic Transmission*. London: Edward Arnold, 1969.

Katz B. *Nerve, Muscle, and Synapse*. New York: McGraw-Hill, 1966.

Seaman P. Membrane actions of anaesthetics and tranquillizers. *Pharmacol. Rev.* 1972; **24**:583–655.

Chapter 2
Neuromuscular junction

STRUCTURE

During development, or on reinnervation, a number of motor nerve terminals may form junctions on each skeletal muscle fibre but soon all disintegrate except one. Polyneuronal innervation is exceptional in human muscle. Within a depression on the surface of the muscle fibre, termed the 'soleplate area', each terminal axon divides into several terminal branches which lose the myelin sheath but remain covered by a continuation of the Schwann cell sheath except on the surfaces facing the receptor surface ('subneural region') on the muscle from which it is separated by a *primary cleft* of about 50 nm (500 Å) width (*Fig.* 2.1). In mammals the terminal branches end in knobs which are normally grouped closely together in a *'plaque'* applied to a discrete region of a muscle fibre. *Terminations 'en grappe'* do not occur in man, with the possible exception of extraocular muscle.

The subneural apparatus does not follow the contours of the nerve terminals but is thrown into folds (*secondary clefts*) radiating out from the sides and deep surfaces of the synaptic gutter or *primary synaptic cleft*. This is not a structure for providing an extensive receptor surface, as formerly thought. *Acetylcholine receptors*, identified by isotope or other labelling of alpha-bungarotoxin, which has a marked binding affinity for these receptors, are restricted to the crests of the sub-synaptic folds (*Fig.* 2.2) and only the mouths of the secondary clefts. There is considerable evidence for cholinergic receptors on the pre-synaptic membrane (nerve terminals) with a modulatory role in neuromuscular transmission. The receptors are conceived as integral membrane proteins with binding sites for acetylcholine which

regulate the opening and closing of channels which traverse the membrane, the whole having a structure shaped like a doughnut. The ligand-activated channel allows passage of ions through the otherwise impermeable post-synaptic membrane.

The molecular structure of the depths of the secondary clefts remains unknown. They contain an amorphous surface material which continues into the primary synaptic cleft. Its nature and function is unknown. It may derive from vesicles described by some authors in the sarcoplasm of the muscle soleplate. The subneural apparatus and the basal lamina in the primary and secondary clefts contain *acetylcholinesterase*, an enzyme which hydrolyses the neurotransmitter acetylcholine. It is not confined to the motor endplate and its exact site of production is unsettled.

FUNCTION

The neurotransmitter acetylcholine is synthesized from choline and acetyl coenzyme A and stored in the distal part of motor nerves. The reaction is catalysed by the enzyme choline acetyltransferase which originates in the soma of the cell and travels down to the nerve terminal by axoplasmic flow. The flow rate is greatly exceeded by the rate of release of transmitter at the nerve terminal so some storage mechanism is required to provide a reserve of transmitter near the release sites.

Coenzyme A (CoA) is acetylated with energy which is usually supplied by glucose and adenosine triphosphate. The enzyme acetyltransferase transfers the acetyl groups to choline to form *acetylcholine* (ACh) which is then stored until required. The mechanism is probably the same as in sympathetic ganglia in

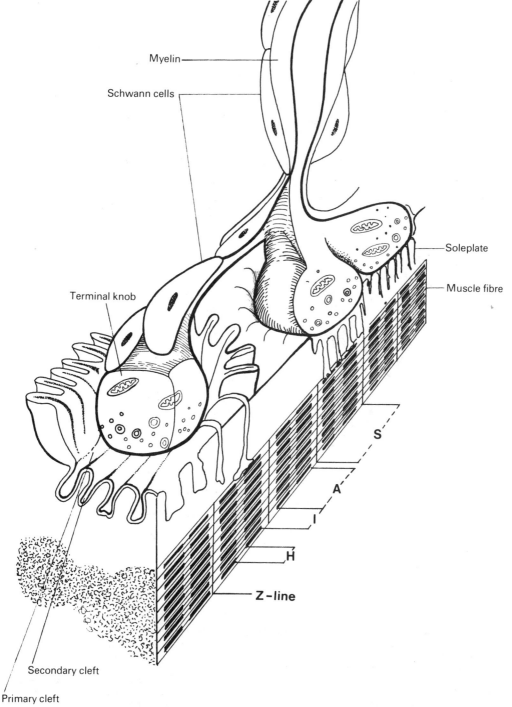

Myelin

Schwann cells

Soleplate

Muscle fibre

Terminal knob

S

A

I

H

Z – line

Secondary cleft

Primary cleft

Fig. 2.1. Terminal of an alpha motoneurone in the synaptic gutter of a striated muscle fibre. The axon loses its myelin sheath just before the terminal arborization. Schwann cells continue to cover the terminal knobs and seal the margins of the primary cleft. In the terminal knob are mitochondria and vesicles containing part of the ACh formed in the soma of the neurone and passed distally in a microtubular system. Vesicles tend to cluster at special release sites opposite the mouths of secondary clefts, where the folds of the sub-synaptic apparatus have high concentrations of ligand-activated receptors. Between receptors and release sites is a fine reticulated basement membrane (not illustrated) formed by extensions of the membrane into the secondary clefts. It carries acetylcholinesterase. Each soleplate supplies one muscle fibre composed of a bundle of fibrils each striated because of overlapping thick and thin filaments at the A band, except for its H zone from which thin filaments are absent. Thin filaments continue through I bands and are anchored at Z-lines differentiating each sarcomere (S), the unit of contraction.

18

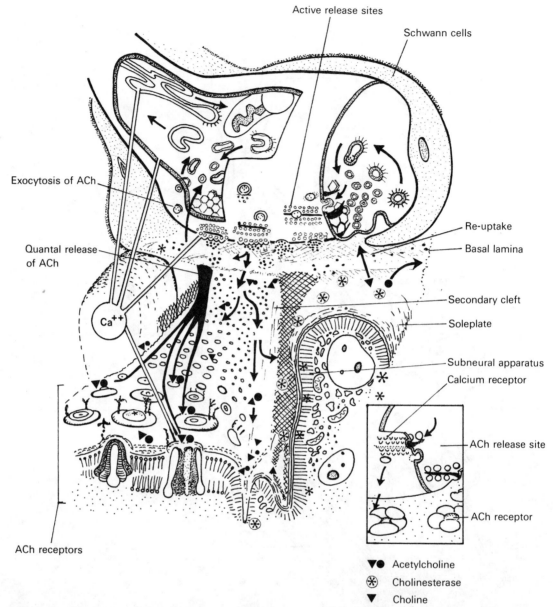

Active release sites

Schwann cells

Exocytosis of ACh

Quantal release
of ACh

Ca⁺⁺

ACh receptors

Re-uptake

Basal lamina

Secondary cleft

Soleplate

Subneural apparatus

Calcium receptor

ACh release site

ACh receptor

◥● Acetylcholine

✳ Cholinesterase

◥ Choline

Fig. 2.2. Neuromuscular junction. A motor nerve terminal knob is wrapped in Schwann cells (but no myelin) which seal
the gap between nerve and muscle and send tongues between them. Basement membrane wrapping Schwann cells meets
basement membrane from the depths of the secondary clefts to form a loose, reticular (? structured) basal lamina between
the nerve ending and the muscle soleplate ridges. Acetylcholine, synthesized in the soma, flows down the nerve and is
incorporated in smooth reticulum which buds off into vesicles, each containing a quota ('quantum') of ACh. Some ACh
free in the cytosol may leach through the cell membrane; more escapes by random exocytosis of vesicles (*upper left*). Most
vesicles move towards the cell membrane and cluster near negatively charged intraterminal dense bands (*upper middle
and insert*), possibly aligned by a hexagonal inner membrane (synaptopore). The folds lie mainly over the mouths of
secondary clefts and extend over the adjacent clefts at right angles to their main axes. On each side of the folds is a
'railtrack area' of twin rows of particles. They are believed to be receptors for calcium. In the presence there of calcium, a
depolarization of the nerve membrane evokes release of a train of vesicles close to this 'active zone' or release site (not
necessarily through it). The membranes of exhausted vesicles are retrieved by internalization either as cisternae (*upper
left*) or as coated-vesicles with markers from the active zone (*upper right*).

which it is believed that ACh is stored in three main compartments: (i) 'stationary ACh' in the pre-terminal part of the axon; (ii) 'depot ACh' (or 'mobilization store') in the synaptic vesicles of the nerve terminal; (iii) 'surplus ACh' in the cytoplasm of the terminal. The nature of the 'stationary ACh' is obscure. It cannot be depleted by prolonged stimulation of the nerve and it is inaccessible to the hydrolysing enzyme acetylcholinesterase which is present in all parts of the neurone. It presumably supplies a back-up store for the synaptic vesicles. 'Surplus ACh' in the cytoplasm of the terminal is, on the other hand, rapidly destroyed by acetylcholinesterase and can only be detected when that enzyme is inhibited. It may re-cycle into the vesicles. These are the sites of 'depot ACh' which is transported from the stationary store. The vesicle is also a site of very active synthesis of ACh and some of this is in a readily releasable form. Electrophysiological evidence indicates that ACh is released from the nerve terminals in 'packets' or 'quanta', suggesting that there is an all-or-none release of the transmitter from vesicles. However, this model is being questioned as evidence accumulates that most of the spontaneous release of ACh is non-quantal.

The vesicles move towards the pre-synaptic membrane of the nerve terminal and tend to cluster at *release sites* ('active zones') opposite the receptors on the sub-synaptic membrane of the motor endplate. In these sites they form an 'immediately available store' of ACh. Some of the vesicles discharge their contents into the synaptic cleft and each quantum activates receptors, producing spontaneous *miniature endplate potentials* (MEPP). The membrane of a discharged vesicle is incorporated into the nerve membrane and moves away from the discharge site, eventually reforming a new vesicle which synthesizes and stores a further supply of transmitter. Some of the ACh liberated into the synaptic cleft is hydrolysed by acetylcholinesterase to form choline and acetic acid which are taken up again by the nerve terminal and supplied to the vesicles for resynthesis of acetylcholine.

In addition to being released spontaneously, the contents of the synaptic vesicles close to the terminal membrane are released when the nerve terminal is depolarized by an action current. The large number of quanta of transmitter released into the synaptic cleft link to ACh receptors, evoking *endplate potentials* (EPP) which are multiples of the MEPP. As only those vesicles near the specialized release sites are affected in this way, less than 1 per cent of the total population of vesicles is released by a stimulus. Thus, despite the slow rate of synthesis there is sufficient store of ACh to permit response to prolonged and frequent stimulation, but this reserve has limits.

STIMULUS–SECRETION COUPLING

The coupling between the nerve terminal action potential and the release of transmitter

---

Fig. 2.2. (contd)

Randomly released vesicles (single quanta) or passively diffused ACh reaches the basal lamina (*middle*). Most is hydrolysed by the cholinesterase which is held there. The choline fraction is taken up by the nerve membrane and re-cycled. A few ACh quanta pass through the loosely structured basal lamina and may activate receptors on the post-synaptic membrane. The brief depolarization resulting is a miniature endplate potential (MEPP). Fewer molecules do not fully activate ion channels but cause brief alterations of ion fluxes ('endplate channel noise'). The probability of sufficient quanta of ACh being released and escaping hydrolysis in the sieve is increased by depolarizing the nerve membrane. The synchronous activation of many receptors causes an endplate potential (EPP) which may be adequate to activate neighbouring sodium and potassium channels with a regenerative action leading to a propagated action potential. Acetylcholine lands on a specific receptor site of specialized receptors arranged in 'herring bone' pattern across the post-synaptic crests. The cationic head of the molecule attaches to specific recognition sites. The closed pore undergoes a conformational change (*bottom left*) permitting rapid flux of Na^+ into and K^+ out of the sarcolemma. It is either hydrolysed in situ or rolls across the crest (possibly stimulating other receptors in passage) and either escapes from the edge of the soleplate area or drops into a transmitter trap in the secondary clefts. The hydrolysing enzyme acetylcholinesterase is formed in the subneural apparatus (*bottom right*). The exact nature of the granules, mitochondria and batonnets of Couteaux is unknown but they appear to synthesize and secrete acetylcholinesterase which is then trapped in the meshes of basal lamina in primary and secondary clefts. It scavenges ACh for recycling and also removes it from receptors which then revert to the resting closed structure.

Inset shows enlarged diagram of pre-synaptic release sites and post-synaptic receptors, with basal lamina removed. The release site has parallel rows of intramembranous particles in the outer face on each side of the dense structure along which are marshalled the vesicles on the inner side.

is uncertain. It is known to be dependent on calcium ions from the extracellular fluid activating voltage-dependent channels on the nerve terminal membrane, a process which can be blocked by magnesium which competes for the same sites. It is possible that the calcium displaces intracellular sodium by joining a carrier molecule.

It cannot be concluded that all the ACh released at the neuromuscular junction is derived from nerve terminals. Observations on denervated muscle and comparison of resting output of ACh with the amount of quantal release estimated from MEPPs indicate that there are additional sources of ACh, possibly from Schwann cells.

The effect of lowering the calcium or raising the magnesium concentration of the fluid perfusing a neuromuscular junction is to reduce the frequency of MEPPs. Excess calcium, however, depresses transmitter release, possibly by inactivating the supposed carrier. Sodium ions competitively depress release of ACh, either by competing with calcium for association with the carrier or by reducing its affinity for calcium. On the other hand, potassium ions tend to depolarize the nerve terminals and thus generate or potentiate a discharge. The potassium liberated from muscle when ACh generates its endplate potential thus potentiates further release of acetylcholine, a positive feedback which is of limited application in the treatment of myasthenia gravis. It has been claimed that the ACh itself, when liberated into the synaptic cleft, reacts with pre-synaptic nicotinic receptors and so potentiates further quantal release and also antidromic nerve action potentials. Acetylcholine in the cleft may depolarize the nerve at more proximal sites, presumably the nodes of Ranvier, particularly in the presence of cholinesterase inhibitors, causing fasciculation and antidromic firing. (Recall that fasciculation implies stimulation of groups of muscle fibres: an immediate pre-synaptic depolarization would excite only one neuromuscular junction.)

EFFECTS OF REPEATED STIMULATION

The amount of ACh released from the nerve terminal depends on the frequency of stimulation. After one synaptic potential further stimuli release progressively smaller amounts of ACh from the immediately available store (estimated from the amplitudes of the resulting endplate potentials). (This is the conventional teaching. It is now suggested that 'tetanic fade' is due to blockade of pre-junctional receptors by the post-junctional blocker, usually tubocurarine required to investigate EPP responses.) The decrement, if it exists in the natural state, has no immediate effect on neuromuscular transmission as, in normal circumstances, the amount of ACh liberated exceeds the amount required to evoke an endplate potential of sufficient amplitude to cause a muscle action potential. This surplus is known as the *safety factor*. It will be referred to again when discussing diseases of the neuromuscular junction. The initial decrement of evoked endplate potentials ('early tetanic rundown') rapidly reaches a plateau level as the immediately available store is sustained by a repletion or '*mobilization*' process — perhaps bringing synaptic vesicles to the release sites. Naturally the rate of mobilization will depend on the frequency of stimulation and also on the availability of calcium ions. The rate is also influenced by hyperpolarizing and depolarizing electric currents and by exposure to an increased concentration of extracellular potassium. With prolonged tetanization faster than 5 per second, the mobilization process gradually drops to a lower level which probably depends on the pre-terminal 'stationary ACh' store which is some 50–100 times larger than the immediately available store. It rapidly restores the mobilization depot stores when stimulation stops.

Release of transmitter depends upon both the frequency and the duration of stimulation and so does the recovery time. A decrementing output from immediate release stores has already been described. The depression of neuromuscular transmission which results is described by some authors as *Wedensky inhibition*. Others use this term to describe the phenomena due to the nerve or muscle refractory period (p. 10). As the term lacks precision it should be discontinued. However, for a shorter time the decrementing output of transmitter is antagonized by a brief potentiating influence of trains of stimuli, since repetitive stimulation appears to facilitate the release of transmitter from the pre-synaptic release sites. In other words the *probability for the release* of quanta of transmitter is increased during repetitive stimulation, but only for a brief period (about 10–60 s in man).

The increased mobilization/release of transmitter is analogous to the *potentiation* that gradually develops during application of a hyperpolarizing current to pre-synaptic terminals which may bring synaptic vesicles up to the release sites by electrophoresis. This effect is negligible with slow rates of stimulation and the effect on depletion of stores is then dominant. This principle is important in electrodiagnostic testing for myasthenia gravis.

Clearly it is not sufficient to have synthesis and vesicular storage of ACh. It is necessary for these vesicles to be brought to strategic release sites confronting the receptors on the junctional folds. The forces regulating this movement are not understood nor their possible disturbance by disease. Whatever the mechanism, it does not stop immediately on discontinuing the stimulation. A stimulus applied after a short rest remains more effective than the first of the conditioning train of stimuli and this *post-tetanic potentiation* subsides comparatively slowly. During this period (10–60 s) there is greatly increased frequency of miniature endplate potentials, suggesting that more than usual synaptic vesicles have been brought up to the release sites. One difficulty is that post-tetanic potentiation has a delayed onset after a prolonged conditioning tetanus, but it must be remembered that the phenomenon is detected by its effect on endplate potentials and so the apparent delay may be due to desensitization of the receptors (*see below*). The antagonistic effect of ACh depletion lasts much longer than the potentiating effect of stimulation, so post-tetanic potentiation is followed by prolonged *post-tetanic depression*. The latter is so long as to raise doubts about transmitter depletion being an adequate explanation. *Receptor desensitization* is certainly an important factor.

Before going on to consider the fate of ACh released into the synaptic cleft, it is worth stressing that the rate of spontaneous release of ACh quanta, as estimated from MEPPs, is controlled pre-synaptically — and only pre-synaptically — by the membrane potential of the nerve terminal.

POST-SYNAPTIC EVENTS

Some of the ACh liberated into the synaptic cleft escapes at the boundaries but the structure of the mammalian neuromuscular junction is particularly favourable to limit this. Some is hydrolysed by acetylcholinesterase within the cleft and taken up for re-synthesis by the nerve terminal. Most of the free ACh binds with receptors in the sub-synaptic membrane of the endplate. It is still debatable whether similar receptors are present on the pre-synaptic membrane, and if so what their function may be.

Specialized receptor structures on the sub-synaptic membrane have been postulated for many years on operational grounds. Identification of acetylcholine receptors (AChR) became possible with the discovery of a polypeptide in the venom of a snake *Bungarus multicinctus*, the Formosan banded krait, which blocks neuromuscular transmission by binding specifically to the post-junctional AChR in an essentially irreversible manner. The toxin, *alpha-bungarotoxin* (α-Bgtx), is easily purified and can be labelled radioactively and in other ways with little reduction in its high specific activity. It can therefore be used to identify specific binding sites which are considered to be on or near the binding sites for acetylcholine. Indeed the strong affinity for receptors is such that a chromatography column carrying fixed α-Bgtx will bind AChR from detergent-treated tissue homogenates (affinity chromatography). Contemporary studies on AChR are based on the understanding that the number of α-Bgtx binding sites is proportional, if not equal, to the number of acetylcholine receptors. Electron microscope autoradiography and histochemical detection of α-Bgtx have localized the main concentration of cholinergic receptors on the crests of the post-synaptic folds and necks of the secondary synaptic clefts. These sites have been correlated with rosette structures identified by freeze-fracture and negative staining of the post-synaptic membrane of electric organs of *Torpedo marmorata*. These are shaped like a doughnut and similar organs are probably present in the sub-synaptic membrane of the muscle endplate.

This is a rapidly advancing field of study, but at present it appears that each rosette consists of a number of subunits and traverses the post-synaptic membrane. In the centre of the rosette is a channel with a mouth, facing the synaptic cleft, which is closed in the resting state but is opened when ACh binds to receptor molecules in the surrounding rosette, thus causing the AChR protein to undergo a conformational change which opens the channel. If conditions are the same as in the electroplaque, it may be necessary for two or more binding sites to be occupied to regulate a single channel. Once the channel has been opened ions flow across the post-synaptic membrane with a direction and intensity which depends solely upon the ionic gradients and electric potential drop across the membrane. Unlike the muscle action potential (p. 3), it has no regenerative link.

The ionic current is normally brief (about 2 ms) as the acetylcholine is rapidly hydrolysed by acetylcholinesterase from the sub-synaptic apparatus, but the resulting *endplate potential* (EPP) declines more slowly due to a passively decaying electrotonus.

Other things being equal, the endplate current increases in proportion to the number of quanta which bind with the reactive zones of the endplate. Unlike the *frequency* of MEPPs, which is controlled entirely by the conditions of the *pre*-synaptic membrane, their *amplitude* is controlled by the properties of the *post*-synaptic element, providing that quantal size remains constant. As the MEPP is the sign of a spontaneously released quantum of ACh binding to a receptor site and opening a channel for ion flow, so the EPP resulting from a nerve impulse is a measure of the number of quanta reacting with the endplate receptors (*Fig. 2.3*).

If the endplate current reaches a critical level it causes sufficient flow through the adjacent resting muscle membrane to generate an action current in it.

ENDPLATE POTENTIALS

Synaptic potentials are distinguished from action potentials by their smaller amplitude, slower time course and, in particular, lack of refractory period. This permits addition of successive synaptic potentials (algebraically in those synapses that have both excitatory and inhibitory functions: no inhibitory potentials have been detected at the mammalian neuromuscular junction).

Spontaneous *miniature endplate potentials* (MEPPs) detected close to the neuromuscular junction result from depolarization of ACh receptors by spontaneously released contents of synaptic vesicles (about 6000 molecules of ACh). They therefore occur randomly, not rhythmically, and the amplitude of each potential is a multiple of a single quantum of ACh since the latter are of uniform size. Coincidence of MEPPs is never sufficient to produce a generator potential adequate to stimulate the muscle fibre.

When, however, the pre-synaptic terminal of a motor nerve fibre is depolarized by a nerve impulse, there is for a brief time a great increase in the release of packets of ACh, producing a depolarization of the sub-synaptic membrane 100 or more times greater in amplitude (but with the same temporal characteristics) as the MEPP. This is the *endplate potential* (EPP). The associated flow of current through the channels may or may not be sufficient to trigger the propagated spike potential of the muscle membrane.

The amplitude of the EPP is (perhaps not universally) affected by the concentration of calcium and magnesium in the synaptic cleft, increasing in proportion to the external calcium concentration. This is antagonized by magnesium ions.

Endplate potentials (and associated *endplate current*) are due to ions moving down their electrochemical gradients, not to an ionic pump. There is therefore no regenerative link and the flow of current does not depend on the level of membrane potential. Inward movement of sodium is mainly responsible, being rather larger than the outward flow of potassium. (Chloride shifts are negligible and other anion flows not significant.) In experimental situations, other cations can be substituted for sodium, eg ammonium and methylammonium ions but not larger. The limiting factor is probably the diameter of hydrated ion compared with the pore diameter of the receptors.

Experiments with continuous electrophoretic injection of ACh on to endplate receptors indicate that the latter become *desensitized* slowly (with a half time of about 5 s) and

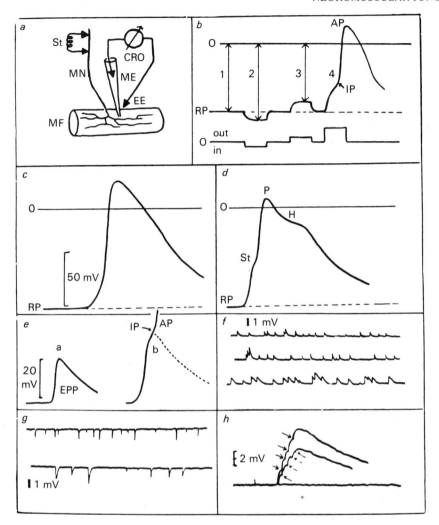

Fig. 2.3. *Endplate potentials of frog muscle.* *a*, Tip of microelectrode in junctional region of a muscle fibre which is stimulated through its motor nerve. *b*, Transmembrane voltage recorded on impalement (1) and with direct stimulation pulses up to critical level (4) for activating the self-regenerating process of the action potential (AP). *c*, Action potential of muscle fibre (direct stimulation). *d*, Action potential of muscle fibre evoked trans-synaptically. *e*, Endplate potential (EPP). In (**a**) there is no action potential as the endplate potential is limited by curare. In (**b**) the endplate potential (dotted) evokes an action potential at threshold level. *f*, Spontaneous miniature endplate potentials (MEPP) recorded within the muscle cell. *g*, MEPP recorded extracellularly. *h*, Two superimposed endplate potentials with inflections caused by lack of synchrony of ACh quanta evoking them (magnesium block).

recover slowly when ACh is no longer applied. This is also found with analogues of ACh such as decamethonium and suxamethonium. Increasing the calcium concentration increases the speed of desensitization and this is antagonized by sodium. A possible mechanism of desensitization is blockage of the open channel by a molecule of the agonist.

GENERATION OF MUSCLE ACTION POTENTIAL

When the endplate potential attains a critical level of depolarization of the sub-synaptic membrane, a *spike potential* is generated in adjacent membrane and propagated as described on p. 6. The receptor structure itself is probably not electrically excitable but the flow of ions through its channel moves the membrane potential towards a new level characteristic of the combined membrane species. Current therefore flows into this 'sink' from neighbouring polarized membrane, depolarizing it. An isolated or brief train of action potentials may follow but this is determined by both the rapidity and the extent of the depolarization and also by the electrical properties of the membrane. Thus an action potential spike 'takes off' at slightly variable points from a series of apparently identical endplate potentials and only if the latter reach a critical amplitude (*threshold potential*) at which the inward sodium current just exceeds the outward potassium and chloride current. The spike usually arises when the EPP is about 40 mV. It starts about 0·5 ms after the onset of the EPP, but the rise time of the latter is not constant.

NEUROMUSCULAR DELAY AND 'JITTER'

The many steps between the impulse in the nerve fibre and the action potential in the muscle fibre (not to speak of the latency of the twitch response) take an appreciable time — about 0·22 ms in mammals. There is sufficient variability at all stages, but particularly in the calcium-coupled release of ACh and in the time course of the EPP and its evocation of a muscle action potential, to give rise to easily measured variations in the time between stimulus and response. *In vivo* it is not possible to determine exactly when a nerve action potential invades the nerve terminal. Consider, however, the situation of muscle fibres belonging to a single motor unit (p. 235). An action potential passing down the axon passes into each of its branches, liberates ACh and stimulates an endplate. Complete synchrony would not be expected as terminal branch conduction times will not be the same to each neuromuscular junction of the unit, but one could anticipate that all muscle spike potentials would be constantly separated in time. However, this is not so. Using selective electrodes capable of recording single muscle fibre potentials, and selecting the action potential of one fibre as a reference point, it is found that the other fibres do not fire with invariant timing,

but with a variability that has been termed '*jitter*'. It is more marked when conditions such as disease interfere with neuromuscular transmission (or terminal branch conductivity) but clearly the exact site of the variable delay cannot be assumed.

Pharmacology of neuromuscular transmission

It is necessary to appreciate that many substances act on more than one part of the synaptic transmission mechanism, and possibly also on nerve transmission or muscular response, and that the relative actions may differ from one type of motor unit to another. Effects vary according to the concentration. The total effect of electrolytes and of 'depolarizing' agents may therefore be different from the anticipated one. For that reason, this section will not be arranged primarily according to the supposed site of action, which would seem to be the logical approach.

CALCIUM

This ion has important actions on both nerve (p. 5) and muscle (p. 74). So far as transmission at the neuromuscular junction is concerned, it has both pre-synaptic and post-synaptic effects. As calcium ions are necessary for the linkage between nerve action potential and ACh release, a decrease of calcium in the synaptic cleft lowers the probability that synaptic vesicles will release their ACh contents. The frequency of spontaneous MEPPs is reduced and the EPP has a lowered quantal content, leading to transmission failure (despite increased excitability of nerve and muscle: this may account for the eventual loss of tendon reflexes in severe hypocalcaemia). High concentrations of calcium depress transmitter release.

MAGNESIUM

This ion appears to compete with calcium for uptake sites on motor nerve terminals. If the calcium ion content of the bathing medium is low, magnesium ions will increase the quantal content of the EPP, but if the calcium content is greater, the competitive effect of magnesium blocks ACh release, ie it opposes the action of calcium and so reduces MEPP frequency and lowers quantal content of EPP.

SODIUM

Sodium ions must pass through the receptor channels to depolarize the endplate, but they also compete with calcium for association with a presumed carrier substance necessary to release ACh from the pre-synaptic membrane and so they depress ACh release.

BARIUM AND STRONTIUM

Both are able to substitute for calcium and so presumably are also competitors. Whether they increase or depress transmission will depend on the calcium concentration.

3,4-DIAMINOPYRIDINE AND TETRAETHYL-AMMONIUM

Both block potassium channels of the pre-synaptic membrane, prolonging the terminal depolarization. This enhances the release of acetylcholine quanta evoked by a nerve impulse. For this reason 3- and 4-aminopyridine are beneficial in Lambert–Eaton syndrome, botulism and neuromuscular blockade caused by aminoglycoside antibiotics.

BOTULINUM TOXIN

This toxin, produced by *Clostridium botulinum*, blocks the release of acetylcholine from nerve terminals (spontaneous or evoked), apparently by obstruction of the release sites. There is progressive reduction of EPP amplitude until inhibition is complete, and MEPPs are reduced in frequency. The effect is partially reversed by calcium ions or 4-aminopyridine. When prolonged, it induces the same post-synaptic changes as denervation, and the nerve terminal responds with ultraterminal sprouting.

HEMICHOLINIUM-3 AND TRIETHYLCHOLINE

These are quaternary ammonium compounds which block neuromuscular transmission mainly by inhibiting the synthesis of ACh by choline acetylase, possibly by blocking the uptake of choline from the external medium. The amplitudes of both MEPPs and EPPs diminish progressively, indicating a change in *quantum size*, presumably due to depletion of the pre-synaptic store of ACh. They also block ACh receptor responses. This action is considered to be less significant than the pre-synaptic one in mammals, although it may be the dominant one in amphibia.

ACETYLCHOLINE

The natural transmitter ACh may be applied to the neuromuscular junction by iontophoresis. Its normal action on ACh receptors post-synaptically and possible pre-synaptic activity are described above. If acetylcholine remains attached to ACh receptors after the initial ionic flux through receptor channels has produced potential changes across the endplate membrane, the receptors will fail to respond to further supplies of ACh. Thirty years ago the blocking effect was considered to be due to prolonged depolarization of the endplate membrane, spreading out to the adjacent excitable membrane of the muscle fibre. The term *depolarization block* derives from that time, though more recent work indicates that the membrane polarization is re-established despite continuing occupation of receptors.

Desensitization of receptors has been demonstrated. Its mechanism is uncertain but may be blockage of the open channel. The activity of ACh attached to the receptors is terminated by its hydrolysis by the enzyme *acetylcholinesterase* (and to a lesser extent by other cholinesterases).

DEPOLARIZING RECEPTOR-BLOCKING DRUGS

Certain mono- or bis-quaternary onium compounds so resemble ACh as to compete with it for attachment to ACh receptors. They successfully open the receptor channels and so depolarize the membrane and produce muscle action potentials and twitches. But they are resistant to hydrolysis by acetylcholinesterase and so persist at receptor sites which are thereby blocked and desensitized after the initial stimulation. Clearly, this desensitization is not a competitive block (*see below*) and so it cannot be reversed by anticholinesterase drugs, indeed these may prolong the block. Eventually the blocking agent is hydrolysed by the other ('pseudo'-) cholinesterases.

Examples of this group of drugs are carbachol, suxamethonium, decamethonium, tetramethylammonium and choline (a breakdown product of acetylcholine). Like ACh, these drugs also have some pre-synaptic action, producing the important clinical sign of fasciculation, and some of them are also weak inhibitors of acetylcholinesterase. Prediction of their pharmacological effect is made more complicated by the observation of differential effects in different muscles and in different species. For instance, administration of decamethonium (C10) in the monkey, dog or rabbit causes increased motor activity then a transmission block which is reversible by ACh. In the cat C10 produces a classic 'depolarization block' in the tibialis and gracilis muscles, while in the soleus it appears to be initially depolarizing and then produces 'competitive block' (sometimes termed '*dual response*'). The differing effects may be correlated with the dominance of one or other type of muscle fibre (which have morphological differences in their endplates). The species differences, related to chain length of the onium molecule, suggest that stimulation may occur if one receptor site is occupied but blockade requires cross-linkage of two receptors. In man, C10 normally acts as a 'depolarizing blocker' but in myasthenia gravis the neuromuscular junctions may be resistant to block and when it does occur the block is of 'competitive' type. Although not investigated by modern techniques, the changed response of the myasthenic junction is likely to be related to the relative poverty of ACh receptors in that disease.

The anaesthetist must be aware that the response to relaxant drugs of depolarizing type is unpredictable in myasthenic patients.

ANTICHOLINESTERASES

Agents that inhibit cholinesterases (particularly acetylcholinesterase) prevent hydrolysis of ACh and so permit longer occupation of receptors by the ACh released from nerve terminals or in the circulation. The main site of action is the motor endplate, but *extra-junctional receptors* exist, near the tendons of many normal skeletal muscles and throughout the muscle membrane in denervated or botulinum intoxicated muscle. Anticholinesterase substances also stimulate pre-synaptically, causing fasciculation.

The prolongation of occupancy of receptor sites by ACh raises the safety factor for transmission and this is beneficial in the treatment of myasthenia gravis or in the restoration of ACh dominance against competitive blocking agents. If carried to excess, so that ACh persists at receptor sites, the endplate remains depolarized or becomes desensitized (*cholinergic blockade*). There are many pharmacologically active drugs, but selection for clinical use is determined by (i) their ability to cross the blood–brain barrier; (ii) their duration of action.

Tertiary amines, obtained from plants, include physostigmine and galanthamine. Their central effects limit their clinical application. The same is true of organophosphorus compounds but the main reason for abandoning these is that the blood level rises cumulatively with prolonged use. This is the major problem in selecting a quaternary ammonium compound although these analogues of physostigmine have little central effect. Edrophonium, administered intravenously, has a peak action too brief (2–10 min) for treatment of myasthenia gravis or curare overdosage. It is used to confirm the diagnosis of myasthenia gravis (brief restoration of muscle power) or to differentiate between underdosage and overdosage of anticholinesterases (no change, or temporary decrease of power due to depolarization block). The test should not be repeated without awareness that residual activity can be demonstrated electrophysiologically for at least 30 min after i.v. injection.

Neostigmine, pyridostigmine and ambenonium are used in the treatment of myasthenia gravis. Bis-neostigmine compounds, though effective, are too cumulative for routine use. For parenteral use, only neostigmine is required by the anaesthetist. In small dosage it will inhibit acetylcholinesterase sufficiently to increase the safety factor for transmission when this is reduced by a competitive-type blocking drug. Bigger doses will stimulate pre-synaptic terminals and cause fasciculation; still bigger doses will cause depolarization/

desensitization block by excessively prolonging the action of ACh on receptors ('cholinergic block').

NON-DEPOLARIZING RECEPTOR-BLOCKING AGENTS

Some completely ionized tertiary or quaternary ammonium salts have a steric resemblance to ACh and bond electrostatically with anionic sites on the ACh receptor molecule but are unable to produce the conformational change required to open the channel and alter the ionic permeability of the endplate membrane. They do not stimulate the receptor but, on the contrary, block it by denying access to ACh. Recent studies suggest an additional blockade of the channel opened by an agonist (ACh).

D-TUBOCURARINE

This is the classic example. As a competitive blocker it is antagonized by raising the concentration of ACh, as by anticholinesterase substances or by ACh releasing agents such as tetraethylammonium ions or calcium. There is some evidence that D-tubocurarine may also have some pre-synaptic action.

Other competitive blocking substances are dihydroerythroidine, gallamine and benzoquinonium (and hemicholinium-3 in high concentration). They have a similar activity. The mean amplitude of the spontaneous MEPPs is reduced and the EPPs are diminished progressively until inadequate to stimulate the muscle action potential, according to the proportion of receptor sites occupied by the competitor.

ALPHA-BUNGAROTOXIN

This example of a snake venom with remarkable affinity for the ACh receptor sites has been discussed above as a useful substance for determining the site of ACh receptors. The latter are blocked by the toxin which is only slowly released by degradation of the receptors. It cannot be displaced competitively and in this way differs from curare-type drugs. It has no pharmaceutical role.

ANTIBIOTICS, ANTICONVULSANT AND OTHER DRUGS

Drugs may block open ACh channels. The reduction of endplate response is usually insignificant unless the safety factor for transmission is low (as in myasthenia gravis). Some drugs (eg alcohols) change the channel properties by alteration of the lipid environment of the ACh receptors.

CATECHOLAMINES

Adrenaline, noradrenaline, ephedrine and isoprenaline have effects on neuromuscular transmission which differ according to their concentration. Thus adrenaline may enhance or antagonize the actions of D-tubocurarine or of anticholinesterases or depolarizing drugs. Too little is known to justify devoting space to this subject but anaesthetists should be aware of the issue and of the possible neuromuscular effect of β-adrenoreceptor blockers. It is probable that the main actions are prejunctional and on the muscle membrane (not sub-synaptically).

HISTAMINE, 5-HYDROXYTRYPTAMINE, PROSTAGLANDINS

There are conflicting reports of stimulant or depressant activity of each of these substances on neuromuscular transmission, and possible species differences.

Further reading

Bowman W.C. *Pharmacology of Neuromuscular Function*. Bristol: Wright, 1980.

Katz B. *The Release of Neural Transmitter Substances*. Liverpool: Liverpool University Press, 1969.

Kelly R.B., Miljanich G. and Pfeffer S. Presynaptic mechanisms of neuromuscular transmission. In: Albuquerque E.X. and Eldefrawi A.T. (ed.) *Myasthenia Gravis*. London: Chapman and Hall, 1983, pp. 43–104.

Peper K., Bradley R.J. and Dreyer F. The acetylcholine receptor at the neuromuscular junction. *Physiol. Rev.* 1982; **62**: 1271–340.

Chapter 3

Neurotransmitters and neuromodulators

Multicellular, and especially multiple-organ, animals require means for communicating between different parts of the body and for co-ordinating their activity, especially for homeostasis. There are two systems which have been developed from the ectoderm — the nervous system and the endocrine system. They are closely related functionally and may be considered as different specializations of a common type of neurosecretory cell. Within the hypothalamus of mammalian brain are cells which secrete peptides. These, passing along a portal vascular system to the anterior pituitary gland, act as releasers for a range of hormones which act directly on cells of all tissues or indirectly via secondary ductless glands such as the thyroid, gonads, adrenal cortex and pancreatic islets. Neurosecretor cells to the posterior pituitary, adrenal medulla and probably the pineal gland release hormones directly, and these are similar or identical to substances recognized elsewhere in the nervous system as neurotransmitters. Neurones which release transmitter substances are, indeed, neurosecretor cells specialized to respond to a limited range of chemical stimuli by secreting their product into a specialized structure to limit the activity to part of the membrane of a target cell.

It is, of course, possible that some of the more diffuse hormonal effects of the prototype neurosecretor have been retained. There is a growing interest in the possibility of neuromodulator activity, as distinct from neurotransmitter activity, for propagation of a quantitative signal.

Many, if not all, conventional hormones act via an intracellular nucleotide mediator ('second messenger') which is commonly adenosine 3′,5′-phosphate, better known as cyclic AMP, a product of the enzymic degradation of adenosine triphosphate by adenyl cyclase. Many peptides and biogenic amines that function as neurotransmitters or neuromodulators also use cyclic AMP as an intermediary. It is not certain that these actions are limited to synaptic membranes. The neurosecretion ('first messenger') links physically with receptor proteins on cell surfaces and stimulates or inhibits the adenyl cyclase reaction which generates cyclic AMP from ATP. Cyclic AMP then interacts with various cellular processes in the effector organ (another neurone, a muscle endplate or a gland) to affect the molecular synthesis of RNA and proteins (in addition to a more general role in carbohydrate metabolism). This is a possible basis for neutrotrophic action.

The best-recognized neurosecretions acting in this way are catecholamines. Noradrenaline, histamine and 5-hydroxytryptamine (5-HT or serotonin) have this property. It may mark them as survivors from the most primitive nervous systems. Their transmitter effects are inhibited by the anti-cAMP actions of prostaglandins of the E series. On the other hand, acetylcholine appears to open conduction channels on receptor membranes (exclusively) without this intermediary and in cholinergic neurones the action of catecholamine–cyclic AMP is on the pre-synaptic release of acetylcholine. Muscarinic cholinergic receptors probably use cyclic GMP (3′,5′-guanosine monophosphate) but nicotinic receptors probably do not. There is a little evidence for a hormonal activity of acetylcholine in ciliary organs, smooth muscle and placenta, but in the nervous system its localized interaction with specialized receptors is found in certain neurones, and possibly in peripheral pain receptors.

THE GENERAL REGULATORY ROLE OF CATECHOLAMINE TRANSMITTERS

In the lower pontine central grey matter there is a compact group of melanin-containing cells, the *locus coeruleus*. From it a dorsally situated *central tegmental tract* and a ventral *medial forebrain bundle* ascend ipsilaterally to the hypothalamus and then by the stria terminalis to the hippocampal formation (*Fig.* 3.1). Some fibres go to the olfactory areas and the cingulum. In short, it is distributed to the hypothalamus and the 'limbic' areas (p. 128). Lesser tracts from the locus coeruleus pass to the non-specific nuclei of the thalamus, the cerebellar cortex, medulla and spinal column.

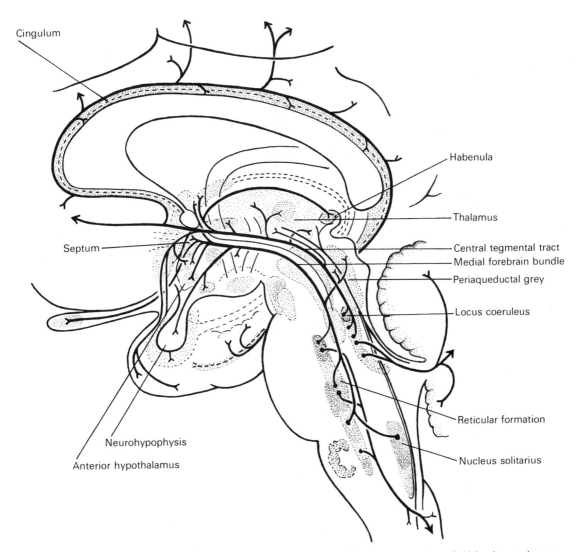

Fig. 3.1. *Noradrenergic systems.* There are two parallel systems. The locus coeruleus (which also projects to the cerebellum) sends fibres to the septum, habenula, non-specific nuclei of thalamus and all forebrain areas through the central tegmental tract and cingulum. It also joins a ventral system projecting through the medial forebrain bundle to the septum, anterior hypothalamus and posterior pituitary. The ventral pathway is probably more dependent on the lateral (ascending) reticular formation of pons and medulla. The secondary distribution by the 'long loops' of the diencephalon is shown in *Fig.* 14.1.

If the system functions as a whole (and this seems likely) it is probably a general activating system. The chemical mediator is *noradrenaline* and the system is associated with 'arousal' of the archipallium. In the neopallium, on the contrary, noradrenaline appears to inhibit neuronal activity. The literature is confusing because of inclusion of data from administration of catecholamines into the circulation, the ventricles and by iontophoresis so that it is

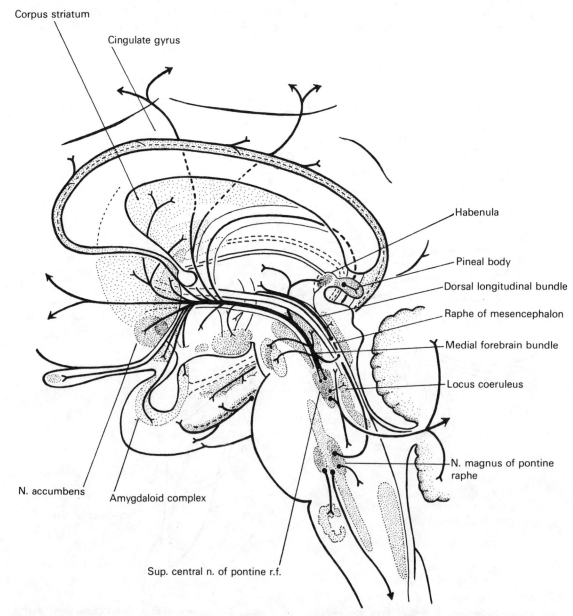

Fig. 3.2. Serotoninergic systems. One originating in the raphe of the pons (which also projects to the medulla and via the inferior olive to the cerebellum) ascends through the mesencephalic raphe of the periaqueductal grey matter through the dorsal longitudinal bundle to the diencephalon. The larger medial forebrain bundle projection, from the superior central nucleus of the pontine reticular formation is widely distributed in parallel with the noradrenergic system (*Fig.* 3.1), but more directly to the neocortex. It also projects to the cerebellum and the locus coeruleus which it may inhibit.

uncertain whether neurones are excited or the receptors on which they terminate.

From the intrathalamic 'non-specific' areas, a projection of arousal signals passes diffusely to the neocortex. This terminal relay is apparently cholinergic. (This may account for the fact that noradrenaline causes electroencephalographic and behavioural arousal when it is injected intravenously, whereas acetylcholine also causes cortical arousal, but only when injected into a carotid artery.) The receptors are muscarinic and can be blocked by atropine or hyoscine. The block may be pre-synaptic as well as post-synaptic since the acetylcholine released from the cortex is increased.

The medial forebrain bundle also contains large numbers of *serotoninergic* neurones originating in the *raphe nuclei* in the midline of the mesencephalon and distributed to the diencephalon and limbic system (*Fig. 3.2*). Unlike the noradrenergic projection there is a group from the dorsal raphe nuclei which projects to the neocortex. Most cortical cells are inhibited by 5-HT but some are excited. Pontine raphe nuclei project to the medulla and spinal cord. If this system also functions as a whole, it is probably hypnogenic. (This is an accepted view, but note that reduction of brain serotonin potentiates thiopentone-induced 'sleep' if the block of the medial forebrain bundle is rostral to its outflow to the septal area.)

The two bundles with reciprocal generalized actions are important with respect to consciousness and sleep (p. 139). They are part of a system of short isodendritic neurones with polysynaptic connections forming a *reticular formation* in the central core of the brain stem (p. 49). These noradrenergic and serotoninergic brain stem systems project and act diffusely.

LOCALIZED TRANSMITTER SYSTEMS

Unlike noradrenaline and serotonin, the local concentrations of adrenaline, dopamine and acetylcholine-containing neurones have a much more topographic projection and some specialized neurones make very localized connections.

ADRENALINE

Some fibres of the central tegmental tract from mid-brain to the periventricular hypothalamus have been shown to liberate adrenaline (acting on both α and β receptors). They project on the nuclei of visceral efferent and afferent systems, especially the dorsal motor nucleus of the vagus nerve (X). Downward-projecting fibres from the tegmentum pass to the lower motor neurones of the sympathetic outflow from the cord. The tegmental centre also seems to inhibit the nearby locus coeruleus.

DOPAMINE

Dopamine, formed from the same precursor as noradrenaline, is released from an important system of neurones connecting the periventricular nuclei of the hypothalamus and the infundibulum to the pituitary gland where they inhibit prolactin secretion. This connection accounts for the clinical use of a dopamine agonist (bromocriptine) in the treatment of certain pituitary disorders. A group of dopamine sensitive neurones in the floor of the IVth ventricle is related to the dorsal motor nucleus of the vagus. It accounts for the emetic effect of some dopamine agonists, including apomorphine.

The other discrete dopaminergic systems of clinical importance are the *nigrostriatal* (from substantia nigra to caudate nucleus and putamen, for motor control — p. 219) and the mesolimbic and mesocortical systems, which arise in the ventral tegmentum of the mid-brain and which are important for higher nervous functions (*Fig. 3.3*). The *mesolimbic system* projects to the amygdala, nucleus accumbens, olfactory tubercle and, via the stria terminalis, to other parts of the limbic area. The *mesocortical system* projects to adjacent cortical areas in the 'smell brain' and lower frontal cortex as well as to the amygdala. They doubtless play a role in the appetite-motivation behavioural patterns discussed in Chapter 14. Many antipsychotic or 'neuroleptic' drugs are believed to act by depletion or blockade of dopamine in these systems which are probably confined to the archipallium. At all of these sites dopamine (as transmitter or in pericellular space) is an inhibitor of tonic activity. It is also the transmitter of an inhibitory interneurone in sympathetic ganglia reducing the depolarizing action of the cholinergic pre-synaptic neurone on the post-synaptic noradrenergic neurone. It would be premature to make the generalization that all dopaminergic neurones are inhibitory.

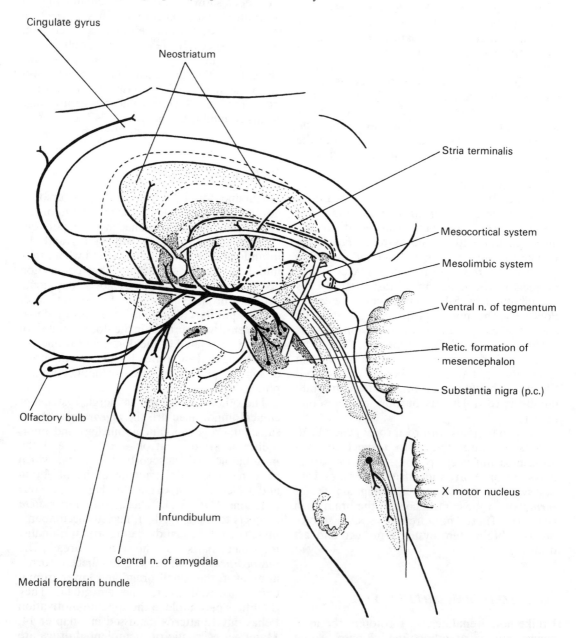

Cingulate gyrus

Neostriatum

Stria terminalis

Mesocortical system

Mesolimbic system

Ventral n. of tegmentum

Retic. formation of mesencephalon

Substantia nigra (p.c.)

X motor nucleus

Olfactory bulb

Infundibulum

Central n. of amygdala

Medial forebrain bundle

Fig. 3.3. *Dopaminergic systems.* Five systems are illustrated. Three are local: within the olfactory bulb; the 'vomiting' centre at the upper end of the motor nucleus of X; a hypothalamic tract which inhibits prolactin secretion by the anterior pituitary gland. A mesolimbic system from the substantia nigra and mesencephalic reticular formation passes directly to the neostriatum (caudate nucleus and putamen) and to the amygdala. A separate mesocortical system from the ventral tegmental area projects by the medial forebrain bundle to the septal area and onwards to the cingulate gyrus, anterior temporal lobe and orbitofrontal cortex.

ACETYLCHOLINE

It may be noted that the topographically distributed dopaminergic systems within the central nervous system synapse with neurones which are almost invariably cholinergic. Acetylcholine-containing neurones are not commonly grouped in discrete bundles and certainly are not diffusely distributed like the catecholamine systems. Cholinergic systems (*Fig.* 3.4) have, however, been identified relaying the effects of the latter, from the non-specific nuclei of thalamus to cerebral cortex (arousal) and from the medial septal area (a terminal of the medial forebrain bundle systems (p. 52 and 128) and the mesolimbic dopamine system), to the hippocampus via the fornix, alveus and fimbria. The habenula — also at the end of a medial forebrain bundle projection (p. 133) — projects to the interpeduncular nucleus of the mesencephalon by a tract (*fasciculus retroflexus*) which contains the highest concentration of acetylcholine in the primate brain.

The identified cholinergic systems account for only a small part of the total choline acetyltransferase (the synthesizing enzyme) in the nervous system. It seems likely that the phylogenetically later development of nervous connections has used synapses of each type, if not randomly, then at least not in discrete bundles. In general, one type of neurone is followed by a different one (eg dopaminergic to cholinergic in the putamen, cholinergic to noradrenergic in a sympathetic ganglion).

The nature of cholinergic action is uncertain. It is usually excitatory and acts on both muscarinic and nicotinic receptors. *Nicotinic receptors* occur on Renshaw interneurones (p. 244), thalamus and cerebellar cortex, but most areas, including the putaminal outflow and the cerebral cortex, have *muscarinic receptors*. Sub-types of muscarinic receptors may account for the striking differences between the actions of atropine, hyoscine and scopolamine and the synthetic anticholinergics used for treatment of Parkinsonism, though all are muscarinic receptor blockers.

The differing affinities of receptor subtypes are equivalent to multiplying the number of transmitters. For these reasons it is not possible to use transmitter type as a guide to the analysis of the structure and function of the nervous system. Neither is it feasible, at present, to identify the neurones responsible for the marked loss of choline acetyltransferase from the brains of demented subjects. Most of the neurones are believed to originate in the nucleus basalis of Meynert in the *substantia innominata*, near the anterior perforated substance (*Fig.* 3.4). Cholinergic activity has been particularly associated with memory and learning (p. 121). The anaesthetist will be aware of the amnesia produced by atropine and scopolamine. As well as lowering the extrapyramidal contribution to muscle tone they cause drowsiness, euphoria and sleep. In higher dosage there is excitement, restlessness, hallucinations and delirium. This is not necessarily a stimulation effect — it could be amygdaloid release associated with blockade of septal output (Chapter 14) (*Fig.* 3.4). The anterior perforated substance is an area where perforating arteries enter the anterior hypothalamus. There is reason to believe that the blood–brain barrier is less complete there, and the vessels include the arterial supply to the portal vessels of the infundibulum and median eminence of the IIIrd ventricle, an area specialized for the release of a spectrum of polypeptides from nerve terminals into blood vessels. Very little is known about neural release of neurosecretions but it has been known for years that the psychic release of pituitary ovulating hormone in many mammals is blocked by anticholinergic and anti-adrenergic drugs. Dopaminergic regulation of neuropeptide release is now well established.

Without question, knowledge of the endocrine functions of the brain is still in its infancy. Secretory functions have been attributed to some specialized collections of ependymal cells such as the *subfornical and subcommissural organs*, and chemoreceptor functions of the ependymal lining of the cerebral ventricles have been proposed by Feldberg.

Transfusion barriers and glial function

Most parts of the ependyma and the external surface of the brain have a *brain–cerebrospinal fluid barrier* owing to tight cellular junctions with intercellular filaments. The *glial tissue* is of three main types, astroglia, oligodendroglia

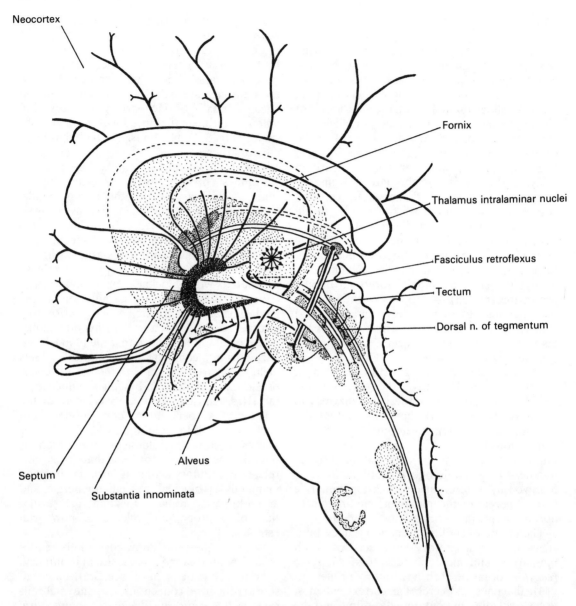

Neocortex

Fornix

Thalamus intralaminar nuclei

Fasciculus retroflexus

Tectum

Dorsal n. of tegmentum

Alveus

Septum

Substantia innominata

Fig. 3.4. *Cholinergic systems.* There are minor cholinergic bundles from the periventricular grey matter and dorsal tegmental nuclei to the intralaminar nuclei of the thalamus (where their relay neurones are diffusely distributed to the cortex, transmitter unknown) and from tegmentum to periventricular nuclei of the hypothalamus. The septal–diagonal band area sends cholinergic fibres to the alvear part of the hippocampus and the posterior cingulate area by the fornix and fimbria, probably a gate control over the perforant pathway from entorhinal cortex through hippocampus to tegmentum and hypothalamus. The habenula–interpeduncular nucleus connection (fasciculus retroflexus) is markedly cholinergic. It relays septo-habenular impulses via the central grey matter to the tectum, controlling eye and head positions. A major diffuse projection, probably to all cortical areas, is distributed from the substantia innominata (nucleus basalis, nucleus accumbens) from the base of the septal region and encapsulating the caudal surface of the striatum and related to the deep aspect of the anterior perforated substance, the neurosecretory area of the hypothalamus, and the amygdaloid complex.

(responsible for laying down spiral sheaths of myelin around axons) and microglia, which has an immunological function. The astroglia is not only a supporting tissue. It plays an important role in the metabolism of the neurones, as an intermediary between blood vessels and neurones, actively transferring material to and from the nerve cells and acting as an important buffer of the internal milieu, especially for ionic flow. Oligodendrocytes (and Schwann cells in peripheral nerves) also have an important nutritive function for maintenance of axonal processes. The foot plates of the astrocytes effectively block spaces between endothelial cells of blood vessels and so constitute a *blood–brain barrier*. In most parts of the central nervous system only material selected by the glial cells can cross the barrier.

There are a limited number of areas without an effective blood–brain barrier. These include the *area postrema* on the floor of the IVth ventricle near the obex, the supraoptic crest and the subfornical organ as well as the pituitary gland and pineal body (which secrete hormones into the general circulation). Possible areas are the anterior and posterior perforated spots, and the ventral surface of the medulla. At these points there is easy access for blood constituents (including hormones and drugs) to enter the brain substance. It is interesting to note their anatomical contiguity with the cell clusters originating the great noradrenaline and serotonin carrying bundles, and possibly the dopamine and acetylcholine systems described above. Anatomically they are sited at the entry to the brain of the great chemosensors (pain, taste and olfaction).

There are some rapid changes of cerebral function caused by circulating hormones, blood gases and drugs which tend to act on these diffuse systems. Some of the chemosensitive areas are known, eg a respiratory and vasomotor area of the brain stem (p. 193), the area postrema and possibly glucose-sensitive areas of the hypothalamus and floor of the IVth ventricle. The glial tissue and neurones have developed in a symbiotic relationship. The neurones are secretory cells which have been specialized for local distribution first and then for transmitting electrical signals over long distances.

The neurone

The terminology of nerve cells and their parts is unsatisfactory. To a purist, the neurone is the whole nerve cell dependent on one nucleus and including its branches. Others restrict the term to the cell body (soma) enclosing the nucleus. In this book we adopt the classic usage — neurone includes the soma, axon and dendrites but it has to be confessed that definitions are difficult. For instance, is every long extension of cytoplasm from the perikaryal region (enclosing the nucleus) to be called an *axon* or only processes conducting centrifugally from the *soma* (cell body) and all processes conducting centripetally to be called *dendrites*? But the apical dendrite of a *pyramidal cell* may be longer than its axon, and in a peripheral afferent fibre the *bipolar cell* is offset from a cell extension conducting first towards and then away from the soma, yet both parts are commonly termed axonal. In *stellate cells* it is impossible to decide on morphological grounds which processes conduct towards and which away from the soma. Indeed, in the Golgi type 2 cell, a common interneurone, the dendrites engage in contacts in which they apparently behave both as dendrites and as axons. Morphological descriptions such as 'basket cell', 'granule cell' or 'stellate cell' indicate ignorance of the exact signal flow. An *isodendritic neurone* is characterized by radiated rectilinear dendrites which branch and rebranch in progressively shorter secondary and tertiary dendrites which overlap with similar dendritic trees of neighbouring neurones, forming a dense formation. This is typical of the central core of grey matter and its limbic extensions. In time it may be possible to identify *receptor* sites and the *axon hillock*, where an efferent branch leaves the soma, but at present the decision on polarity of the cell parts is difficult for the smaller cells which may have thousands of processes. In this book, where we use the term 'dendrite' we imply that it has receptor sites and conducts centripetally: an 'axon' has few if any receptors but may conduct either centrifugally (efferent neurones) or centripetally (afferent neurones). The surface of the dendrites of some neurones is increased by branching and by small 'thorns' or spikes, presumably representing discrete receptor sites. An 'efferent axon' terminates in endings that are rounded, clubbed or with elaborate end-feet (*boutons terminaux*).

AXONAL FLOW

From the perikaryal region, cytoplasm flows distally into the processes and within them can be recognized *neurofilaments* and *neurotubules*. Their function is uncertain, but the latter probably act as channels for flow of substances from the nuclear area to the periphery including precursors of neurotransmitters and, possibly, trophic substances for the next neurone or, in the case of neurones entering peripheral nerves, the muscle or gland end-organs. (The evidence for neurotrophic substances is inconclusive.)

SYNTHESIS OF TRANSMITTER

The neurone contains microsomes like other cells, eg Golgi apparatus, endoplasmic reticulum, mitochondria. The specialized terminals contain unique *synaptosomes*, usually vesicular. For good (but not definitive) reasons the vesicles are considered to contain thousands of molecules of a transmitter substance, synthesized in the whole neurone from chemical precursors and packaged in remarkably regular amounts in the vesicles ('quanta'). The mechanism of storage in granules is prevented by the alkaloid reserpine and by tetrabenazine in neurones synthesizing noradrenaline, 5-hydroxytryptamine and dopamine. (Stores depleted by activity are not replenished.) Guanethidine and bretylium act similarly on peripheral nerve terminals, apparently failing to cross the blood–brain barrier.

In most cases a neurone synthesizes and stores only one neurotransmitter. Recently some neurones have been identified which apparently produce two, but as a general rule it is possible to define a neurone by the type of transmitter released from its terminal(s), eg acetylcholine, noradrenaline, dopamine, serotonin (5-hydroxytryptamine), gamma-aminobutyric acid (GABA) and others. It has been proposed that the granular storage sites

for catecholamines are relatively non-specific and that '*false transmitter*' may be formed in some metabolic diseases or by drugs (eg alpha-methyldopa and other hypotensive agents). Until recently, all neurotransmitters seemed to be amines, but it is now known that many neurones secrete peptides — eg substance P, enkephalins etc.

SPONTANEOUS RELEASE OF TRANSMITTER

There is a slow turnover of neurotransmitter from the nerve terminal at rest — some molecules leaching through the terminal membrane, others being released as whole quanta when vesicles move towards the membrane and release their contents by exocytosis ('spontaneous discharge'). The vesicular membrane then passes back into the cell for recharging with transmitter. Unlike the molecular release, the quantal release occurs only at specialized structures (*synaptopores*) arranged as a hexagon around electron-dense points in the membrane.

ACTIVE RELEASE

If the terminal membrane is abruptly depolarized by an action potential passing centrifugally along the axon, large numbers of vesicles are discharged from the synaptopores at the *release sites*, but only if extracellular calcium is present and passes into the nerve terminal. (The popular vesicular hypothesis is under attack and it has to be stressed that there is no unequivocal evidence. Acetylcholine may be quantally released through a gated channel, both voltage- and calcium-dependent.) If the extracellular calcium is deficient, or if magnesium or certain other ions compete with it, the action potential does not cause the conformational change required to permit egress of transmitter in quantal amounts. The electrogenic mechanism is also blocked by subthreshold depolarization such as by the action of another neurone terminal on receptors proximal to its own terminal. This is the mechanism of *pre-synaptic inhibition* which is widely used in the nervous system (p. 45).

Note that the nerve's own action potential is essential for release of quanta of transmitter, but the *probability* that it will do so is determined by the calcium gradient and the resting potential of the terminal membrane. Transmitter release is potentiated by some simple amines. Amphetamine and tyramine promote release of noradrenaline; ephedrine promotes release of both adrenaline and acetylcholine. It is possible that these sympathomimetic chemicals may potentiate locally released noradrenaline by retarding its re-uptake mechanism into the nerve terminal. As this action saturates, the pharmacological effect may gradually disappear (*tachyphylaxis*).

Neurotransmitter synthesis

The known amine transmitters are formed from simple precursors under enzyme control:

$$\text{AcCoA} + \text{Ch} \xrightarrow{\quad(1)\quad} \text{ACh}$$

$$\text{Glu} \xrightarrow{\quad(2)\quad} \text{GABA}$$

$$\text{Tyr} \xrightarrow{\quad(3)\quad} \text{Dopa}$$

$$\text{Dopa} \xrightarrow{\quad(4)\quad} \text{Dopamine}$$

$$\text{Dopamine} \xrightarrow{\quad(5)\quad} \text{Noradrenaline}$$

$$\text{Trp} \xrightarrow{\quad(6)\quad} \text{5HT}$$

where AcCoA = acetyl-coenzyme A; ACh = acetylcholine; Ch = choline; Glu = glutamic acid; Tyr = tyrosine; dopa = 3,4-dihydroxyphenylalanine; dopamine = 3,4-dihydroxyphenylethylamine; Trp = tryptophan; 5HT = 5-hydroxytryptamine. The enzymes are: (1) choline acetylase; (2) glutamic acid; (3) tyrosine hydroxylase; (4) aromatic amino acid decarboxylase; (5) dopamine hydroxylase; (6) tryptophan hydroxylase.

The water-soluble enzymes are either free in the nerve cytoplasm or in vesicles. The transmitter survives for a short time and, if not liberated, is then degraded by specific enzymes, acetylcholinesterase (hydrolysis of ACh), GABA transaminase (transamination reaction of GABA with α-ketoglutarate to form glutamate), or a monoamine oxidase (noradrenaline oxidized). (Methylation of noradrenaline by catechol *O*-methyl transferase probably does not occur within the neurones.)

The transmitter which escapes from the terminal enters a narrow cleft — the *synaptic gap* — where it passes across *receptor sites* on the post-synaptic membrane before disposal. Molecules of transmitter which bind and link two adjacent receptors cause a conformational change of pores in the post-synaptic membrane, allowing the ionic shifts which trigger a *post-synaptic potential* in the lower order neurone, in the same way as at the neuromuscular junction (p. 22). The further fate of the chemical depends on the type of synapse. In the neuromuscular junction some of it leaked away, the rest was hydrolysed by the anticholinesterase enzyme in the sub-synaptic apparatus. This does not happen with central synapses, and probably not in peripheral autonomic ganglia. In these sites the degrading enzyme is within the pre-synaptic neurone. These types of pre-synaptic neurones have *re-uptake sites* similar to the post-synaptic receptors which trap molecules of transmitter substance and ingest it by pinocytosis. It is not known whether it is directly incorporated into empty vesicles or, as seems likely, broken down by the degrading enzyme and added to the precursor store for re-synthesis.

The re-uptake mechanisms are important targets for pharmacological blockade (eg cocaine and tricyclic compounds such as imipramine). The evidence for existence of re-uptake sites is strong for dopaminergic and noradrenergic neurones but not satisfactory for cholinergic neurones, which may take up choline liberated in the synaptic gap. Nevertheless, pre-synaptic acetylcholine receptors may exist and some workers suspect that even the neuromuscular junction may have such a mechanism. There is also uptake by glial and Schwann cells surrounding the synapses. Unfortunately it is not possible to settle this by identifying the site of degrading enzymes as, in contrast to the biosynthetic ones, they are widely distributed in the neuronal cytoplasm and in the *synaptic gap substance* — ie between the pre-synaptic release grid and the organized receptor sites.

Note that an anticholinesterase allows ACh to have prolonged and cumulative action at endplates and central synapses, but monoamine oxidase or catechol *O*-methyl transferase inhibitors do *not* allow synaptic accumulation of noradrenaline. To achieve that it is necessary to block the re-uptake process with cocaine or inhibitors such as desipramine.

The biological purpose of so many transmitters (and they are certainly not all known) is unknown. In general acetylcholine is excitatory and GABA and glutamate inhibitory, but this is not absolute. Another observation difficult to explain is that it is exceptional for a chain of neurones to use a single transmitter type — for instance a dopaminergic neurone synapses with a cholinergic or noradrenergic neurone, rather than with another dopaminergic. These facts constitute a formidable problem for pharmacological interference with synaptic functions.

The post-synaptic effects are essentially like those described at the muscle endplate but the latter is a comparatively simple form of synapse. So far, we have written as though all cholinergic or adrenergic synapses were the same apart from their chemical specificity. It is becoming apparent that each of the transmitter amines can link with a number of similar but not identical sites. These are identified by their different affinities for substances which bind to them (*ligands*) either inducing the necessary conformational change to open the pores (*agonists*) or occupying the receptor sites but failing to open the channels (*antagonists*). Some agonists first open the channels, stimulating the post-synaptic neurone, and then persist in their occupation as they are not degraded or removed by the uptake system ('depolarizing antagonists'). The natural agonist may act in this way, and block further transmission if its occupancy of receptors is prolonged by inhibiting the degrading enzyme. For instance, anticholinesterases first increase the efficacy of small numbers of quanta of

acetylcholine and then cause depolarization block. This is well seen in the neuromuscular junction where anticholinesterases potentiate the effect of spontaneously released ACh quanta to cause fasciculation and antimyasthenic potentiation, and then cause a depolarization ('cholinergic') block (p. 25). The same sequence is supposed to happen with central cholinergic synapses, but only in response to anticholinesterases which can penetrate the blood–brain barrier. These include physostigmine and organic phosphorus compounds, but not neostigmine, pyridostigmine or edrophonium in normal doses. (It is necessary to point out that this statement assumes a synaptic or post-synaptic action of acetylcholinesterase similar to that in the neuromuscular junction. This widely accepted belief may be questioned.)

Receptor subtypes

CHOLINERGIC RECEPTORS

Since the early experiments on chemical transmission it has been known that there are at least two types of cholinergic receptor — nicotinic in skeletal muscle, muscarinic in autonomic ganglia and in the central nervous system. There may be more: these names have been given in recognition of ligand-binding differences using alkaloids available to the early experimenters. Atropine blocks muscarinic but not nicotinic receptors, D-tubocurarine blocks both.

ADRENERGIC RECEPTORS

Responses to catecholamines are mediated by highly specific adrenoceptors on cell surfaces. These bind the catecholamines with high affinity. The agonist-receptor binding changes the fluidity of the cell membrane and activates a *second messenger* system. Membrane-bound adenylate cyclase when activated by an agonist ligand stimulates the conversion of adenosine triphosphate to cyclic AMP which then activates intracellular protein kinases: the latter phosphorylate enzymes which cause relaxation of smooth muscle cells (β -adrenoceptor), or they inhibit the second messenger system and reduce cyclic-AMP levels (α_2-adrenoceptor). The α_1-adrenoceptors probably have a direct effect on calcium ion flux across the cell membrane. Thus the same ligand may produce radically different effects at different synapses. An approximate classification of receptor types is given by the rank order of potency of several agonists and antagonists.

Alpha-adrenoceptors, which mediate smooth muscle contraction, respond to adrenaline, noradrenaline and isoprenaline in that order of potency, and are blocked by phentolamine and phenothiazines. α_1 receptors are post-synaptic, α_2 receptors pre-synaptic and so inhibitory.

Beta-adrenoceptors, which mediate relaxation of smooth muscle, respond to isoprenaline, adrenaline and noradrenaline in that order of potency and are blocked by propranolol. Within the beta-type receptors there are subgroups (β_1, β_2 etc.) so that certain antagonists have selective activity.

Receptor blockade does not block the re-uptake mechanism so *increased output* may occur and be disclosed when the blocking drug is withdrawn. The central and some of the peripheral actions of all the amines are reduced by barbiturate anaesthesia. The receptors are not confined to nervous tissue, muscle or secretory glands. Cholinergic and adrenergic receptors (and no doubt the others described below) are found on other tissues such as lymphocytes and polymorph leucocytes and fat cells.

HISTAMINE

Histamine and its receptors are best known for their immunological function in leucocytes, mast cells and smooth muscles. There is good, but not definitive evidence for a neurotransmitter function in the central nervous system. Subtypes are already identified. The H_1 type is present on blood vessels and the H_2 type mediates gastric secretion. The H_1 type is blocked by classic 'antihistamines', and the H_2 type by cimetidine. The sedative effects of H_1 blockers suggest that these receptors are present in the brain. Histamine stimulates arousal.

DOPAMINE, SEROTONIN, GABA, GLYCINE, GLUTAMATE, TAURINE

These, and possibly other, amino acids are examples of other neurotransmitters which will be introduced in later pages. It is probable that they also have receptor sub-types. Multiple serotonin receptors have been identified recently. The 5-HT$_2$ receptor involved in blood pressure regulation has a specific antagonist, ketanserin. Many of the central and peripheral actions of 5-HT are blocked by lysergic acid diethylamide (LSD). *Homocysteic acid* and other acidic amino acids are excitatory to many interneurones and may be natural transmitters.

REGULATION OF RECEPTOR NUMBERS

The number of specific receptors and their localization on receptor membranes is regulated by hormonal mechanisms and also by the transmitter itself. A high concentration of agonist reduces receptor numbers (down-regulation) and desensitizes them. A low concentration induces increased numbers (up-regulation) and sensitivity of receptors. This *'denervation hypersensitivity'* is important in disease of the nervous system and responses to drugs. Knowledge about hormonal control of receptor density is still rudimentary.

Paradoxically, a prolonged increase in the activity of the cholinergic nerves supplying terminal adrenergic nerves or adrenal chromaffin cells induces increased activity of the enzymes required for synthesis of the adrenergic transmitter. Prolonged stimulation of peripheral motoneurones reduces atrophy of muscle. These observations of trans-synaptic induction by acetylcholine as a first messenger are important with respect to memory and learning (p. 121) and may make it unnecessary to postulate *neurotrophic factors*. (One of us has described neurotrophic factors as the aether or phlogiston of neurobiology.) The matter is by no means settled. A *nerve growth factor* has been isolated which promotes growth of peripheral sympathetic neurones and dorsal root ganglia. Others generated by astroglia have been suggested. Nerve growth factor is obtained from the saliva of adult male mice and from some snake venoms. Other tissue products such as the prostaglandins, insulin, steroids and other hormones from ductless glands are important controllers of neurone metabolism and cell surface phenomena such as stimulus–secretion coupling. They cannot be considered as neuromodulators in the accepted sense, but account for some behavioural differences between young and old, and male and female.

Neuromodulators

It is possible that some of the biogenic amines, especially dopamine, 5-HT and the amino acids (especially glutamate) act diffusely as hormones in the brain, modifying excitability but not essential links in the transmission of signals between neurones. While the well-established transmitters may be either excitatory or inhibitory according to the synapse involved, GABA and glycine are invariably inhibitory. It is almost certain that many peptides have a neuroregulatory action though it remains possible that some of these are transmitters in the original sense of the word. The peptides that are largely confined to the hypothalamo-pituitary axis (p. 251) and may only act as neurohormones are beyond the scope of this book.

Angiotensin directly influences stimulus–secretion coupling in the terminals of adrenergic nerves. Peptides that are widely distributed in the nervous system include substance P, methionine enkephalin, leucine enkephalin and small quantities of the hypophyseal peptides.

SUBSTANCE P

Substance P is an undecapeptide of known structure (it has been synthesized). It is released by a calcium-dependent process and is unevenly distributed, features suggesting that it is a true neurotransmitter. Particularly high levels are found in the dorsal horn, trigeminal sensory nucleus, substantia nigra, interpeduncular nucleus and medial hypothalamus. Its synthesis in dorsal root ganglia, localization in dorsal horn synapses and overlap with opioid receptors suggest that it is associated with the first synapse for pain fibres (p. 62).

ENKEPHALINS

These are pentapeptides which bind to the same receptor sites as morphine and other opiates, suggesting that they are endogenous substances which block transmission of pain signals. Since their discovery many other transmitter sites have been found, indicating a wider role. There is a high concentration in the limbic system, hypothalamus and periaqueductal grey matter as well as in laminae I and II of the dorsal horn (p. 62). (So it may be difficult to dissociate euphoriant and analgesic effects of opiates.) Analgesia may be induced in experimental animals by stimulating neurones of the periaqueductal grey matter. This is attributed to release of endogenous opiate-like peptides. There is evidence that acupuncture (and some placebos) release central met-enkephalin and beta-endorphin. The site of release is uncertain, and the type of peptide released seems to depend on the frequency of the stimuli. Other neurotransmitters such as serotonin are also liberated. The matter is further discussed in the chapter on pain (p. 68). Enkephalins may inhibit the interaction of catecholamines with their receptors. At present they appear to be confined to short-axon interneurones with axo-axonic synapses.

ENDORPHINS

Endorphins are endogenous peptides with chain length longer than the enkephalins. α, β and γ types are segments of the β-lipotrophin molecule which is probably their precursor. The major stored product is β-endorphin, most abundant in the basal hypothalamus. They are extremely potent analgesics, reversible with naloxone, but their physiological function may be more closely related to the appetitive drives of the hypothalamus and limbic system (Chapter 14). Naloxone is an antagonist to some of the enkephalins and endorphins, but not all.

It is unfortunate that the term 'opiate receptor' is likely to persist for historical reasons. Clearly there are endorphin or enkephalin receptors, with a number of subtypes. As with adrenoceptors, a number of related agonists bind to them with differential potencies and they have their own favoured antagonists. Since an antagonist may be used to displace an agonist according to the law of mass action, the anaesthetist should be aware of the principle receptors and their ligands. Martin's classification of receptors according to their affinity for narcotic analgesic substances has practical value. This grouping includes three main classes:

μ *receptors*: Agonists have morphine-like actions. There is supraspinal analgesia, with euphoria, and addiction. Respiration is depressed.

κ *receptors*: Agonists have nalorphine-like actions. Analgesia is of spinal type, associated with sedation and anaesthesia.

δ *receptors*: Agonists have nalorphine-like actions. There is dysphoria and hallucinations. Respiration is stimulated.

The endorphins are degraded by a number of peptidases and these are inhibited by some D-amino acids.

Without question, any future edition will have more to say about these important substances. In the meantime, it is necessary to warn the reader that amino acids and peptides have hormonal as well as transmitter actions. Acetylcholine is involved in the release of the catecholamines from chromaffin cells, histamine from mast cells and thiamine from neurones. Even simple chemicals may have important generalized actions. For instance, the potassium in glia acts as a 'buffer' for ionic shifts during neuronal activity and released potassium may account for *spreading depression* in the cerebral cortex. Meanwhile, all we know with reasonable certainty is the molecular biology revealed by microelectrodes in or near nerve cells and synapses.

Post-synaptic potentials

Microelectrode studies show that when a neurotransmitter is released into a synaptic space and binds with post-synaptic receptors it triggers ionic shifts which either depolarize or hyperpolarize the post-synaptic membrane. The first type is associated with stimulation of the post-synaptic neurone and the depolarizing potential change recorded is described as an *excitatory post-synaptic potential* (EPSP). The hyperpolarizing type gives a potential change in the opposite sense and is associated with depression of the post-synaptic neurone. Its potential change is described as an *inhibitory post-synaptic potential* (IPSP). These are due to properties of the receptor cell. It is not possible to predict the transmitter involved, though ACh is commonly excitatory and GABA inhibitory.

The amplitude and time course of the post-synaptic potentials are determined by the quantity of transmitter liberated into the synaptic cleft and the speed of its removal. Since this is determined by the number of quanta released by one or more terminals, the synaptic content and its potential are additive. The addition is algebraic, ie convergence of excitatory and inhibitory neurones will counteract each other.

Chemical synapses have a significant *synaptic delay* of about 0·3 ms (mainly in mobilizing the transmitter). This is appreciably reduced in *tight junctions* for which there is evidence that the transmission process is mediated directly by the current flow from the pre-synaptic element. In mammals they are less prominent that in lower vertebrates, but their existence is probable. An artificial electrical synapse may be formed by close juxtaposition of demyelinated segments of axons, so that current flow from one active neurone may stimulate the other. This *ephapse* is a possible mechanism for pain and paraesthesia in causalgia, stump neuromas and multiple sclerosis.

It is important to appreciate that the neurone conducts 'all or none' impulses over long distances (intensity being signalled by a frequency code), but at the chemical synapse this is converted to an *amplitude* code which is directly related to the total input to a synapse. This in turn determines the *rate* of firing of 'all or none' impulses in the next neurone. The signal is transmitted with little or no decrement. This is one advantage in having a synapse. It is now necessary to consider other advantages.

Further reading

Brigew A., Kosterlitz H. and Iversen L. (ed.) *Neuroactive Peptides*. London: The Royal Society, 1980.
Chouchkov C.N. Cutaneous receptors. *Adv. Anat. Embryol. Cell. Biol.* 1978; **54**: 1–62.
Cooper J.R., Bloom F.E. and Roth R.H. *The Biochemical Basis of Neuropharmacology*, 4th ed. New York: Oxford University Press, 1983.
Martin W.R., Eades C.G., Thompson W.O. et al. The effects of morphine- and nalorphine-like drugs in the nondependent and morphine-dependent chronic spinal dog. *J. Pharmacol. Exp. Ther.* 1976; **197**: 517–32.

Chapter 4
The principles of organization of the nervous system

A unicellular organism such as amoeba reacts to appropriate stimuli. The same cell both detects chemical molecules in the water and moves pseudopodia towards or away from them. In principle, a more elaborate nervous system for a multicellular organism could use directly coupled sensor–effector modules, perhaps connected by a nerve net or syncytium. It could have useful integrative properties. However, as the action potential generated at one point in the net could propagate in all directions, the excellent 'local sign' (p. 58) of the receptors would immediately be lost. Impulses conducted over long distances would tend to die out.

These disadvantages are absent from nervous systems with polarized relays. A local depolarization of one part of a nerve cell (neurone) including its processes, will propagate in all directions on the membrane of that neurone except that post-stimulus refractoriness prevents it from retracing its course immediately. If it then reaches a synapse, the signal can only be passed forwards since synaptic transmission is polarized (from a pre-synaptic neurone to a post-synaptic neurone). It functions like a valve. The name of Ramon y Cajal is honoured for espousing the *Neurone Doctrine* in preference to a syncytial net.

Additional advantages accrue to a nervous system with synapses. The next neurone in the chain generates its own action potential at full amplitude, acting like a 'booster station' in a transmission line. This makes it possible to transmit a signal over long distances without decrement, by using a frequency code in which *frequency* of 'all or none' nerve impulses is simply related to the depolarization pressure on a receptor surface of the neurone. The transmission across the synaptic gap may be either chemical or electrical by a process which is *not* pulsed but which has its amplitude determined by the frequency of impulses in the pre-synaptic neurone. The synaptic change, generally (? always in man) a neurotransmitter package of precisely determined amount, activates the post-synaptic membrane and evokes there a post-synaptic potential.

Excitatory and inhibitory synapses

This biological development was extremely important, since the different areas of the post-synaptic membrane may carry receptors for different neurotransmitters. One of these may depolarize and another one hyperpolarize the receptor membrane, one exciting and the other inhibiting the post-synaptic neurone. The post-synaptic membrane undergoes potential changes like those described in Chapter 2 for the endplate of muscle. Synaptic potentials that excite the post-synaptic neurones are termed *excitatory post-synaptic potentials* (EPSP), though they may not reach stimulation threshold but only *facilitate* other depolarizing potentials. Those that suppress the post-synaptic neurones are termed *inhibitory post-synaptic potentials* (IPSP). Almost invariably EPSP depolarize and IPSP hyperpolarize. *Pre-synaptic inhibition* is an exception. The transmitter depolarizes an excitatory nerve ending and so reduces its effect on a receptor cell (*Fig. 4.1*).

The decay of post-synaptic potentials is longer than that of action potentials. Prolonged EPSP following a single activating stimulus evoke repetitive firing of the next neurone (eg in spinal Renshaw cells). The IPSP is almost a mirror image of the mono-

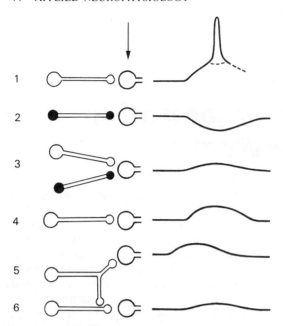

Fig. 4.1. *Inhibition.* The post-synaptic potential of a cell (*arrowed*) recorded when it is activated by: 1, An excitatory synaptic knob. The EPSP is adequate to generate a spike potential. 2, An inhibitory synaptic knob generates an equal hyperpolarization causing *post-synaptic inhibition.* 3, Coincident activity of converging excitatory and inhibitory cells produces no PSP or an EPSP below spike threshold. 4, This excitatory synaptic knob evokes an EPSP insufficient to fire a spike but facilitatory to any other excitatory input. 5, Post-synaptic neurone 5 has a sub-threshold EPSP when the excitatory pre-synaptic cell fires. 6, A branch of the latter cell has a terminal knob near the synaptic knob of an excitatory pre-synaptic neurone which it depolarizes and this reduces the transmitter released from the latter which is now ineffective on the post-synaptic neurone. This is *pre-synaptic inhibition.*

synaptic EPSP recorded from the same neurone but it has a longer latency and decays more rapidly. (This contributes to the '*rebound*' commonly seen after inhibition of a neurone driven by both excitatory and inhibitory inputs.) Whether a transmitter causes excitation or inhibition depends on the type of post-synaptic *receptor* and its site on the receiving neurone and not on the chemical nature of the transmitter.

The principal difference between inhibitory and excitatory receptor channels is that sodium ions pass through excitatory channels and not through inhibitory channels. Conductance in the latter depends mainly on potassium and

chloride ions as the channel is too small for hydrated sodium ions. A neurone may have more than one type of receptor for the pre-synaptic transmitter (eg Renshaw cells have both nicotinic and muscarinic cholinergic receptors). For this reason it is incorrect to use the term 'inhibitory transmitter' despite the fact that GABA and glycine usually involve inhibition.

Both types of post-synaptic potential are graded, according to the total amount of transmitter substance captured by receptors. The summed potentials must depolarize the post-synaptic membrane by a certain amount (*threshold*) to activate the regenerative process responsible for the 'all or none' spike potential of the neurone (p. 3). The depolarization spreads electrotonically across the neuronal membrane, eliciting a spike from that part which has the lowest threshold. This is usually the *axon hillock* or initial segment of the axon in those cells which have a long axon. (There is no favoured zone in stellate cells.) It has been suggested that the actual receptor sites are not electrically excitable.

SUMMATION

Two or more neurones may converge on to one synapse. Their depolarizing/hyperpolarizing pressures sum algebraically. The post-synaptic neurone responds to the summed signals. It is 'ignorant' of the source and acts as an *integrator.* Convergence of neurones on to common lower-order neurones permits *summation in space or in time* (p. 46).

CONVERGENCE

Convergence is assisted by dispersing the receptors on the *soma* of the neurone and on specialized branching processes, *dendrites*, sufficiently close to the soma for the dendritic current to complete its circuit through the soma membrane.

On the other hand, a neurone may have one or more long axonal processes, and each axon may branch ('collateral', or 'terminal'). Thus activity of one neurone may be transmitted to more than one lower-order neurone.

DIVERGENCE

Divergence results in signal amplification (by recruitment of additional neurones) and to generalization of a response to a stimulus which was originally local. It has been believed that each neurone produces only one type of neurotransmitter (Dale's law). There is recent evidence that this is not universal, but as a general rule it is only possible to convert an excitatory signal to an inhibitory one (as seen by the receptive neurone) by having an *intercalated neurone* (interneurone) producing a different neurotransmitter. An extension of Dale's principle, that successive neurones in a chain always produce different chemicals, is no longer accepted, but that arrangement is certainly common. The interneurone may be *recurrent* to the first order neurone soma or its neighbours, as in the Renshaw loop (p. 244).

The properties of (i) making the signal line unidirectional, (ii) boosting signal strength for long transmission, (iii) integrating by convergence and (iv) causing multiple responses by divergence, are important advantages well illustrated in the sensory pathways of the spinal cord and brain stem. The fact that opposing effects (facilitation and inhibition) can be summed, adds important versatility to the nervous system. The following are some of the more elementary functions possible.

COINCIDENCE DETECTION

Consider two excitatory neurones converging on a common post-synaptic neurone which has a threshold requiring EPSP from *both* pre-synaptic neurones before it will fire action potentials. The post-synaptic neurone then signals 'coincidence' of activity in the pre-synaptic neurones. One of them could be used as a 'trigger'. If one neurone is carrying signals reporting the contemporary environment and the other is from some sort of 'memory store', the coincidence recorded by the post-synaptic neurone constitutes a *recognition* signal (p. 118).

GATE CONTROL

Alternatively, if one of several pre-synaptic inputs is essential for the post-synaptic neurone to respond, that pre-synaptic neurone can control all transmission from the remaining pre-synaptic inputs. This 'gate control' as it is called is most powerful when the controlling neurone actively inhibits the synapse and only allows transmission when the IPSP is withdrawn. The inhibition may be either post-synaptic or pre-synaptic. *Pre-synaptic inhibition* results when the inhibitory neurone acts on a neighbouring neurone near its terminal, preventing it from releasing its neurotransmitter. In this particular type, the inhibitory process is not one of hyperpolarization. On the contrary, the excitatory synaptic knob is depolarized and consequently its spike potential is diminished and so the output of transmitter substance is decreased. This is particularly valuable for gate control purposes since the post-synaptic neurone retains its normal excitability. It is well-recognized in the substantia gelatinosa (p. 63). It appears to be a more effective method at this level than in higher levels of the brain. The inhibitory transmitter is probably GABA. At this site the inhibition is potentiated by a number of general anaesthetic agents and not by strychnine and other convulsants with the possible exception of metrazol.

DIRECTION-SENSITIVE NEURONES

As the receptive surface of many neurones is distributed over dendrites, each with branches and *spines* receiving excitatory transmitters from discrete nerve terminals, an additional refinement is possible. A stimulus moving across the receptive fields of a group of neurones projecting sequentially to a dendrite may provide temporal and spatial summation to excite the cell, but only when the receptors are activated in the correct serial order (*Fig. 4.2*). The group of receptors, and hence the cell on which they converge, is then sensitive to a linear stimulus orientated in one direction. A variant is a *movement-sensitive neurone*. Neurones of this type almost certainly exist in the retina and visual cortex (p. 97) and probably cutaneous mechanoreceptors converge on similar neurones in the spinal cord.

There is some evidence for conduction in dendrites. This raises the possibility that a group of terminals contacting a dendrite will only summate their influences if applied in the

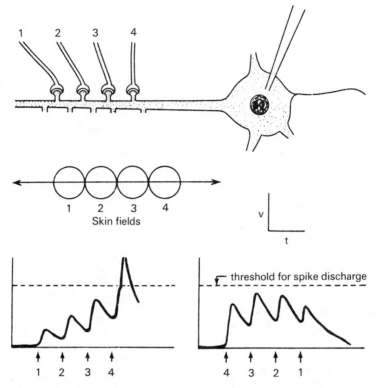

Fig. 4.2. Detection of serial order of dendritic activation. A stimulus moving across a receptor field (skin, retina, organ of hearing etc.) activates afferent neurones in serial order (1–4). With the synaptic arrangement on a dendrite as shown, the threshold for excitation of the post-synaptic cell will only be reached if the pre-synaptic neurones are activated in the correct serial order and time intervals. A stimulus moving across the receptor field in the opposite direction is ineffective as the spatial summation provided by inputs 3,2 and 1 is inadequate to depolarize the cell.

correct order. A neurone with this property would be a detector of serial order and hence *time-sensitive*. This property would account for some of the functions of the temporal lobes (p. 106) and the cerebellum (p. 230) and the function may be widespread.

The summed dendritic potentials (and their spikes in some cases) generate spike responses from the *axon hillock* of the neurone soma. There is a fascinating field of microcircuitry of the soma and its dendritic tree, and the effect of different neurone geometries which promises to be important for full understanding of neuronal function. It is not required for a presentation of this type, but necessary for using electrical field studies to interpret the anatomy and function of cell groups in grey matter. The extracellular potential changes associated with pyramidal shaped cells are less symmetrical than those around stellate cells.

For this reason most of the activity recorded by extracellular electrodes in or on the cerebral cortex is due to the more or less synchronized activity of pyramidal cells with particular orientations and groupings. Synchronous activity in many dendrites arranged in a parallel formation (as in the hippocampus) gives a symmetrical potential field which can be recorded from wide areas of the brain. The 'waves' recorded are not necessarily more significant than other dendritic potentials from less favourably oriented cells.

Modality and local sign

The versatility of the central nervous system as a computer depends on the convergence, divergence, gating and summation properties of synapses just described. But a coincidence detector transmits a signal which no longer has modality specificity or sign of its origin. Signal intensity depends on *recruitment* from numerous parallel neurones ('*a tract*') more than on *frequency* coding. The redundancy of neurones also provides a safety factor for injury or disease. This compounds the difficulty of retaining the purity of the message transmitted and relayed from booster stations.

The solution adopted in the evolution of the nervous system is to 'crispen' or sharpen the signal by surrounding a group of active fibres with others conveying inhibitory signals to lower order neurones which would receive their excitatory input from receptors some distance around the field of primary stimulation. This *surround inhibition* heightens spatial contrast and is renewed at each relay stage — spinal, thalamic and cortical. It is evoked by collateral branches from conducting axons to fringe synapses. In addition, *corticofugal inhibitory fibres* from the receiving areas of the cortex regulate the afferent bombardment at all levels. Examples will be presented in the following chapters. The important point to be made here is that an afferent signal can be routed through synapses like a railway train through points in the permanent way. This is under cortical control. Nevertheless, by repeated use an alternative route may be established as the 'usual' route. *Facilitation* by repeated usage is undoubtedly one mechanism for memory and learning (p. 117). It probably depends on frequent re-establishment of synaptic connections, which are always breaking down and regenerating.

MULTIPLE CHANNEL LINKAGE

Multiple channel linkage is another fundamental feature of higher nervous systems. Elementary descriptions of the nervous system commonly illustrate simple input–output neuronal arcs with one or more intercalated neurones. The human nervous system is not structured in that way. Most input–output connections are multiplied by parallel circuits with more and more relays, ie a monosynaptic arc is backed up by polysynaptic arcs, sometimes with the intercalated neurones at considerable distances (cerebral or cerebellar cortex), presently termed '*long loop*' reflex arcs. This arrangement has two important

consequences. The efferent response is spread out in time as well as in space after a temporo-spatially limited input. Secondly, the additional synapses permit modulation of the response (facilitation, inhibition, gating) by neural activity elsewhere in the nervous system, or by hormones. To illustrate this important principle, examples will be described in the chapters on reflexes (p. 155) and the vestibular system (p. 173), but it is of general application. The relatively long time-constant of synaptic transmitter action may also generate repetitive firing of post-synaptic neurones, one type of *after-discharge* which also prolongs the response to a brief afferent signal. This also depends on the different accommodation and adaptation properties of different parts of the neurone, described in the last chapter, modifiable by altering the chemical environment.

Distributed neuronal systems

A consequence of the *plasticity* and multiplicity of function provided by a synaptic system, as distinct from a fixed network, is that neurones are used for many functions. (We do not know whether there is time-sharing or simultaneous, ie coded, utilization.) The nervous system therefore uses the same elements for a number of functions and the neurones involved form anatomically *distributed systems*. This gives rise to difficulty in describing the functional systems. It will be necessary to ascend and descend the nervous system many times in the following chapters. A concept of anatomical *levels* is too simplistic.

It is useful to have an outline model to bring some semblance of order into the approach. In the following chapters we will describe the afferent side of the nervous system, from receptors via peripheral and central conducting axons to their cells in the cerebrum where the fact that receptors have been stimulated may be 'perceived'. For convenience, the information processing known as 'cross-modality linkage', memory storage, learning and the nature of conscious awareness will then be discussed, followed by the efferent or 'motor' side of the nervous system. The control of the oxygen and pH of the internal milieu in a multicellular organism requires a feedback regulating system

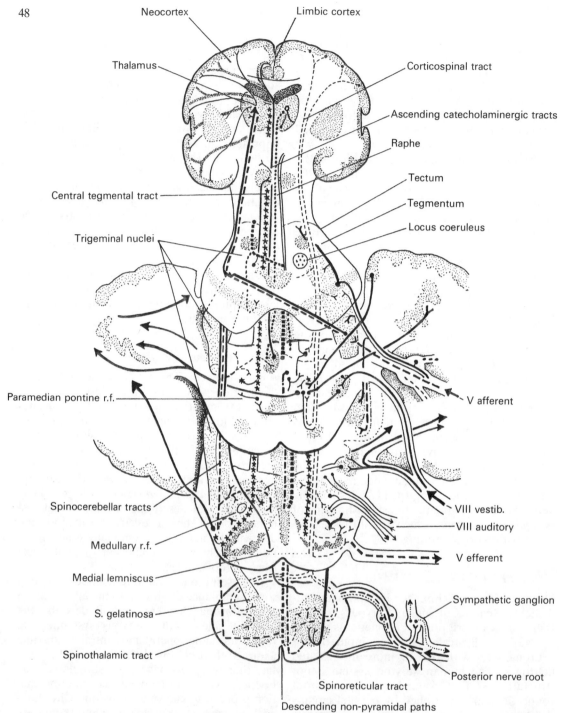

Fig. 4.3. The continuity of grey matter from spinal cord to diencephalon; transverse sections at cord, upper medulla, pons and mesencephalon, with coronal section of cerebrum. The substantia gelatinosa (*left*) continues upwards and expands to form the descending and main nuclei of V (*light grey*), extending to its mesencephalic nucleus. The central grey core continues upwards as the raphe nuclei as far as the thalamus with lateral specializations in the pons and medulla for the motor automatisms, modulated by major inputs from V and VIII (*right*). Paramedian pontine reticular formation is connected bilaterally with the cerebellum which also receives vestibular and spinal inputs recurrent to the mid-brain. Major ascending tracts are spinothalamic and lemniscal crossing and ascending to thalamus; a corticospinal pathway is sketched. These are in the outer areas (homologous with the spinal white matter). The horns of the cord grey matter are

between chemoreceptors and a gas-exchange device, gills or lungs. The system for regulating cyclic motor outputs with 'off switches', limiters, phase spanning neurones and feedback control modulated by extrinsic inputs (Chapter 20) is a paradigm for the cerebellum which is elaborated from it.

The conventional method for presenting the afferent or sensory nervous system is that adopted by Sherrington — interoceptors, exteroceptors and 'special senses'. We propose an alternative classification which highlights the central distribution rather than the site of receptive fields and which may have phylogenetic significance.

CHEMORECEPTORS

Present already in unicellular organisms (p. 43), chemoreceptors of astonishing variety are used for detection of molecules in the environment (smell and taste) and in damaged tissues (pain). The hypothalamus and some specialized organs such as the carotid bodies have neurones which are influenced by changes of pH and of temperature, as well as of osmotic changes in the blood. The mechanism by which temperature is transduced by heat and cold receptors is uncertain. There is evidence that they do so by virtue of their small size and active Na^+–K^+ pump which is highly temperature-dependent. Perception of light (vision) is due to photochemical changes caused by wave energy selectively filtered by specialized non-neural structures. The stimulus to the nervous system (in the retina) is chemical.

Brain stem reticular formation

The most primitive chemoreceptor systems (smell, taste and a major part of pain) project to the 'oldest' part of the brain, the archipallium, directly or via the hypothalamus and amygdalo-septal nuclei (Chapter 14). They have simple receptor organs, commonly only free nerve endings, project centrally by small nerve fibres, relay from cells with extensively intermingled axons and dendrites and have reflex connections with a small fibre efferent system. It is necessary, immediately, to discount the notion that this is a 'primitive' system in man. It is the essential input for survival behavioural patterns and the higher functions of emotion, memory, learning and motivation (Chapters 13 and 14). Furthermore, it is this system which provides most of the input to the arousal systems (reticular formation and septal area) which control consciousness and awareness without which the rest of the nervous system is an automaton. The 'isodendritic core' has been postulated as essential for human mental functions, carrying cholinergic neurones from the striatum, septal area and brain stem reticular formation to layer V of the cortex. The receptors on the pyramidal cells of that layer are muscarinic, blocked by atropine. Thalamocortical neurones are not cholinergic.

This small fibre isodendritic system of the central core of neurones is slowly conducting, not discriminative and with little preservation of topography. An important advance must have been the evolution of parallel, larger fibred, oligosynaptic pathways from, for instance, pain and visual receptors to a greatly enlarged head ganglion of the mechanoreceptors, the thalamus, with cross-modality linkage to afferents of the latter system which has good topographic representation.

There was little interest in, and certainly no understanding of the anatomy and function of the central core of the neural axis until the recognition some 30 years ago of the important 'arousal' mechanism (Chapter 15). It appeared to be an undifferentiated network of short intercommunicating neurones which could not have local sign or, presumably, specialized function. That this was mistaken is clear from the meticulous studies of modern anatomists, histochemists and electrophysiologists. A glance at some known anatomical connections (*Fig. 4.3*) suggests a complexity beyond comprehension but some principles of organization can be extracted by closer examination.

Fig. 4.3. (contd)
homologous with afferent and efferent cranial nerve nuclei. The descending control from diencephalon to the central core is by the central tegmental tract to the inferior olive and spinal projections from the tectum, tegmentum, red nucleus and vestibular nucleus. The ascending chemoreceptor fibres of the spinoreticulo-thalamic tract and Vth nerve send excitatory collaterals into the central core which project major catecholaminergic bundles to the diencephalon and parts of thalamus, the arousal mechanism.

The central core consists of three concentric layers from the grey matter of the spinal cord caudally to the periventricular zone of the cerebrum rostrally. The grey matter is the site of multiple synaptic contacts (and therefore important for integration) by short unmyelinated neurones which are commonly regarded as intercalated (hence *interneurones*) between afferent fibres from peripheral receptors and efferent fibres to effector organs. With the evolution of the forebrain the main receptor and efferent neurones have additional oligosynaptic connections to and from the forebrain by fast conducting myelinated fibres in a peripheral zone of white matter. These bypass the central core but the latter remains an important though slow and poorly localized route for afferent and efferent signals concerned with self-preservation and thermal regulation. Later chapters will develop the theme of alternative route sensory systems gated by efferent control from the higher nervous system and of modulation of the excitability of the somatic efferent system to muscles by brain stem projections to the spinal interneuronal pool. Most of the latter are in less rapidly conducting, thinner myelinated fibres lying between the grey core and the circumferential fast conducting fibres. The latter are collected into recognizable bundles (*tracts*).

In the spinal cord the grey matter has its main pool of interneurones (inhibitory and facilitatory) in Rexed's lamina VIII surrounding a central canal, and the cells to which 'warning' afferents project are grouped in a dorsal (posterior) horn while efferent cells (motoneurones) are in somatotopically arranged groups in the anterior horn. Efferents to the organs for body homeostasis (autonomic, Chapter 27) are in an intermediate horn at restricted levels of the spinal cord. These specialized cell clusters are broken up at brain stem levels by the increasing abundance of white matter bundles but homologies of the posterior and anterior horns form the *nuclei* of the cranial nerves. The continuity is well seen in the long nuclear mass of the afferent fibres of the trigeminal nerve (V), the main cutaneous receptors for the leading segment of animals less evolved than bipedal man. *Fig.* 4.4 shows the structural continuity between the *substantia gelatinosa* of the posterior horn at cord level and the descending nucleus of V in the brain stem from medulla through pons to mid-brain (mesencephalon).

The most central grey matter continues up to the walls of the IIIrd ventricle of the brain where specialized chemosensitive areas develop in the hypothalamus. Between cord and hypothalamus the *central grey matter* is more or less prominent at different levels of the *diencephalon* and brain stem. The caudally projected cell groups of the base of the posterior horn of the cord are represented by major cell groups in the *raphe* (near the midline), small in the medulla but increasing in size and importance in the pons and mesencephalon. They supply important regulatory fibre bundles to the diencephalon (Chapter 25) and to the cerebrum (*telencephalon*, the brain for distance receptors) (Chapter 14–16).

The caudally projected cell groups of the base of the anterior horn are represented in the brain stem by less compact cell groups in the tegmentum and tectal plate which project caudally by short chains of neurones homologous with the *propriospinal fasciculi* surrounding the spinal grey matter, and by the slowly conducting myelinated 'inner ring' tracts, lateral reticulospinal from the medulla, anterior reticulospinal from the pons, tectospinal from the tectum and vestibulospinal from the ponto-medullary junction. Some neurones are facilitatory, others inhibitory. In the medullary reticular formation these tend to be grouped separately (Chapter 22). Specialized neurones in that area may rhythmically switch from one to the other for motor automatisms such as respiration (Chapter 20) and gait (Chapter 21).

This zone of the reticular formation provides chemosensitive feedback loops from the periphery. The most primitive (but still a major driving force for movement stimulation) are blood gas and pH receptors and from taste and smell receptors (Chapter 20): taste impulses project to the nucleus solitarius (*see Fig.* 20.2) and smell to the olfactory bulb and then by multiple routes (Chapter 14) to the ventral tegmental nuclei of the mesencephalon. Chemoreceptors in the retina transduce light waves (Chapter 10) and project via diencephalic areas controlling circadian rhythms and by the superior colliculus to the upward projecting

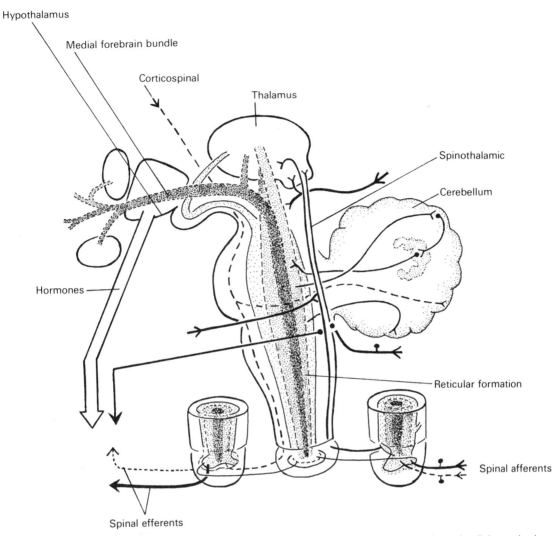

Hypothalamus

Medial forebrain bundle

Corticospinal

Thalamus

Spinothalamic

Cerebellum

Hormones

Reticular formation

Spinal afferents

Spinal efferents

Fig. 4.4. Simplified diagram to show continuity of the central grey core and the anterior–posterior and radial organization from spinal cord to diencephalon, continuing forwards through the medial forebrain bundle. Corticospinal projections run anterolaterally and spinothalamic connections dorsolaterally. The mid-grey shading represents the bases of the horns of the cord and the reticular formation of the brain stem, the lightest shading the efferent (anterior) and afferent (posterior) cranial nuclei, including those of the tegmentum and tectum. The hypothalamus and associated structures secrete hormones into the bloodstream (*open arrow*).

tegmentum of the mid-brain. These inputs from cranial nerves I and II are not shown in ·*Fig.* 20.2. The diagram indicates important inputs from somatic and visceral chemoreceptors ('pain' and (?) temperature) by the massive V nerve input to the pons and by collateral fibres from the *spinothalamic tract* which is also intimately mixed with direct *spinoreticular* fibres originating in the dorsal horns.

An accessory control of late evolutionary development is an input from mechanoreceptors in the inner ear [VIII], (*a*) vestibular to the medullary tegmentum and more directly caudally by the *vestibulospinal tract* to the anterior horn, and (*b*) acoustic via the trapezoid body to the medullary tegmentum where its relay upwards provides important arousal stimuli (Chapter 15). The pontine and lateral medullary reticular nuclei modulate and integrate segmental body movements and have developed important higher control in the paleocerebellum (Chapter 23), to which later evolution has added inputs from the major mechanoreceptors, vestibular (Chapter 18) and proprioceptive from muscles and joints (Chapter 9). This late development was not significantly incorporated into the ascending upper part of the reticular formation. The largest fibres entering dorsal nerve roots ascend the spinal cord white matter posteriorly and relay from the gracile and cuneate nuclei of the medulla directly to a head ganglion in the *thalamus*, without sending collaterals into the ascending arousal system. At that level they converge on fast auditory and visual afferents ('distance receptors') for relay to the *neopallium* where later specialization of the relationship of the body to extracorporeal space is elaborated (Chapter 12). For manipulation of the extracorporeal environment, a fast corticospinal efferent system projects down the outer white ring directly to the motoneurone pools (Chapter 24). The necessary postural adjustment is interpolated by the cerebellum, basal ganglia (Chapter 24) and direct cortico-ponto-reticular and 'extrapyramidal' corticospinal fibres (*see Fig.* 20.2).

The whole forms an efficient and adaptable machine for moving to or from a stimulus (*reflex*) and for postural adjustment. The most important feature of the evolution of the forebrain, however, is that it has developed by modification and outgrowth of an older cerebrum, the *archipallium*, which has reciprocal feedback (controlling) connections with the hypothalamus. This 'inner brain' has visceral afferent input and olfaction (I) and taste (VII, IX) as its distance receptors and so it has been known in the past as the 'smell brain' (*rhinencephalon*). It regulates the activities for preservation of self and species (Chapter 14). With the lowered importance of these functions in higher, mobile, animals other related functions have developed so that a need has been felt for an alternative name. This area of cortex and its subcortical nuclei is now described as the *limbic system* as it forms a ring around the cerebral peduncle and interhemisphere commissures (such as the *corpus callosum*). This is an example of the conservation of structure in phylogeny, but modification of

function by new connections. These vary considerably between species. The principle of conservation makes it reasonable to extrapolate to man most of the findings of mammalian physiology but it must never be forgotten that man probably has unique synaptic connections. This is especially evident in the development of certain integrative areas of the neocortex and its connections with the limbic cortex through the hippocampus, inferior parietal cortex and orbital area of the frontal lobe. The development of these *association areas* and particularly of the *frontal pole*, along with, but in control of, the limbic cortex provides the substratum for higher nervous functions including mind (Chapters 12–14) but only when the cortex is aroused and that is still at the mercy of the midline system from hypothalamus down to pons (Chapter 15).

This is, clearly, regional specialization of function, but the nervous system works as a whole. Even the reticular network has its own well-defined longitudinal connecting bundle to the 'non-specific nuclei' of the thalamus, the *central tegmental tract* (*Fig.* 4.3). The upward messages from the mesencephalon are distributed by discrete fibre bundles to the posterior hypothalamus and thalamus (*dorsal longitudinal fasciculus* and *medial forebrain bundle*), mammillary bodies and anterior hypothalamus (*mammillo-tegmental bundle*) and to the preoptic area, amygdalo-septal complex, limbic area (by elaborate loops — the Papez circuit) and to the (neo)thalamus and neocortex by the medial forebrain bundle. These bundles also convey fibres from the areas mentioned back to the mid-brain tegmentum (Chapter 25). A large nucleus ascending in the anterior white matter from pons through midbrain to diencephalon is the *substantia nigra*. It is reciprocally connected with the *neostriatum* for motor control (Chapter 24) and this is probably a specialized development of a projection system between the mammillary peduncle and medial forebrain bundle, dopaminergic pathway from ventral tegmentum of the mid-brain to the preoptic and limbic areas (*mesolimbic*) and frontal cortex (*mesocortical*) which are particularly important in the human brain (*see Fig.* 3.3).

Although the neopallium has developed as two hemispheres (with contralateral contact with the environment), they are interconnected by large *commissures* (corpus callosum, anterior, posterior and habenular). The limbic areas are continuous across the midline (induseum griseum; *fornix*), and at all levels in the reticular formation and cerebellum and spinal cord there are connections by laterally running collaterals and reciprocal interneuronal connections. The fast conducting myelinated tracts are mainly unilateral, but the central core functions as a balanced whole using the principle of reciprocal inhibition (p. 159).

The lessons from the synoptic view of the nervous system are

1. functional 'systems' are analytical isolates from a versatile interactive machine: neurones may be a 'common path' for many functions;
2. there are no discrete 'centres' linking input to output. These are 'distributed systems' utilizing all levels of the nervous system in parallel, not serially.

The most recent evolutionary development, reaching its acme in man, is the granular cortex of the frontal pole. It receives no direct thalamic input but integrates thalamic and limbic signals. How it enables intelligent anticipation of the future is discussed in Chapter 13.

The various afferent systems are connected to the motoneurones of bulbar and spinal centres (*lower motor neurones*) by more and more elaborate reflex arcs with output from the afferent relays at all levels from the dorsal horn of the spinal grey matter to the brain stem, thalamus and cerebral cortex, with specialized 'long loops' through two important (but anatomically rather similar) integrating circuits based on the vestibular and proprioceptive systems, the cerebellum and basal ganglia respectively.

The cerebral cortex areas for cross-linking *afferent* signals have *command* neurones which can entrain the lower reflex arcs and a number of automatisms (gaze control, gait, respiration and others). This structure for *goal-directed movements* is under the further control of the motivation drives and the frontal lobe in 'voluntary' movement, at first directed by the distance receptors of olfaction, vision and hearing, but eventually put at the control of the somatosensory areas of the cortex for manipulative exploration of the environment. The necessary inhibition of postural and withdrawal reflexes, and the requirement for a fast conducting (large fibre, oligo- and mono-synaptic) pathway, is provided by the *pyramidal tract* from a fronto-central part of the cortex — a specialized but not exclusive efferent system of *upper motor neurones*.

Finally, we resume the story of the automatic systems for controlling behaviour (somatic), hollow organ volume and glandular secretion (autonomic) and hormonal balance, ie the outflow from the hypothalamus and tegmentum, by a slow conducting small fibre system of neurones. Whereas the large fibred reflex system to skeletal muscles is 'open loop', the small fibred autonomic system to smooth muscle and glands has reciprocal feedback. It is 'closed loop' and hence *homoeostatic*. Similar closed loops, entirely neuronal-synaptic, probably exist within the central nervous system to stabilize the spontaneous activity which is characteristic of central (but not of peripheral) neurones.

Further reading

Edelman G.M. and Mountcastle V.B. *The Mindful Brain*. Cambridge, Massachusetts, London: MIT Press, 1978.

Granit R. *The Purposive Brain*. Cambridge, Massachusetts, London: MIT Press, 1977.

Sherrington, Sir Charles. *The Integrative Action of the Nervous System*. Cambridge: Cambridge University Press, 1947.

PART 2   The Afferent Nervous System

Chapter 5
Sensation

The personal nature of sensory experience, the variability of behavioural responses to standardized stimuli and the inability of non-human animals to communicate experience are sufficient reasons for the uncertainties about the physiology of sensation. Few would dispute that the awareness of the body and its relation to external space results from processing by the central nervous system of nervous impulses initiated by transducers responding to physical or chemical stimuli, but it remains uncertain whether receptors are specific for a unique type of stimulus ('modality specific') and have point-to-point representation between periphery and cerebral cortex ('*local sign*'), or whether the nature of stimulus and its point of application are signalled to the higher nervous system by a pattern of impulses in time and space, the transducers (receptors) being responsive to a variety of stimuli. There is no reasonable doubt that many internal receptors within muscles and probably all of the distance receptors of the so-called special senses are truly modality-specific. There is therefore a prima facie case for expecting that this should also be true of receptors monitoring stimuli applied to the body surface, but if these are late biological developments it may not be so. Modality specificity of cutaneous receptors is denied by many authors, but is being increasingly accepted.

INTEROCEPTORS

Some receptors transduce information about the posture of the body (proprioceptors), deriving information about the length of muscle, position or displacement of joints. These are therefore mechanoreceptors. Others transmit impulses about painful or pressure stimuli arising within the body, and are not essentially different from similar receptors on the surface.

EXTEROCEPTORS

Exteroceptors of the integument respond to stimuli interpreted psychologically as touch, pain, warmth and cold. Vibration receptors are both deep and superficial.

There is no real distinction between interoceptive and exteroceptive sensation and yet the receptors identified by the histologist look quite different. There are good reasons for stating that the specialized receptors described by the anatomist — Meissner corpuscles, Merkel discs, Pacinian and Krause endbulbs — free nerve endings and nerve networks are modifications imposed by the site of the endings in, for instance, different layers of hairy or glabrous skin. But nobody can be confident about this. The Pacinian corpuscle seems as well suited for detecting changes of pressure, and the basketwork ending round a hair follicle for detecting hair movement, as is the annulospiral ending of the muscle spindle as a detector of length difference between extra- and intrafusal muscle fibres. These familiar endorgans, however, represent points on a spectrum of endorgans which vary widely from one place to another. Furthermore, the innervation of the skin is not static. The distribution and morphology of the nerve endings alter with age, and in response to injury. Most authors consider that the Pacinian corpuscle is relatively stimulus-specific (to deformation) and that pain is signalled by free nerve endings but there is no proof that they are the sole receptors for these stimuli. The morphology of cold receptors has been found to differ from that of the free nerve endings, but as for warmth, no stimulus-specific endings have been identified.

The Pacinian corpuscle is probably unique in having a single axon linking it to one sensory neurone. Other sensory neurones branch terminally to a group of nerve endings (of a single type for each neurone), so that each nerve cell has a *receptive field* overlapping with the receptive fields of other neurones.

It would be impertinent for non-specialists to adopt a firm point of view on this controversial subject. The present trend is to group receptors according to anatomical similarities rather than differences, and to describe their functions according to their responses to precise stimuli rather than to a supposed sensation. A recent morphological classification of human receptors (by Chouchkov) is:

Epidermal:	Free endings
	Hederiform endings (Merkel's discs)
Dermal:	Free endings
	Hairs
	Encapsulated
	(*a*) without a lamellated inner core (Ruffini)
	(*b*) with an asymmetrical lamellated inner core (Meissner, Krause, Golgi–Mazzoni)
	(*c*) with a symmetrical lamellated inner core (Pacinian).

From the functional point of view, a single criterion is not sufficient to categorize a sense organ in the skin. Factors taken into consideration are preferential sensitivity, size and nature of receptive field, high or low threshold, type of discharge at rest and on activation, rapid or slow adaptation and conduction velocity of the associated nerve fibre. Some of the preferential sensitivity may be attributed to the transducer action of structures such as different types of hair and hair follicles. A useful functional grouping is (i) mechanoreceptors, (ii) thermoreceptors and (iii) nociceptors.

MECHANORECEPTORS

Mechanoreceptors detect displacement of tissue. They can be further subdivided into slowing adapting units which detect position (Type II) and velocity (Type I) of stimulus, rapidly adapting units which detect velocity and very rapidly adapting units which detect transient displacements. Some respond to displacement of a single hair, others ('field units') only to displacement of groups of hairs. Low threshold C fibre mechanoreceptors have not been identified in man and it is possible that there may be other species differences.

THERMORECEPTORS

Thermoreceptors are preferentially receptive to cold or to warmth. Both have a resting discharge so that an appropriate change of skin temperature reduces the firing rate of one type as well as increasing the firing rate of the other.

NOCICEPTORS

Nociceptors are receptors signalling potentially dangerous stimulation of the tissue. There are three main groups: (i) mechanoreceptors with a threshold at least five times greater than the mechanoreceptors transducing displacement; (ii) mechanical/thermal receptors; (iii) polymodal receptors responsive to mechanical, thermal and chemical stimuli. The nociceptors supply unmyelinated C fibres as well as myelinated fibres. In man the C fibre polymodal nociceptors are believed to account for most if not all of the unmyelinated units in the distal skin of the limbs. The range of fibre diameter with sufficient differences of threshold and conduction velocity give rise to detectable elevations of the compound action potential (p. 12) and to recognizable 'first pain' and 'second pain' (Aδ and C fibres respectively).

SPECIAL SENSES

The distance receptors of the cranial nerves are specialized modifications of receptor types present in the peripheral nervous system. They appear to be modality-specific but, like those just described, usually have receptive fields. Point to point representation is achieved by central recognition of overlap, and inhibition of fringe zone responses. Quite possibly the same principles apply to the undefined cutaneous receptors just described.

The basic similarity between 'special' and 'general' sensory organs allows us to recognize the same general principles of function. It is unlikely that cutaneous or periosteal vibration receptors differ materially from the hair cells of the organ of Corti and vestibular endings in the inner ear. Smell and taste clearly use chemoreceptors and it is likely that pain endings do likewise. Vision uses an interesting transposition from wave energy (light) to chemical energy by transforming chemical substances (eg visual purple) in the retina. Similar chemical intermediaries might be postulated for perception of warmth and cold but even the receptors have not been identified.

The appropriate stimulus (and, unfortunately, a range of stimuli used by the experimentalist) causes production of a *receptor potential* by depolarization of the receptor. This spreads electrotonically along the axon and, if the intensity is adequate, initiates 'all or none' spike responses at the first node of Ranvier, the frequency depending on the degree of depolarization of the receptor.

ADAPTATION

Adaptation occurs if the stimulus is maintained, the end organ becoming repolarized and the nerve therefore firing more slowly until it ceases. Rate of adaptation to a steady stimulus is rapid for touch, less so for pain and much less for muscle spindles and cold receptors. Conversely, a rapidly applied stimulus is more effective. These characteristics are quantitatively similar to the accommodation of axons (p. 10) but modifications of the receptor environment undoubtedly play a role by modifying the intensity of the stimulus applied to the receptor membrane.

Modifications may be mechanical (eg deformation of the capsule of a Pacinian corpuscle) or chemical (eg potassium, histamine, acetylcholine and serotonin applied to the skin). Hyperaemia of the skin can lower the threshold for prick, pressure and thermal stimulation. The sympathetic innervation may provide an inhibitory control over the somatic sensory thresholds as sympathetic block often causes a temporary increase of sensation. Recent work by Nathan suggests that peripheral sympathetic blockade stops chronic pain when it has a hyperpathic element, possibly by inactivating the beta group of sensory nerve fibres.

Activation of adjacent receptors or nerve fibres from the same somatic area may summate, inhibit, or alter the quality of experienced sensation (eg a 'cold' stimulus may be experienced as 'hot'). Whether or not these observations may be considered to support a 'pattern' view of sensation, clearly it is technically difficult to study receptors in isolation except for mechanoreceptors and some of the special senses. Specificity may be present but impossible to detect in the conditions of the experiment.

The transducer properties of receptors depend on variations in at least six properties — thresholds to mechanical distortion, negative and positive temperature change and chemical change and also peak sensitivity to temperature change, curve of response to different strengths of stimuli, and rate of adaptation to stimulation. There are probably a multitude of different kinds of specialized receptors and the conventional 'four modalities' of perceived sensation is a simplification forced on us by the difficulty of describing actual experience. If this concept is correct, a receptor may transduce two or more kinds of energy, but clearly one of these may have a lower threshold or evoke a neural firing pattern more suitable for onward transmission at 'filters' in the central nervous system, such as pre-synaptic terminal arborizations (*see* pp. 21, 43 on post-tetanic potentiation, pre-synaptic inhibition and synchronization) to recognition cells tuned to particular temporal and spatial patterns (possibly more than one pattern). In most circumstances, one, the *adequate stimulus*, would be expected to produce impulses more easily than others. The classification of the impulse patterns in time and also in space within the nervous system is a discriminative function of the highest parts of the nervous system, thalamus and cortex. It is on this classification that perception and response depend.

In later sections it will be shown how the afferent signal is modified by the central nervous system, not least to maintain a constancy in the face of sensory adaptation. The different modalities of sensation will be discussed separately but some general principles require preliminary discussion.

FECHNER'S LAW

This is a psychophysical 'law' derived from observation. It states that the quantity of a sensation is proportional to the logarithm of the stimulus — ie when stimulus strength increases in geometric progression, the 'quantity' of sensation increases in arithmetical progression. It is not an exact formula but adequate for practical purposes. Impulse frequency in a primary afferent neurone is almost proportional to the logarithm of the stimulus. There is, however, growing support for a power function law as more accurate — equal stimulus *ratios* produce equal sensation ratios.

It is a general principle, associated with adaptation, that a receptor responds best to abrupt stimulation, with a high-frequency discharge which slows to a low-frequency constant discharge proportional to the maintained stimulus. (This principle should be remembered in clinical testing of sensation, including joint movement.) Many, possibly the majority, of sensory receptors/fibres exhibit spontaneous activity. When a stimulus is abruptly withdrawn the firing rate drops briefly to zero before gradually returning to the resting level of spontaneous discharge, a form of 'biological noise' about which there has been considerable speculation as a source of 'tonic energizing influence' on the nervous system, and in particular on the reticular formation of the brain stem.

Another principle is that there are overlapping *receptive fields*, both large and small, each with its greatest sensitivity at the mid point of the field. Permutations of overlapping fields permit localization as efficiently as single point representation with the added advantage that the same apparatus can be used in numerous combinations without sacrifice of discrimination. Furthermore, intensity of signal can then be indicated by the number of channels recruited as well as by frequency — a principle well understood in the control of muscle. Indeed, facilitation and inhibition of sensory signals may depend more on recruitment than on frequency. It is even possible that one nerve fibre can transmit several messages at the same time.

SUMMATION

The importance of both frequency and recruitment can be seen in the phenomenon of summation of subthreshold stimuli. If a cutaneous area is identified as the centre of a peripheral sensory neurone field (commonly known as a 'touch spot', 'pain spot' etc.) and this point is then stimulated appropriately with a stimulus of just subliminal strength, no sensation will be perceived unless that stimulus is rapidly applied to the same spot or an identical stimulus to a neighbouring area.

In the first case, *summation in time*, the depolarization of the receptor is increased to a level that triggers action potentials. In the other, *summation in space*, there is either additional depolarization of receptor on a different branch of the axon or recruitment of receptors of neighbouring axons with overlapping receptive fields. On the other hand, two or more stimuli applied simultaneously may inhibit each other.

REFERRED SENSATION

The observation that pain and paraesthesiae resulting from lesions in the peripheral nervous system can be prevented by blocking the relevant nerves distal to the lesion suggests that a continuous stream of subliminal impulses enter the nervous system from the periphery which can be summated with impulses arising locally in the nerve. Similarly, subliminal impulses from two or more peripheral sensory fields converging on a common axon, either primary or secondary, may summate sufficiently to cause central transmission of a suprathreshold message. The nervous system will give the summated signals the local sign of the receptor field which normally dominates its input and hence pain will be 'referred' to that site even if the pathological increase in signal activity arises from a less usual receptive field, but the pain can nevertheless be reduced or abolished by lowering the input of subliminal afferent firing from the site of referred pain by local anaesthetics or by cooling the painful area which is not the seat of pathology.

LOCALIZATION

It will be apparent that the ability to localize stimuli or to discriminate two simultaneously applied stimuli will vary with the size of receptive field as well as with discreteness of central (mainly cortical) representation. Thus the limen for two-point discrimination varies according to the region stimulated and also according to the modality. Variations with age and after injury demonstrate that the sensory innervation of the skin is a dynamic process. Like the motor units (p. 235) the 'sensory units' probably undergo cycles of breakdown and regeneration. Tactile localization is extremely poor before puberty and in old age, but the superior plasticity of the immature nervous system is shown by the better functional recovery after nerve section in the child than in the adult.

At first sight it might appear that overlapping of receptor fields of sensory units would prejudice localization compared with a 'point-to-point' system linking skin receptor with cortical sensory neurone. Observation shows that in areas like the fingertips with good localization, there is a high degree of overlap, with dense innervation, and vice versa in areas with poor spatial discrimination such as the back of the trunk. This is not a problem if localization is based on the central nervous system detecting coincidences and differences between overlapping sensory units, and their temporal patterns would add another dimension of discrimination. Additionally, one of a group of overlapping receptor fields may be 'selected' for attention if its neurone (primary or secondary) is facilitated or its neighbours inhibited (*surround inhibition*) and this is a well-recognized property of sensory systems in the spinal cord and cerebrum (*Fig.* 5.1). The principle of discrimination by overlapping fields of different sizes and surround inhibition is well authenticated in vision.

Sensory nerves and dorsal roots

As the afferent nerve fibres from skin and deep tissues run centrally, they are collected into peripheral nerves, at first sensory and then mixed with motor fibres distributed to the same anatomical territory. Before reaching their cell bodies in ganglia, they regroup into dorsal nerve roots entering the spinal cord segmentally in zones related to the body segments from which the somatic tissues migrated with their nerve fibres during

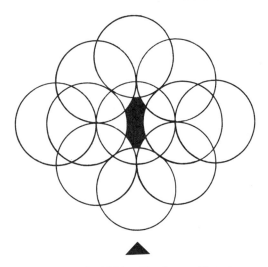

Fig. 5.1. Surround inhibition. The diagram illustrates some overlapping receptive fields. If all afferent neurones respond to a localized stimulus but are mutually inhibitory, only the neurone receiving from the black area will transmit a maximum signal. Surround inhibition of this type is repeated at each relay nucleus, thus sharpening the signal relayed forwards.

embryological development. As muscle does not necessarily migrate along with overlying integument, the myotomes do not lie deep to the dermatomes from the same segment. Consequently, pain, spontaneous or referred, in muscle and other skeletal tissues, is not obviously related to dermatomal patterns.

Early studies on laboratory animals, by cutting three dorsal roots above and below an intact one, or clinical studies on herpes zoster in man, have provided dermatomal maps. Recent work by Denny-Brown and colleagues has shown that the dermatomes overlap and axons of a single dorsal root may spread over at least five segments of the body. Various manipulations on the tract of Lissauer (where dorsal roots enter the cord) suggest that the apparent size of the dermatome, and possibly the quality of the sensation experienced from it, is determined in part by a synaptic interaction of primary afferent fibres. The concept of segmentation, appropriate enough for nerve roots, is too simplistic for the spinal cord.

Each dorsal root breaks up into small fascicles before entering the cord and it has been said that these show some rearrangement of fibres according to their diameter, with the

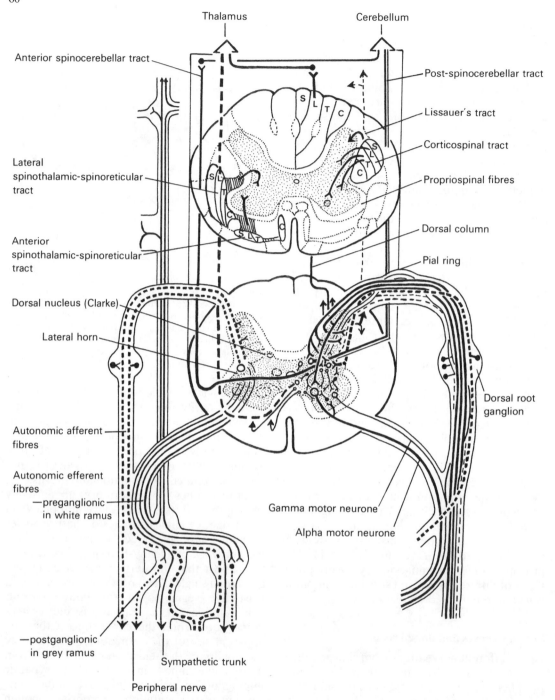

Thalamus

Cerebellum

Anterior spinocerebellar tract

Post-spinocerebellar tract

Lissauer's tract

Corticospinal tract

Lateral spinothalamic-spinoreticular tract

Propriospinal fibres

Anterior spinothalamic-spinoreticular tract

Dorsal column

Pial ring

Dorsal nucleus (Clarke)

Lateral horn

Dorsal root ganglion

Autonomic afferent fibres

Autonomic efferent fibres

—preganglionic in white ramus

Gamma motor neurone

Alpha motor neurone

—postganglionic in grey ramus

Sympathetic trunk

Peripheral nerve

Fig. 5.2. *Integrative functions of spinal cord.* Somatic (*right*) and autonomic (*left*) afferent fibres entering the spinal cord by dorsal nerve roots. In the peripheral nerve and root they have no regular position until the pial ring, shortly before entering the cord, where the small fibres group laterally to enter the tract of Lissauer. They pass up and down that tract and enter the dorsal horn at a number of laminae. A and C fibres transmitting thermal sensation and pain from somatic and visceral areas relay to the contralateral spinothalamic–spinoreticular tract and ipsilaterally in the thoracic and upper lumbar cord to efferent autonomic neurones (*left*) for local and distant distribution in the visceral sympathetic chain (*see Fig.* 26.2) and in peripheral nerve trunks to blood vessels and skin (*see Fig.* 26.3).

larger axons in the central and medial parts of the rootlet and the small myelinated and unmyelinated fibres on the lateral side (*Fig. 5.2*). These small fibres pass into the tract of Lissauer at the apex of the posterior horn. The large fibres have their cell bodies in the dorsal root ganglion, but these small fibres have their cell bodies in the cord. Not all anatomists accept this rearrangement of fibres according to size in the nerve rootlets, but the concept of *size ordering* within the spinal cord is fundamental to the understanding of modern views about the afferent pathways in the spinal cord.

Before turning to that subject, it should be recorded that certain *ventral* nerve roots are known to have a large number of afferent fibres, mainly unmyelinated. This should be remembered when evaluating the results of dorsal rhizotomy.

A major proportion of the dorsal root fibres, mainly group I fibres from muscle and joint receptors with a proportion of low threshold mechanoreceptors from the skin, pass dorsally without further relay into the dorsal white column of the cord, ascending to the *dorsal column nuclei* of Goll and Burdach in the medulla oblongata. Others pass anteriorly in the grey matter of the cord to the *anterior horn* where monosynaptic connections are made with motoneurones for segmental reflexes controlling muscle length and tension (*see Fig. 17.1*). The remainder of the dorsal root fibres, including most of the smaller myelinated and all the unmyelinated fibres, synapse in the grey

matter of the dorsal root entry zone, either the *substantia gelatinosa* or the more medial *dorsal horn* of the grey matter. The secondary neurones cross the midline either directly or after passing up or down the cord for a few cord segments in the *tract of Lissauer*. Some are distributed to motoneurones or grey matter interneurones as the substratum of the protective reflexes (p. 61). Others link cord segments by the intrinsic *propriospinal pathways* applied to the central core of grey matter. The majority pass cranially in the lateral and anterior white columns. The conventional description of their grouping into recognizable tracts is questioned (p. 64).

THE DORSAL HORN OF THE SPINAL CORD GREY MATTER

The dorsal horn of the spinal cord grey matter is an exceedingly complicated zone of nerve cells, interneurones and fibre connections, too complicated to represent in detail in a book of this type. Its importance as the gateway for afferent impulses entering the cord and as a site for integration and feedback control of sensory input makes a simplified presentation essential.

The laminar arrangement of dorsal horn cells described by Rexed is considered to have functional significance. The laminae are numbered I–VI concentrically centripetally. Lamina I, the marginal cell layer, receives collaterals from Lissauer's tract (mainly propriospinal axons connecting cord segments) and projects

---

Fig. 5.2. (*contd*)

Larger somatic afferent fibres enter the cord in a medial bundle. The Ib fibres terminate in the more central laminae of the dorsal horn in (*a*) Clarke's nucleus, for relay to the ipsilateral posterior spinocerebellar tract, and (*b*) the lateral part of the base of the dorsal horn to relay to the contralateral anterior and lateral spinothalamic tracts. (*c*) Some Ib (A) fibres pass with a central bundle of fast conducting (Ia, A) fibres to the dorsal column for passage upwards to their first relay in the dorsal column nuclei (*see Fig. 9.2*). Many relay by the contralateral anterior spinocerebellar tract to the inferior olive (*see Fig. 23.1*).

A major group of Ia (A) fibres from primary spindle receptors ends monosynaptically or after internuncial relay (*see Fig. 17.1*) on anterior horn cells, the alpha motoneurones for type I efferent fibres (*right*). Interneurones (facilitatory and inhibitory) relay segmental and descending extrapyramidal fibres to slow gamma motoneurones. The descending extrapyramidal motor control is shown separately in *Fig. 17.1*. The crossed corticospinal tract input is indicated in the upper spinal segment. The monosynaptic input is probably restricted to distal limb muscles. The top of the diagram indicates convergence of second order lemniscal afferent fibres to the contralateral thalamus (*see Fig. 8.1*). Spinocerebellar fibres converge to the ipsilateral cerebellum.

Intersegmental connections (trains of short neurones) pass caudally as well as rostrally in the propriospinal fibres surrounding the grey matter, in the substantia gelatinosa (Rexed lamina II) and in the tract of Lissauer. The extramedullary sympathetic chain does not project back into the cord. It receives descending neurones from hypothalamus (ipsilateral) and reticular formation (bilateral) (*see Fig. 25.1*) in cord areas cross hatched. Note the convergence of autonomic and reticulospinal projections on the major relay area for pain sensation (*see Fig. 6.1*) and thermoregulatory reflexes.

to the thalamus and to other regions of the cord. Laminae II and III constitute the *substantia gelatinosa* which receives coarse collaterals of primary afferent fibres from hair follicles, and fine fibres from the same sources as the marginal cell layer (predominantly propriospinal). The neuropil of lamina II contains structures termed *glomeruli* which appear to be extremely complicated synaptic structures with probably integrative functions, probably acting on large cells in the deeper laminae of the dorsal horn including laminae IV, V and VI which project via the contralateral side of the cord to the thalamus.

At this important synaptic area on the central projection of afferent signals, there are numerous opportunities for interaction by pre-synaptic and post-synaptic actions, particularly of interneurones excited by cutaneous and muscular afferents and also by axons descending from higher parts of the nervous system (lamina V). Lamina VI includes cells forming *Clarke's column*, receiving afferents from muscles and joints and relaying their signals to the *ventral spinocerebellar tract*.

The enormous potential for facilitation and inhibition with either selection or summation of incoming signals suggests that the dorsal horn is a site for 'volume control' of afferent signals according to the state of excitability of higher centres, and also for selective 'gating' of the type of signal to be passed forwards in the communication channels. For instance, the traffic of impulses entering the cord in small nerve fibres of the dorsal root could be suppressed if inhibitory interneurones were activated by collateral branches of large afferent fibres. There is also increasing evidence that peripheral sympathetic (noradrenergic) nerves and circulating noradrenaline enhance the responses of receptors for pain (man) and cold (frog). Surgical or chemical (guanethidine) block of adrenergic action has been investigated for treatment of pain.

Further reading

Chouchkov C.N. Cutaneous receptors. *Adv. Anat. Embryol. Cell. Biol.* 1978; **54**: 1–62.

Hallin R.G. and Torebjork H.-E. Studies on cutaneous A and C fibre afferents, skin nerve blocks and perception. In: Zotterman Y. (ed.) *Sensory Functions of the Skin in Primates*. Oxford: Pergamon Press, 1976, pp. 137–48.

Rexed B. Some aspects of the cytoarchitectonics and synaptology of the spinal cord. In: Eccles J.C. and Schade J.P. (ed.) *Progress in Brain Research. Organization of the Spinal Cord*. Amsterdam: Elsevier, 1964, vol. 11, pp. 58–92.

Schmidt R.F. (ed.) *Fundamentals of Sensory Physiology*, 2nd ed. New York: Springer-Verlag, 1981.

Chapter 6
Pain

From this chapter on, the physiology of the afferent pathways will be described mainly in terms of conduction velocity of groups of nerve fibres rather than of supposed specificity of sensory modality. Nevertheless, the protective value of appreciation of noxious stimulation, and the particular importance of pain to the anaesthetist, justify special consideration of the experience of pain.

We have already drawn attention to uncertainty about the existence of specific receptors and peripheral nerve fibres for transducing and transmitting signals associated with appreciation of pain. We cannot be certain about different experiences reported as being painful. The common clinical test of ability to distinguish 'sharp' from 'blunt' using a pinprick involves Aδ fibres but is commonly called 'first pain'. A stronger stimulus with a pin evokes a delayed or 'second pain' involving C fibres (p. 13). The Aδ 'first pain' fibres are involved in the afferent limb of the protective reflexes (p. 162) and may be selectively damaged by lesions at the dorsal root entry zone such as tabes dorsalis and in the dorsal root ganglia in herpes zoster (as the soma of the C fibre neurones is in the dorsal horn, not in the ganglion). Much of the confusion in human studies and their correlation with studies on animals which cannot communicate if an experience is truly painful, is due to failure to discriminate between Aδ and C fibre responses. The uncertainty about central pathways is fundamentally due to the same reasons — the impossibility of confirming objectively such a subjective experience as pain, and the conflicting results of stimulation and ablation 'experiments' of human disease and its surgical treatment. Not least of the problems is that the afferent signals relayed from the dorsal horn are controlled by descending influences which are largely dependent on such matters as emotional set, alertness and attention.

SUPRASPINAL CONTROL OF AFFERENT INPUT

Descending influences include the pyramidal tract, by pre-synaptic depolarization of primary afferent fibres as well as facilitatory and inhibitory actions on interneurones. If the human is the same as other primates, other pathways include a dorsal reticulospinal and raphe-spinal system which provide tonic inhibition of spinal flexion reflexes (*Fig.* 17.2). Damage to this probably contributes to paraplegia in flexion. Similarly, vestibulospinal and cerebellar projections are not only to the anterior horn, but to primary afferents from muscle (group Ia) and also from the skin as they enter the dorsal horn.

The *interneurones* of the dorsal horn are strongly influenced by anaesthetic drugs. Their action is not confined to the brain. But cells in the dorsal horn respond to a wide range of stimulus intensity applied to the skin, rather than specifically to noxious strengths.

GATE THEORY OF PAIN

On clinical grounds Noordenbos (1959) suggested that synaptic transmission in a system activated by small afferent fibres can be inhibited by large fibre activity. The idea was developed by Melzack and Wall (1965), who proposed that the substantia gelatinosa constituted a 'gate control system' to control afferent input before it affects the *first central transmission (T) cells* in the dorsal horn. According to this idea the gate is kept partly open by tonic activity in small fibres but closed by input over large fibres which (in addition to exciting T cells) excite interneurones which cause pre-synaptic inhibition of all dorsal root input fibres and which also have collaterals ascending to the dorsal column for switching on the descending control system just described. It was further postulated that the excitation of the large fibre system is short lasting compared to the small fibre system. Thus a prolonged stimulus would cause adaptation of the large afferents and the continuing small fibre activity would 'open the gate', allowing the T cells to send signals up the spinothalamic pathways to be interpreted as pain. In fact this would be facilitated by collaterals of the small fibres inhibiting the tonic activity of substantia gelatinosa neurones, so causing *pre-synaptic disinhibition* of the T cells.

The gate theory of pain has been widely publicized but, at least in its original form, it is not consistent with a number of experimental and clinical findings (see the critical review by Nathan, 1976). We suggest that the apparent anomalies are due to the fact that there are (at least) two pain systems with different properties. Loss of large fibre control, with release of small fibre pain would admirably account for post-herpetic neuralgia with severe pain in an 'analgesic' area. (The special liability of the trigeminal nerve territory suggests this as a site for detailed investigation.)

Ascending pathways in pain sensation

From clinicopathological studies of spinal cord disease and spinal cord 'tractotomies' followed up over a number of years, it appears likely that the central projection of the dorsal horn cells receiving nociceptive afferent impulses involves fibres throughout most of the ventrolateral white matter of the cord (*Fig.* 6.1). There are no 'pure' tracts carrying fibres subserving only one sensory modality. Nevertheless, groupings of fibres, and the obvious necessity of having some landmarks to describe the position of major groupings, justify the use of familiar anatomical names such as *spinothalamic tract* although it also contains the *spinoreticular* fibres. Axons of many dorsal horn cells decussate through the anterior white commissure in the same or in a nearby segment

of the cord and ascend to the thalamus in the ventrolateral white column without further synapse. Other fibres pass to the thalamus *bilaterally* via relay(s) in the reticular formation and mid-brain tectum. Phylogenetically, the direct spinothalamic pathway (which also projects bilaterally) is a late development. In the spinal cord it is close to or mixed with the spinoreticular projection. It is the target for destruction in the operation of spinal tractotomy for relief of pain, but the eventual recurrence of pain suggests that the indirect pathways (which may even include the polysynaptic propriospinal fibres adjacent to the central grey matter) play some role in the transmission of impulses from nociceptors. Between the inferior olive and the thalamus the reticular projection runs more medially (*Fig.* 6.1). Mesencephalic tractotomy limited to the spinothalamic fibres abolishes sharp pain but not diffuse pain. Major differences between species make it difficult to draw conclusions about the 'pain pathway(s)' in man from experiments on laboratory animals. The human subject probably resembles other primates in having an approximate somatotopic organization of the spinothalamic fibres (caudal body parts represented dorsolaterally or laterally, and rostral parts represented ventromedially or medially in the ventrolateral column of the cord) but, contrary to previous ideas, the spinothalamic tract does not form a compact bundle. Its fibres are distributed throughout the ventrolateral white matter, and this plus the indirect pathways referred to above accounts for the inadequate relief of pain unless cordotomy is so extensive as to risk cutting downward projecting fibres involving bladder and limb control. The most anterior spinothalamic fibres, in the ventral part of the cord, have been considered to transmit tactile impulses but anatomical separation of touch and pain/thermal sensation fibres probably does not occur.

The spinothalamic tract ascends through the brain stem, gradually approaching and eventually intermingling with medial lemniscus fibres, and gives *collateral branches to the lateral reticular formation* in the brain stem. Their important role in the 'alerting system' of the brain will be discussed in Chapter 15. The spinothalamic fibres project to well-defined

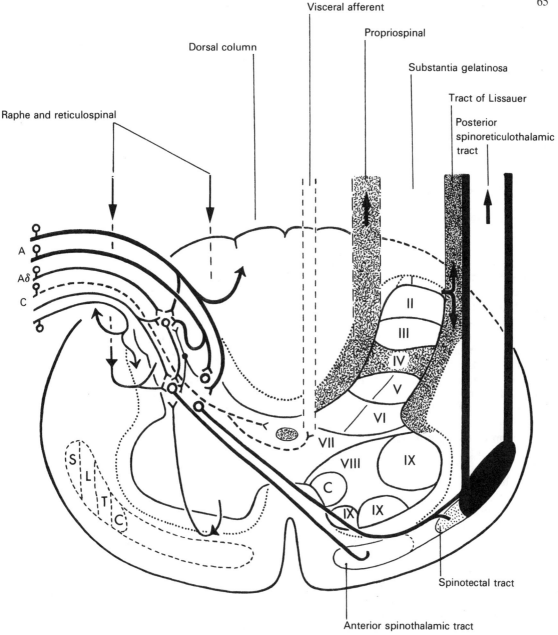

Fig. 6.1. Spinal pathways for impulses from nociceptors. The small C and A fibres regroup to the lateral side of the dorsal root before entering the cord and pass to Rexed laminae III–V. Those from the viscera (*dashed*) relay or pass directly to the intermediomedial nucleus bilaterally. Those from somatic tissues relay across the anterior white commissure to the anterolateral white column (uncrossed fibres omitted from diagram). They ascend in the anterior spinothalamic, spinotectal and a combined spinoreticular and posterior spinothalamic tract (*black*) which carries most of the fibres subserving fast pain. Second order neurones from many of the C fibres ascend bilaterally in Lissauer's tract and upward extension of lamina IV and the propriospinal fasciculi (*grey*). The right side of the diagram illustrates the continuity of the substantia gelatinosa (II, III) with the trigeminal nucleus of the brain stem, and the intermediomedial nucleus with the solitary tract nucleus. The nociceptor afferents and their relay neurones in the dorsal horn receive gating control (mainly inhibitory) from collaterals of the larger A group afferents (medial side of entering root) and from descending fibres from the raphe and ponto-medullary reticular formation. Segmental efferent connections are shown in *Fig.* 17.1.

parts of the *thalamus* — the ventrobasal complex, the posterior nuclear group, including the medial geniculate body, and the intralaminar nuclei (*Fig.* 6.2). Here also there are some species differences and the data for man are somewhat scanty.

The posterior thalamic nuclei project 'third order' neurones to specific modules of cells in the post-central gyrus and other sensory areas of the cerebral cortex as described in Chapter 12 and the intralaminar nuclei project widely over the cerebral cortex. As the first and second order neurones include large and small fibres, and the second order projections are both direct and indirect, the signals reaching the thalamus and relayed to the cortex are desynchronized and prolonged in time even after a brief stimulus. There is limited evidence from cerebral lesions in man that pain impulses are projected to the primary sensory area of the neocortex (SmI) but no satisfactory evidence regarding the supplementary sensory areas SmII and MsII shown tentatively in the diagram. From the septal nuclei fibres are relayed by various pathways to the hippocampus and from there to the limbic cortex (Chapter 14). Thus the cortical appreciation of 'slow pain' is not neocortical: the cortical projection of the spinothalamic tract from the ventrolateral thalamus adds local sign but it is questionable if it contributes to the analysis of pain other than its 'sharpness'. However, the cingulate gyrus, septum and amygdala project to the inferior frontal lobe of the neocortex. If these fibres are sectioned (pre-frontal leucotomy or cingulectomy) the psychological importance of pain as a threat to future well-being is removed. It is a clinical tradition that pain is 'appreciated' at the thalamic level but quality and quantity of pain are 'discriminated' in the cortex, where the impulses are also integrated with those of other sense modalities. This is largely due to the observation that analgesia rarely results from suprathalamic lesions. Nevertheless it is doubtful whether any sensations enter consciousness at thalamic level and there is no part of the thalamus which is functionally independent of the cortex. Some examples of loss of pain sensibility after parietal lobe damage, and pain as an epileptic aura suggest that the cortex is at least involved in appreciation of some aspect of pain, an appreciation which is modified by tactile and pressure impressions and the state of activity of other cortical centres. Thus, prefrontal leucotomy increases the 'pain tolerance ratio' though it does not abolish its perception. A similar principle may be involved in the use of chlorpromazine and similar drugs along with true analgesics in the treatment of chronic pain syndromes (but cf. pain as a conditioned response, p. 135).

An interpolation of clinical data suggests the following model (*Figs* 6.1, 6.2). A C fibre chemoreceptor system with poor local sign ascends bilaterally in the fasciculus proprius of the spinal cord, as short chains of intercommunicating neurones to the lateral (afferent) reticular formation to the pons and then by the central tegmental tract to the intralaminar nuclei of the thalamus, hypothalamus and septum with a primitive higher control from septum to amygdala, hippocampus and fornix back to hypothalamus and thalamus. (The pathways are described in Chapter 25.) Pain associated with stimulation of this system has an aching quality, poor local sign and may be poorly lateralized. It is characteristic of visceral pain but persists in the mesenchymal tissues. Its upward projection to subthalamic areas gives this pain a linkage with other small fibre afferent systems experienced as nausea, unlocalized and poorly differentiated sensations of hot and cold, and a marked efferent autonomic response. The higher 'centres' of this system may be involved in headache, and particularly that type known as migraine. The input areas are, we propose, involved in the aching somatic pains familiar to the physician and which are alleviated by factors dispersing local accumulation of chemicals, ie movement, massage, heat, vasodilatation (including the effect of guanethidine?). It is this system which may be influenced by acupuncture.

An additional, A delta fibre mechanoreceptor and possibly a different C fibre chemoreceptor system (spinothalamic and spinoreticular) projects more directly to the 'specific' thalamus. It has good local sign, rapid conduction, evokes somatic motor response (withdrawal) and is not significantly influenced by physical dispersion of algesic chemical substances, vasodilatation or antiprostaglandin drugs. This is the pain familiar to

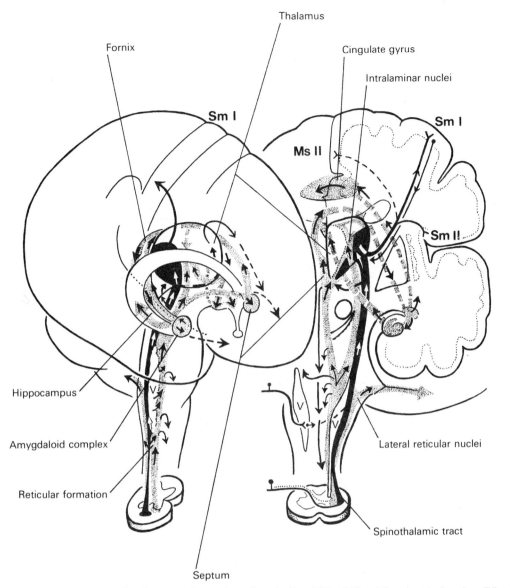

Fig. 6.2. Central connections of nociceptor pathways from the spinal cord (*Fig.* 6.1) and the trigeminal nucleus (V). The left hemisphere is shown in coronal section and the right as seen through the hemisphere obliquely from the front to show the brain stem overlaid by the amygdaloid complex and the hippocampus which runs forward and medially to join the diencephalic termination of the mesencephalon at the hypothalamus and septum. The thalamus lies medial to the hippocampal formation and above the hypothalamus. Its VPL nucleus (*black*) receives the spinothalamic (lemniscal) fibres and has limited relay of tertiary neurones to the primary (SmI) and secondary sensory areas (SmII and the adjacent mainly motor area MsII). Some spinotectal fibres relay in the superior colliculus to the same area of the thalamus.

The grey shading represents the upward projection of the small fibre system (shown in *Fig.* 6.1) in the lateral (afferent) medullary reticular formation. Much of this ascending traffic is relayed into the cerebellum from the lateral reticular nucleus (*see Fig.* 23.1). The remainder passes up the central tegmental tract, with numerous collateral branches to the efferent reticular nuclei. The ascending system of short neurones splits into a number of bundles (Chapter 3). For central appreciation of pain, and integrated response to it, the two main routes are to the intralaminar and reticular nuclei of the thalamus (as an important general arousal system) and through the mid-brain raphe to hypothalamus and septal nuclei, each projecting onwards to the anterior thalamus and thence to the cingulate gyrus.

From the septum further relays pass by stria terminalis to the amygdaloid complex and dentate gyrus of hippocampus. From there they enter the cingulate cortex directly and around the fornix–mammillo-thalamic route. The limbic cortex is thus the main integrative area for 'small fibre' pain sensation. It further projects, along with the septum and amygdala, to the orbitofrontal cortex for delayed behavioural responses (Chapter 12).

the trauma surgeon. It requires limitation of movement, and centrally acting narcotics or blockade of afferent nerves. It is investigated by applying sharply defined stimuli to the skin and experiments confined to that aspect tell only a little about pain as a whole. The larger fibred system exerts some inhibitory control over the small fibred system at the dorsal horn, reticular formation and thalamus and these controls may be regarded as 'gates' since they are threshold controllers.

Reference has already been made to the control of pain-responding cells in the dorsal horn by impulses conducted in large nerve fibres, acting via pre-synaptic inhibition of the primary afferent input, disinhibition of inter-neurones and feedback from medullary centres. It is reasonably certain that similar modulation of the second order neurones occurs at the thalamus, and feedback inhibition of thalamus by cortex is important. The 'thalamic syndrome' of spontaneous and prolonged pain with elevated threshold may be due to interference with this type of control since it occurs with lesions immediately above and below the thalamus as frequently as with localized thalamic damage.

The unpleasant quality and persistence of a type of pain occurring with lesions of peripheral nerves or thalamus, the protopathic pain of Henry Head, were indeed attributed by that author to a 'release' mechanism, but the term protopathic (and its antithesis — epicritic) is best abandoned because certain assumptions required by Head's theory cannot be supported.

Studies on inhibitory control of the thalamus using adequate pain stimulation are difficult since the spinothalamic volley is inhibited at dorsal horn level by corticofugal impulses from the sensorimotor cortex as well as from the brain stem (p. 63).

There is a system of neurones in the *periaqueductal grey matter and the raphe nuclei* of the brain stem which appear to be of special importance in controlling the response to noxious stimuli. Stimulation of these areas produces behavioural signs of analgesia and their destruction causes increased responsiveness to noxious stimuli (*hyperalgesia and dysaesthesia*). Many of the neurones involved are serotoninergic and may be stimulated by opioid drugs (p. 40).

Current speculation postulates that the central nervous system has an *intrinsic analgesia system* using three transmitters — 5-hydroxytryptamine (serotonin), dopamine and a morphine-like transmitter (p. 40). A suggested circuit involves activation by spinothalamic neurones of endorphin-secreting cells acting on the periaqueductal and periventricular grey matter serotoninergic cells projecting to raphe nuclei and reticular formation which have descending inhibitory control on the dorsal horn input. These descending fibres are in the dorsolateral white column and may be the same as those responsible for tonic inhibition of the flexion reflex pathways (p. 163).

A *spinoreticular tract* in the ventrolateral white matter of the spinal cord carries impulses from cells of the deeper laminae of the dorsal horn to a number of reticular nuclei in the medulla and pons, and to the raphe nuclei. Unlike lower animals, it appears to be unilateral and largely uncrossed in primates. There is, of course, no evidence that these neurones mediate pain as a sensation though they respond to noxious stimulation. They may be on the afferent limb of the flexion reflex arc and some fibres are relayed to the cerebellum rather than to the thalamus. The importance of spinoreticular fibres in arousal and aversive behaviour is also discussed elsewhere. At this point the important thing to stress is that stimulation of nociceptive nerves and their endings causes not only pain but reflex responses (sweating; the flexion reflex) and strong motivational affective responses involving the amygdala and limbic system (*see* p. 135 on pain as a conditional or learned response, and on asymbolia for pain).

Although it is conventional to discuss these separately, it is becoming evident from the recent growth of interest in pain and its management that the subjective phenomenon described as pain can be substantially modified by altering the somatic and autonomic motor responses and, particularly, the behavioural reaction by psychotherapeutic as well as by pharmacological measures, or by various methods of 'large fibre stimulation' by electrical pulses applied to skin, nerve or dorsal column. The empiric nature of these measures makes it particularly difficult to analyse the effects of acupuncture. Statements that this treatment stimulates release of endogenous endorphins depend on circumstantial evidence which is not entirely convincing (p. 40).

Chemical aspects of pain sensation

The receptors giving rise to sensations of pain are all nociceptors: the converse is not necessarily true. There are some detectors of tissue damage which do not, at least at threshold levels of response, activate second order 'pain' fibres though they may activate pain-related responses such as the autonomic and flexion reflexes described in Chapters 25 and 17. Some mechanoreceptors produce signals interpreted as pain. Nevertheless, the majority of pain receptors are probably chemoreceptors. The nature of the receptors is undetermined. There may be many (in analogy with the chemoreceptors for taste sensation), as a number of algesic substances have been identified, presumably released from damaged tissue. These include KCl, H^+ ions, serotonin, histamine and bradykinin. Bradykinin also potentiates prostaglandin E2 and other derivatives of arachidonic acid which *sensitize the receptors* to other algesic agents. It has been postulated that a major part of the action of certain analgesic drugs (acetylsalicylic acid, ibuprofen, diclofenac, indomethacin, phenylbutazone) is to inhibit the enzyme cyclooxygenase which converts arachidonic acid to prostaglandins, prostacyclins and thromboxanes. Prostaglandins are released from fat by noradrenaline and this could be related to the *hyperpathia* and *allodynia* of some chronic painful states which may be relieved by sympathetic blockade or by infusion of guanethidine though vasodilatation cannot be dissociated. (Hyperpathia is a painful syndrome, characterized by delay, over-reaction and after-sensation to a stimulus, especially a repetitive stimulus. Allodynia is a state in which pain is caused by a stimulus which does not cause pain in normal skin.) Expression of alpha-adrenergic receptors on sprouts from injured nerve fibres may also account for sensitivity to locally released noradrenaline in causalgia and stump neuromas as well as ephaptic stimulation (p. 70).

Corticosteroids interfere with the production of arachidonic acid from phospholipids. Some of the analgesic effect may be indirect, by altering the calibre and permeability of capillaries in the damaged tissue. This is a rapidly developing field of pharmacological research and the concepts outlined here are provisional.

There is also no certainty about the neurotransmitter released on dorsal horn neurones by Aδ and C fibres of the dorsal nerve root (which may be different for each fibre type). There is growing evidence that a transmitter is substance P, and possibly also glutamate. *Substance P* is an undecapeptide also found in the intestine (like many of the peptides believed to be active in the central nervous system). The same neurotransmitter is present at other central synapses, for instance the striatonigral fibre system. It is by no means certain that it is the excitatory transmitter of the first afferent synapse of either of the pain pathways: like some other peptides it may be a *modulator* of neuronal excitability. It is found in laminae I and II of the dorsal horn but is absent if the unmyelinated neurones of the dorsal root ganglion are absent (rats treated neonatally with capsaicin), so it is likely to be related to C fibres. There is no specific antagonist, but the inhibitory neurones of the substantia gelatinosa and the descending fibres from the raphe nuclei and periaqueductal grey matter may release *serotonin* and/or an *enkephalin* (dynorphin). The receptors for the latter ('opioid receptors') could account for the analgesia produced by peridural injection of morphine.

It is increasingly likely that endorphins (the endogenous chemical substances binding with opioid receptors) are the transmitters at a number of the synapses in the central pain-modulatory mechanisms such as the spinothalamic projections on the periaqueductal and periventricular grey matter, but these synapses can be stimulated by similar exogenous chemicals such as morphine and its congeners. Clinical experience suggests that morphine does not inhibit the affective response to painful stimuli which may be due to action on opioid receptors which have been identified in the locus coeruleus, striatum and hypothalamus.

There are a number of *endorphin peptides*,

including the enkephalins and β-endorphin, and their synaptic specificity has still to be determined. Currently it would seem that short acting enkephalins are probably neurotransmitters, while longer acting peptides such as β-endorphin have a general modulatory ('hormonal') effect on the nervous system. It is fashionable to attribute the claimed analgesic effects of acupuncture, hypnosis, transcutaneous and nerve stimulation and similar procedures to 'endorphin' release. Naloxone appears to be an antagonist to enkephalins, a possible explanation of its action as a narcotic antagonist.

The *serotoninergic central inhibitory neurones* are perhaps equally important. (Recent evidence suggests that raphe spinal neurones contain substance P as well as 5-HT, the first demonstration of two neurotransmitters in one neurone.) Depletion of central serotonin levels has been suggested to play an important role in chronic pain (and its associated depression). There is some clinical evidence that tertiary amine tricyclic antidepressant drugs have analgesic properties. Dopamine, noradrenaline and β-endorphin are also involved in pain control. The exact role of each remains to be defined.

The interplay between psyche and soma in the behavioural response to pain and indeed in its generation is beyond the scope of this book, but that is not to minimize its importance or to deny the possibility that psychological factors may modify levels of central neurotransmitters through the hippocampal loops outlined in *Fig. 6.1.* It is well known that peripheral block of pain nerve fibres (by local analgesia, nerve or root section), cordotomy or even thalamotomy are less effective as pain becomes 'chronic'. Many writers have postulated 'central' changes induced by prolonged activation of distal pain pathways without being able to suggest an acceptable mechanism. Conversely, it is well known that acute tissue damage may be apparently pain-free until the excitement of battle or sport is over. The possible gate-closing effect of activity in large fibres is the rationale for transcutaneous stimulation by electricity and for various locally applied 'counter-irritants'.

Possible mechanisms for chronic pain in peripheral nerve disorders have been sug-gested. Neuralgic pain of this type may be considered a paraesthesia of those nerve fibres normally involved in the centripetal transmission of impulses interpreted as painful. As with other forms of paraesthesia (p. 8), a damaged zone of axonal membrane may constitute a generator of iterative action potentials.

CAUSALGIA

Causalgia is the term used for a pain with 'burning' qualities associated with incomplete lesions of certain sensory nerves, notably the median and sciatic, especially in their proximal parts. It differs from the neuralgic pain just described in being increased by any circumstances causing discharge of associated sympathetic nerve fibres (eg emotional reactions), responsive to cold and relieved by sympathectomy or adrenergic blocking drugs. A favourite explanation is that an artificial synapse (termed an *ephapse*) may be formed at the site of injury so that action potentials in closely adjacent nerve fibres, particularly if unmyelinated, cause local circuit currents which generate action potentials in the damaged sensory nerve fibres.

A similar mechanism has been suggested for the pain that may persist or recur after cordotomy for peripheral pain. An excitable focus in the central nervous system has been postulated to result from retrograde and transneuronal changes in the secondary and tertiary pain neurones, with hypersynchronization at that area because of lack of disturbing impulses to upset the synchrony. Speculation such as this is rendered unnecessary by advances in knowledge of the inhibitory mechanisms, but speculation is inevitable since chronic pain cannot be investigated in experimental animals and the human subject with chronic pain is hardly capable of objectivity.

Itch, tickle and qualities of pain

The subjective nature of pain, and the limitations of experiments on human subjects, account for large areas of uncertainty. Various authorities regard itch and tickle as the same or different sensations and one, both, or neither as a subsidiary of pain. The analogy with taste suggests that different chemoreceptors of essentially the same type may be involved, rather than intensity of stimulation.

There is increasing evidence for a central enkephalinergic mechanism for some kinds of itch. Naloxone suppresses the itching in the trigeminal area which is commonly induced by intrathecal opioids and it may suppress generalized itching caused by liver disease or by butarphanol. With other morphine-like analgesics itching may, however, be due to release of histamine from mast cells in body tissues. Local release of *histamine* is undoubtedly associated with sensation of itch.

The reflex motor response (rhythmical scratching automatism) is quite different from the withdrawal reflex induced by pain. It is probably organized in the medulla in association with the trigeminal sensory nucleus, at the upper end of a spinotrigeminal chain of interneurones from enkephalin receptors in the substantia gelatinosa of the dorsal horn of the spinal cord (*Fig.* 6.1).

It is also uncertain whether pricking, burning, cutting and stabbing types of pain are related but separate sensations, or differ only in intensity and temporospatial pattern of stimulation. The dull aching pain aroused by stimulation of viscera is thought by most authorities to differ from cutaneous pain and may be conveyed by a separate system of nerve fibres, mainly if not exclusively unmyelinated as discussed above. The adequate stimulus is commonly distension of a hollow viscus or blood vessel but it is uncertain whether the receptors are mechanoreceptors, another variety of chemoreceptor, or both. Even the aching type of pain in somatic tissues and especially migraine pain, tend to be throbbing in nature.

The relationship between pain and temperature sensations is also difficult to define. With increasing heat stimulation, the sensation of warmth passes insensibly to one of pain, and with increasing cold, a sensation of 'paradoxical warmth' is experienced before cold-pain. Nevertheless, it is now accepted that there are separate receptors for thermal sensations, projecting to related parts of the diencephalon.

Further reading

Bowsher D. Termination of the central pain pathway in man: the conscious appreciation of pain. *Brain* 1957; **80**: 606–22.

Corregal E.J.A. Neurophysiology of pain — present status. In: Crue B.L. (ed.) *Pain, Research and Treatment*. New York: Academic Press, 1975.

Fields H.L. and Basbaum A.I. Brainstem control of spinal pain-transmission neurons. *Ann. Rev. Physiol.* 1978; **40**: 217–48.

Freeman W. and Watts J.W. Pain of organic disease relieved by prefrontal lobotomy. *Proc. R. Soc. Med.* 1946; **39**: 445–7.

Hockaday J.M. and Whitty C.W.M. Patterns of referred pain in the normal subject. *Brain* 1967; **90**: 481–96.

Kerr F.W.L. Neuroanatomical substrates of nociception in the spinal cord. *Pain* 1975; **1**: 325.

Loh L., Nathan P.W., Schott G.D. et al. Effects of regional guanethidine infusion in certain painful states. *J. Neurol. Neurosurg. Psychiat.* 1980; **43**: 446–51.

Marshall J. Sensory disturbances in cortical wounds with special reference to pain. *J. Neurol. Neurosurg. Psychiat.* 1951; **14**: 187–204.

Melzack R. and Wall P.D. Pain mechanisms: a new theory. *Science NY* 1965; **150**: 971–9.

Nathan P.W. The gate-control theory of pain. A critical review. *Brain* 1976; **99**: 123–58.

Nathan P.W. and Smith M.C. Spino-cortical fibres in man. *J. Neurol. Neurosurg. Psychiat.* 1955; **18**: 181–90.

Noordenbos W. *Pain*. Amsterdam: Elsevier, 1959.

Wall P.D. The gate control theory of pain mechanism. *Brain* 1978; **101**: 1–18.

Chapter 7

Thermal sensation and regulation of body temperature

Although temperature variation may alter the discharge of mechanoreceptors, it is likely that thermoreception depends on the activity of specific receptors, separate for cold and warmth. Sensation of coldness is not merely an absence of warm sensation.

WARMTH

The morphology of cutaneous warm receptors is unknown; they are probably free nerve endings. Their discharge slows with cooling and increases with warming the skin, but ceases when heat activates pain receptors. There are also *polymodal nociceptors* with unmyelinated axons which respond to noxious mechanical, thermal and chemical stimuli.

COLD

Specific cold receptors (as distinct from polymodal nociceptors) are found at the tips of papillae in the dermis, as a swelling containing microsomes at the end of fibres which are chiefly myelinated in man. In addition to cold perception some, which may have special discharge characteristics, serve thermoregulation by reflex vasoconstriction, piloerection and shivering. ·

Passing centripetally in a peripheral sensory nerve, with cell body in the dorsal root ganglion, the fibres for warmth and cold enter the spinal cord and are relayed centrally with the spinothalamic fibres responsible for pain (*see Figs* 6.1, 6.2). There is some evidence for a differential distribution of pain and thermal fibres in the anterolateral column of the spinal cord (temperature sensory fibres lying deep to the pain fibres) but they are probably inter-mixed. Anterolateral cordotomy in man usually causes loss of pain and thermal sensations in the same areas. The alternative pathways described for pain (p. 64) may be involved in the temperature regulation system but are probably not involved for *thermal sensation* as thermanaesthesia is usually permanent after cordotomy although pain recurs. Presumably the substantia gelatinosa and other synaptic stations are under inhibitory control like that described for pain pathways. Surprisingly, the effect of opioids on thermoregulation has not been extensively investigated, a subject of some concern to the anaesthetist.

The primary afferent fibres for cold and warmth have static discharge rates at particular temperatures but there would be little value in stabilizing the firing rates of second order and subsequent neurones as the thermoreceptors adapt (p. 57) within about 30 seconds. In addition to the static response, specific thermoreceptors have a dynamic response in which the rate of firing is proportional to the amplitude of a step or ramp change of temperature (experienced as sensations of cooling or warming). The intensity of heat or cold is judged on a basis of both number of warm/cold units recruited and their firing rates during the dynamic response, integrated at the second order neurones. Decussating in the cord with the spinothalamic tract pain fibres, the termination of these axons is uncertain but they presumably end in the thalamus and, either directly or indirectly, in the thermoregulatory area of the hypothalamus (p. 73). Thermoreceptors in the abdominal and thoracic viscera contribute to thermoregulation but not to thermal sensation. The latter is mediated by the thalamus: there is no evidence for cortical representation.

THERMOREGULATION

A simple domestic central heating system keeps house temperature regulated within a comparatively restricted range of temperature by sensing the temperature of a central living area or of the water in pipes returning heating water to the heat source, a boiler of some sort. The control depends on the absolute temperature reached at the sensing transducer. More sophisticated systems measure the temperature gradient between the central reference point and others outside the house ('frost booster') or in individual rooms and instruct the boiler to boost its output before the living area cools off, and/or boosts the temperature locally by turning on a radiator or closing a vent (as in greenhouses).

Thermoregulation in the human resembles the latter system in that it gives very precise regulation of body core temperature based on central and peripheral thermodetectors, and also regulates heat loss locally. In normal circumstances, the *autonomic control* is brought into play when behavioural *thermoregulation* is insufficient. The comatose or paralysed patient depends on the regulatory mechanism.

The regulatory mechanism is reflex. The core temperature of the body, as indicated by the blood temperature, is sensed by thermoreceptors in the *anterior hypothalamus* (and possibly in the medulla and spinal cord). Some authorities consider that the entire brain stem from the septal-preoptic region through the caudal posterior hypothalamus senses temperature and integrates thermal afferent pathways. Thermoreceptors may also be located in or near the large blood vessels, the walls of the gut and the carotid baroreceptors and chemoreceptors (their interaction has been postulated in heat syncope). The deep body thermosensors probably account for some of the unexpected sudomotor and vasomotor thermoregulatory responses in paraplegic patients.

Temperature gradients across the skin detected by the warmth and cold receptors described above, provide a sensory input analogous to the frost warning and local thermometers of the advanced domestic system. Just as the effect of the latter depends on the pre-set response level of a thermostat, so the response of the physiological system depends on the 'set-point' of a *central thermoregulatory control* which is believed to be located in the *posterior hypothalamus* and dependent on the ratio between sodium and calcium ions. From experimental injection of substances into the lateral ventricle of the cat and monkey, it appears that 5-HT entering the IIIrd ventricle produces a prolonged rise in body temperature and noradrenaline has the opposite effect. (It is not known whether they act as neurotransmitters or by adjusting the blood flow through the thalamus.) Prostaglandins of the E series have also been implicated. The connections between the primary thermal afferent fibres and the hypothalamus probably ascend from the dorsal horn via the mid-brain raphe nuclei and reticular formation to the hypothalamus (*see Fig. 6.2*), the terminal fibres secreting 5-HT and noradrenaline. Integrating pathways in the hypothalamus use acetylcholine. It is postulated that 5-HT is the final mediator by which pyrogens such as proteins and bacterial toxins cause fever. Their action is blocked by antipyretic drugs such as aspirin and by general anaesthesia.

The posterior hypothalamic thermoregulatory centre controls the core temperature by adjusting the balance between heat loss and heat gain, provided that skin temperature is not grossly abnormal.

Heat loss is promoted by the control centre activating a cholinergic neuronal system in the medial anterior hypothalamus which projects via relays in the brain stem and anterolateral grey matter of the spinal cord to *cholinergic* sympathetic nerve fibres which cause dilatation of skin vessels in the trunk and *eccrine sweating*, and the somatic response of *panting* in extreme cases. Extremity blood vessels dilate passively by decrease of sympathetic activity. For effective cooling by sweating, the humidity of the environment must be sufficiently low to allow evaporation.

Heat gain is promoted by the control centre activating an adrenergic neuronal centre in the medial posterior hypothalamus. By similar medullary and spinal cord relays, it activates the sympathetic *adrenergic* neurones to conserve heat by causing vasoconstriction of skin and mucosal vessels, and piloerection. The somatic responses are *shivering* (asynchronous then synchronous muscular contractions) inaugurated by rubrospinal and tectospinal pathways, and noradrenaline-stimulated metabolic responses designed to increase the rate of body metabolism, especially of carbohydrate (by thyroxine) and of brown fat. The metabolic responses collectively described as *non-shivering thermogenesis* are more important in the long term, coupled with reflex and voluntary efforts to reduce the surface area by crouching and to reduce heat loss by insulation (body fat and clothing). *Behavioural responses* also actively heat the body externally and internally by hot drinks and muscular exercise. Non-shivering thermogenesis may be blocked by an adrenergic β-receptor blocking agent: cooling then immediately evokes shivering.

Despite the central control, *peripheral reflex regulation* may be locally effective. Thus even the overheated subject may show local vasoconstriction, piloerection and generalized shivering in response to cold stimulation of the skin. The subjective feeling of bodily warmth or cold depends more on skin temperature than on core temperature, possibly to encourage appropriate heat conservation behaviour before the core temperature changes. Sweating is an exception to this — it is more responsive to rise in core temperature than to skin warming. Thermal comfort is a complicated subject involving core temperature and differential rates of cooling or heating local areas of skin. Although we cannot elaborate on it, the matter is of some importance in the recovery room or intensive care unit.

Shivering, and possibly other aspects of thermogenesis, is inhibited by area 4 of the cerebral cortex. The cortex may also be implicated in the poorly understood phenomenon of *acclimatization* (toleration of either hot or cold climate, but not of both simultaneously). Increased or decreased release of central or peripheral neurotransmitters (eg noradrenaline) may be involved, but this seems to be a likely role for neuromodulators such as peptides. The body's response to change of environmental temperature is obviously influenced by insulation (subcutaneous fat, hair) and the amount of brown fat tissue. The set point of the central regulator changes with a *circadian rhythm*, lowest in early morning, highest in late evening (and thus subject to 'jet lag' phase shift) and it changes independently with sleep. The variation between upper and lower temperatures tolerated without invoking the feedback control is greater in old age so the danger of both hypothermia and hyperthermia is increased. The control system of the neonate is remarkably mature though the fluctuations of body temperature are greater than in the adult but the effector systems are relatively less efficient with respect to body size (and in the first few hours of life metabolism is depressed). When central regulatory control is severely compromised by general anaesthesia or in coma, or if the compensatory mechanisms are damaged (spinal cord transection, peripheral neuropathy, myxoedema), the body becomes poikilothermic, ie it passively assumes the temperature of the environment.

The important role of muscles will be obvious. Heat is generated by shivering and by active exercise, and the muscles contain a major part of the body's glycogen reserves. The risk of hypothermia is therefore increased in muscular dystrophy as well as in paralysing diseases. Conversely, hyperthermia is a hazard in certain disorders of muscle, including a small proportion of patients with congenital myopathy and myotonia and a rare mitochondrial disorder. A familial disorder, transmitted by autosomal dominant inheritance with variable penetrance and without recognizable clinical evidence of muscle disease, has been termed *malignant hyperthermia*. A rapid rise in body temperature (up to 1°C every 5 minutes) with lactic acidaemia combined with respiratory acidosis from overproduction of CO_2, hyperkalaemia, raised serum creatine kinase and myoglobinuria, is provoked by inhalational anaesthetics (halothane, ether, cyclopropane, methoxyflurane, enflurane) or by depolarizing relaxant drugs such as succinylcholine. These factors appear to cause abnormal release of calcium ions from the sarcoplasmic reticulum of muscle which activates breakdown of glycogen and also ATP splitting with uncontrolled muscle contraction and uncoupling of oxidative phosphorylation. Abnormal contracture of muscle strips in response to halothane and/or caffeine is used as an *in vitro* test. The response is limited by dantrolene given intravenously (1–2 mg/kg repeated 5–10 min up to 10 mg/kg). This drug blocks the release of calcium ions from the sarcoplasmic reticulum. The other calcium-inhibitor drugs described on p. 9 do not have this action. It is also necessary to combat the metabolic acidosis with sodium bicarbonate and the respiratory acidosis with mechanical hyperventilation.

In all types of hyperthermia, heat loss must be promoted by encouraging vasodilatation and evaporation from the skin (eg by rubbing with wet towels and keeping the skin moist) while actively cooling the body. Surface-applied ice is often counterproductive by reflexly inducing vasoconstriction and shivering.

Halothane commonly produces postoperative shivering.

Less obvious factors leading to increased risk of hyperpyrexia are congenital or acquired anhydrosis and inhibition of sweating by ganglionic blocking drugs and by the anticholinergic drugs used in the treatment of Parkinsonism and bladder disorders.

Further reading

Benzinger T.H. Heat regulation: homeostasis of central temperature in man. *Physiol. Rev.* 1969; **49**: 671–759.

Hardy J.D., Gagge A.P. and Stolwijk J.A.J. (eds.) *Physiological and Behavioural Temperature Regulation.* Springfield, Ill.: Thomas, 1970.

Hensel H. *Thermoreception and Temperature Regulation.* London: Academic Press, 1981.

Zotterman Y. (ed.) *Sensory Function of the Skin in Primates.* Oxford: Oxford University Press, 1976.

Chapter 8
Contact sensations

It is increasingly acknowledged that the classical modalities of cutaneous sensation are somewhat artificial isolates from a wide range of sensory experiences. Some aspects of pain-related and thermal sensations have already been discussed. This chapter will deal with some sensations which include touch, pressure, vibration and tickle, evoked by innocuous contact stimulation of the skin. Blends of these with the pain and thermal groups give sensations of wetness, smoothness etc. (Even the place of the sensation called 'heat' is disputed.)

The contact group of sensations result from stimulation of *mechanoreceptors*. Many of these have now been differentiated and classified according to their rate of adaptation to a maintained stimulus and their response to 'static' displacement or velocity ('dynamic'). Two slowly adapting mechanoreceptors signal both position and velocity.

Type I slow-adapting receptors are associated with Merkel cell complexes in the epidermis. They have small receptive fields with sharp borders. In some animals they are in structures described as tactile domes but these are difficult to define in man. Indentation of the skin causes an irregular dynamic response followed by a static response which adapts slowly to a silent state.

Type II slow-adapting receptors are in the dermis and have been identified with Ruffini endings. Unlike the type I endings they show a background discharge. They have large receptive fields with poorly defined borders. When the overlying skin is displaced there is a dynamic followed by a slowly adapting static response of regular rhythm.

Cutaneous *velocity detectors* comprise a number of recognizable types (at least 5) which include hair follicle receptors and Meissner's corpuscles in non-hairy (glabrous) skin, each apparently tuned to different frequencies of movement and with different thresholds. Some are activated by movement of single hairs, others, known as *field receptors*, are excited by brushing large numbers of hairs, probably deforming the underlying skin. Psychophysical studies on man with microelectrodes permitting recording from and stimulation of single intact nerve fibres indicate two fast-adapting receptors, type I from Meissner's corpuscles and type II from Pacinian corpuscles and Golgi–Mazzoni receptors. Some of the types described in laboratory animals (eg the C mechanoreceptors with unmyelinated afferent fibres) have not been identified in human skin.

Some mechanoreceptors in skin detect only transient deformation. They include some hair follicle receptors and the Pacinian corpuscles in subcutaneous tissue. The latter may be protected from simple deformation by its capsule which filters out all but fast displacements such as vibration. At rates of oscillatory stimulation less than 40 Hz the sensation is experienced as '*flutter*'. Experiments with local anaesthesia of the skin suggest that two different peripheral receptors are involved, one for frequencies below 60 Hz ('flutter') and one for higher frequencies (experienced as a sensation of *vibration*). These endorgans adapt rapidly and, within limits, permit discrimination of frequency of stimulation. This is an unusual property since, in general, frequency change is correlated with intensity of stimulation. This clearly demands further investigation as in the analogous situation of the organ of hearing, frequency discrimination is based on selective stimulation of receptors. It is possible that recruitment is more important than frequency for signalling intensity in the afferent nervous system. Experiments on intact nerve in man (recording from single units) and recording of sensory nerve potentials in peripheral neuropathy and during recovery from a local nerve block indicate that a few afferent fibres suffice to mediate touch at threshold. A single impulse in a single type I fast-adapting unit can be appreciated (in man) as a sensation of touch. A type I slowly adapting unit requires a train of impulses. The threshold for perception, however, depends on the locality of the receptor. Normal sensory thresholds are reached when the evoked sensory nerve potentials are only 40 per cent of normal (even after allowing for temporal dispersion of unit responses). The clinical implication of this is that sensitivity can be normal even when most of the sensory fibres are lost. A moment's reflection will make it obvious that sensation is not necessarily impaired by reduction of the conduction velocity of sensory nerve fibres. However, it is impossible to appreciate time relationship and synchrony of stimulation of a group of endorgans unless conduction velocity remains normal. For this reason alone, vibration/flutter sensation is particularly vulnerable to the effects of ageing or disease.

Temporal relationships of signals from anatomically related endorgans are also important for discriminative aspects of sensation. On recovery from peripheral nerve injury the threshold to testing with cotton wool or a pinprick may return to normal or show only a little elevation. This is adequate for the protective function of sensation, including withdrawal reflexes, but tactile gnosis of the hands will be seriously impaired unless *two-point discrimination* is restored to near normal. The role of afferent inhibition in sensory discrimination is discussed below, but at this point it is necessary to draw attention to the importance of overlapping sensory fields, so that discrimination is highest in those areas of skin with a high density of innervation from multiple neurones. Reinnervation by sprouting may restore threshold but will not achieve normal sensory discrimination, especially if motor recovery is imperfect (*see* p. 94).

The afferent fibres connecting the cutaneous mechanoreceptors are predominantly fast conducting Aα fibres. Smaller diameter fibres, including unmyelinated C fibres, are involved to some extent. All have their neurone soma in the dorsal root ganglion appropriate to their dermatomal origin (or its homologue in the trigeminal nerve) and pass into the cord by the posterior nerve roots (some fibres enter by the anterior roots) to be relayed by second order neurones mainly according to the fibre size rather than to the type of receptor. It is probable that the large primary afferents release glutamic acid and some of the small primary afferents release substance P or somatostatin. The inhibitory interneurones with which they are associated in the dorsal horn probably release gamma-aminobutyric acid (GABA).

DORSAL HORN

As discussed in Chapter 6 on pain sensation, Aδ and C fibres probably relay mainly in lamina I through interneurones of the *substantia gelatinosa* and laminae IV–V to the contralateral ventrolateral column of white matter in the cord, passing to the thalamus (*spinothalamic* and related tracts). Many of the larger diameter and C fibres from the skin relay in laminae IV–VI. Those with small receptive fields and short latencies (presumably most important for sensory discrimination) end in the more superficial laminae. Conversely the direct input from proprioceptors is mainly into lamina VI (p. 87). Afferent fibres from different types of receptors converge on the second order neurones, making the dorsal horn an important site for sensory integration. A current controversy concerns a proposal that the dorsal horn laminae are connected as a cascade system.

It will be noted that the so-called spinothalamic tract contains second order neurones activated by cutaneous mechanoreceptors as well as by nociceptors. This is the basis of the clinical teaching that 'part of touch is carried by the spinothalamic tract'. Few of the pain fibres go to the anterior spinothalamic tract. A second group of A fibres terminate in *Clarke's column* upon neurones giving rise to the *spinocerebellar tract* and hence not involved in conscious appreciation of sensation (p. 225). The large afferent fibres have an additional fast conducting pathway in the long dorsal column systems (fast with relation to other cord pathways; the conduction velocity is slower than that of the peripheral axons).

The *dorsal column* afferent fibres are both first and second order neurones, all originating from mechanoreceptors, cutaneous and deep, including muscle. The first order neurones are ascending branches of primary afferent fibres. As they enter the cord in the lateral bundle of the dorsal root they turn medially into the dorsal column without relaying in the dorsal horn. Their cell body is in the dorsal root ganglion and there is no synapse at that point. It is less well known that the dorsal column also has second order neurones ascending from cells in the dorsal horn and projecting to the dorsal column nuclei of Goll and Burdach by the *dorsolateral fasciculus*. Furthermore, only a fraction of the dorsal column fibres run all the way to these nuclei. Others terminate in higher segments of the cord grey matter (eg lower limb afferent fibres project to the neuronal machinery controlling the forelimb) and others travel only one or two segments up or down the cord. The long fibres have some topographical organization, those entering from the most caudal segments being displaced medially by fibres entering at higher levels.

These long fibres terminate in the *dorsal column nuclei* of the medulla oblongata — the nucleus gracilis (Goll), nucleus cuneatus (Burdach) and lateral cuneate nucleus (Monakow). The second order neurones from the lateral cuneate nucleus pass into the inferior cerebellar peduncle and so to the cerebellum (p. 225). The gracile and cuneate nuclei are relays for the dorsal column primary afferent fibres to second order neurones which decussate to form the *medial lemniscus* running rostrally to the contralateral thalamus (*Fig. 8.1*).

The dorsal column–medial lemniscus pathway is considered to be an important fast conducting channel for signals from mechanoreceptors in skin, joints and muscle spindles and some visceral afferents (including bladder afferents near the midline).

In clinical practice, a dorsal column lesion is considered to cause ipsilateral loss of vibration and muscle-joint sensation with some loss of touch, especially the discriminative aspects. Indeed it has been called the pathway for discriminative sensation. It is accordingly surprising that dorsal cordotomy (in attempt to relieve phantom limb pain) causes transient reduction of sensation of touch, passive movement or two-point discrimination, but no loss of vibration sensation, supporting similar observations on laboratory animals. In the cat (but not the rat) section of all the cord except the dorsal column is said to spare all forms of sensation (tested by operant conditioning) including tactile discrimination, but orientation and arousal reactions are lacking. It is suggested that all modalities of sensation are represented in the dorsal column but that ventral column fibres passing to the reticular formation are necessary for arousal.

Evidence on the human is scanty. The so-called 'posterior column degenerations' (eg Friedreich's ataxia, tabes dorsalis, subacute combined degeneration) are due to lesions of the primary afferent neurones. Nevertheless most authorities accept an important role of the dorsal column for the sensations of vibration, limb movement and for tactile discrimination requiring sequential or spatio-temporal analysis. This sensory information may play an important part in the selection of appropriate motor programmes (p. 236). Tactile discrimination is perhaps specially associated with those dorsal fibres travelling up in the dorsolateral fasciculus of Lissauer at the root entry zone, a second order pathway which arises in or near Clarke's column of lamina VII.

Although situated in the brain stem, it will be obvious that the dorsal column nuclei bear the same relation to large fast conducting peripheral sensory neurones as does the dorsal horn to the smaller slower conducting afferent fibres. It is not surprising to find that the dorsal column nuclei are not simple relays to second order neurones but have pre-synaptic inhibition and control by interneurones of a type similar to the dorsal horn. The relay cells are easily excited by the primary neurones.

The transmitter at the synapse is probably glutamate. Inhibition of the dorsal column nuclei (both pre- and post-synaptic) is attributed to GABA. (Extracellular accumulation of K^+ released by activated neurones cannot be excluded as a cause of primary afferent depolarization responsible for pre-synaptic inhibition.)

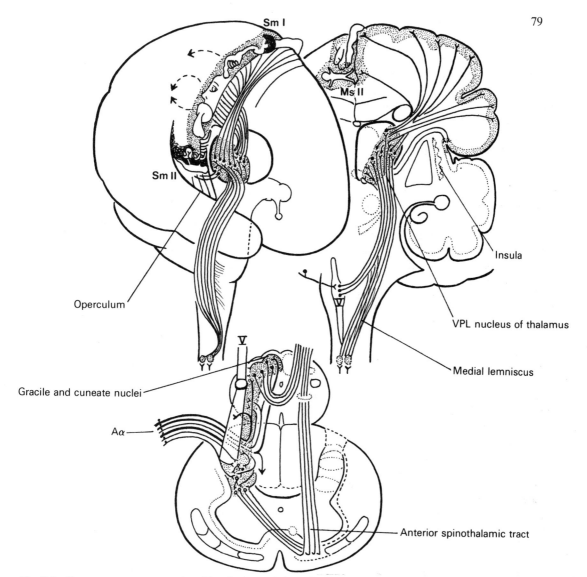

Fig. 8.1. *Cutaneous contact sensation.* The figure excludes Aδ and C fibre contributions relayed in the posterior spinothalamic tract (*Fig. 6.1*). Also omitted are inhibitory fibres from all relay areas (medulla, thalamus, cortex) which descend to the previous input synapses along with corticofugal fibres in the pyramidal tract and reticulospinal inhibitory projections to the base of the dorsal horn.

First order A alpha-gamma neurones terminate in laminae IV–VI, possibly converging on a cascade of interneurones many of which are inhibitory. The medial bundle of A alpha fibres enter laminae III–V at several levels up or down a grey column which condenses at its upper end as the gracile and cuneate nuclei of the dorsal column. They all relay in the dorsal column nuclei, decussate in the lower medulla and ascend as the medial lemniscus, closing up with second order neurones of smaller A group fibres which decussate in the cord and ascend in the anterior spinothalamic tract. Regrouping in the upper medial lemniscus (joined by similar crossing projections from the principal sensory nucleus of V) allows somatotopic projection to the posterior ventral nuclei of the thalamus (face medially, other areas laterally) with a small inferior group which relays bilateral impulses to the secondary sensory area (SmII). A similar projection to supplementary motor area (MsII) ends above the limbic cingular gyrus and at the lower end of the medial surface extension of the post-central gyrus which is the primary somaesthetic area (SmI). A somatotopic representation (homunculus) of half of the body is shown (according to Penfield). Inferior to the large tongue representation the teeth, larynx and abdominal viscera are represented in the parietal operculum of the Sylvian fissure which has been opened to show the continuity with the secondary sensory area (SmII) and with the visceral sensory area of the insula. The urogenital viscera have their sensory representation at the other end of the primary sensory strip where it passes into MsII, in relation to a medial frontal area which controls bladder continence. Commissural connections are not shown (SmI to contralateral SmII) and only the main projection to parietal association cortex is indicated.

The *inhibitory input* to laminae IV–VI of the dorsal horn and the dorsal column nuclei comes mainly from the lower reticular formation and the sensorimotor cortex. Pyramidal tract fibres inhibit these nuclei directly and also indirectly via the reticular formation. The cerebral cortex and the arousal system therefore have connections enabling them to modify or focus the sensory input being projected to the thalamus. The functional significance of this is not clear. It could contribute to programmed movement by preventing it from being disrupted by peripheral feedback, or, by filtering out sensory input which is already predictable from the motor programme, it could sharpen the significance of additional un-programmed sensory information.

This raises the interesting questions how does the nervous system select from the afferent bombardment those signals of immediate relevance, and how can it detect the locus of a peripheral stimulus which activates receptors of many overlapping first order neurones which then relay to second order neurones, many of which accept converging signals from a number of first order neurones? Localization is best in areas like the fingertips with a high density of cutaneous receptors with much overlap. The general principle adopted by the central nervous system is known as *surround inhibition* and this is well seen in the gracile nucleus. The activity of many of its cells can be inhibited by stimuli applied to the areas surrounding their peripheral receptive fields. Convergent neurones summate their depolarizing pressure on the next neurone in a chain. If it is also divergent, there is an avalanche cascade of spreading excitation with mass response but no local sign. To prevent this, many neurones have collateral branches to inhibitory interneurones so that those fringing a neurone receiving convergent inputs will be excited while lateral, surround, or 'fringe' neurones will be inhibited. A neurone receiving stimuli from receptors near the centre of its receptive field will therefore be favoured for onward transmission compared with those that are stimulated near the periphery of their receptive fields and indeed the latter will be inhibited, so 'focussing' the stimulus. Conversely, other neurones show *surround facilitation*. Those showing surround inhibition and

facilitation are probably also the cells that are inhibited and facilitated respectively by feedback from the cerebral cortex, a mechanism for cortical selection of the sensory message by modification of the spatial contrast achieved by the surround system of inhibition and facilitation. An additional advantage is that *contrast enhancement* occurs which increases the signal to noise ratio of a communication system.

Is there any biological advantage in an overlapping and convergent collecting system which can be 'crispened' when the organism is alerted, and focused to suit the behavioural circumstances? What advantage is there over a point-to-point transfer of information from periphery to cortex? The overlapping-convergent system has the great advantage of integration of stimuli from a wide area (*see* spatial and temporal summation, p. 44) which is valuable for initial detection and regional localization of cutaneous stimulation. The alerted animal then automatically sharpens the signal by first suppressing fringe responses and then, by some value judgement, ignoring or enhancing significant signals isolated from background noise. Within this general system some neurones have wide receptive fields, others have small ones. It would clearly be advantageous if reflex movement could bring the small field neurones towards the stimulus. This certainly happens with vision and it is likely that the same principle is used for tactile discrimination (*see* p. 114). Dorsal column lesions produce a severe disorder of exploratory movements and of 'anticipatory' motor behaviour.

MEDIAL LEMNISCUS

The second order neurones of the gracile and cuneate nuclei project to the thalamus as a bundle of axons, the medial lemniscus, which decussates to the medial anterior part of the contralateral half of the medulla, dorsal to the pyramidal tract fibres. As it ascends to the thalamus the bundle rotates and moves laterally in the pons and mid-brain, gradually merging with the spinothalamic tract. Unlike the latter, the medial lemniscus does not give off collaterals to the reticular formation. A somatotopical organization of fibres is maintained throughout its course including the fibres from the main sensory trigeminal nucleus of the contralateral pons which join it at that level. The spinal lemniscal fibres enter the *nucleus ventralis posterior lateralis (VPL) of the thalamus* and the trigeminal fibres more medially in the nucleus ventralis posterior medialis (VPM), in the same parts of the thalamus which receive spinothalamic projections from the same body segments. The distribution of spinothalamic fibres is, however, not restricted to the thalamic areas receiving medial lemniscus fibres.

In some animals a third afferent projection system has been described, the *spino-cervico-thalamic system*, in which dorsal root fibres relay from the dorsal horn up the lateral part of the dorsal column to a lateral cervical nucleus in the upper cervical spinal cord and relay from there to the contralateral thalamus. There is increasing evidence for its presence in man. In the cat it is activated by A and C fibres from the skin and by high threshold muscle afferents, which apparently converge on to the cervical nucleus cells, suggesting a role in pain mechanisms and in tactile roughness discrimination. Like the spinothalamic and medial lemniscus systems, this pathway is also controlled by neurones descending from the cerebral cortex and brain stem, both inhibitory and facilitatory, but inhibition is not of the surround type and receptive fields are large proximally and relatively small distally. The impression is of a general detection system for nociceptor impulses from the skin and muscles, more suitable for subserving the protective reflexes than for sensory discrimination.

Quite recently yet another pathway, the *spinomedullo-thalamic*, has been described, apparently serving only the lower limbs, and projecting via the same dorsolateral fasciculus of the cord and the medial lemniscus. Its input is predominantly from low-threshold muscle and joint afferent fibres.

The role of these dorsolateral tracts in man is unknown but it is necessary to be aware of their existence as they may be responsible for the surprising retention of tactile and proprioceptive sensibility after dorsal column lesions.

It will now be evident to the reader that no modality of sensation has a unique pathway to the thalamus. The nociceptors make most use of the ventrolateral ('spinothalamic') and dorsolateral white columns of the cord. The mechanoreceptors use both pathways though those from muscles and joints ('proprioceptors') use mainly the dorsal column, but there are plenty of neurones on which both nociceptors and mechanoreceptors may converge. It is little wonder, then, that the paraesthesiae associated with partial lesions or disinhibition of central afferent pathways differ from normal sensation (descriptions such as 'wet', 'clammy', 'clamp-like' and others are common).

FLUTTER–VIBRATION SENSATIONS

The ability to detect the nature of an oscillating stimulus indicates that the mechanoreceptors stimulated are rapidly adapting, their signals are transmitted by afferent nerve fibres of virtually identical conduction velocity (otherwise the temporal characteristics of the stimulus would be lost during centripetal transmission), and relayed through a limited number of synapses with transfer functions which do not summate the signals. (At most synapses changes in frequency are proportional to intensity of stimulation.) Presumably vibration–flutter intensity is signalled by recruitment only. These characteristics are found in the large A fibres passing without relay into the dorsal column to the medial lemniscal system. There are two classes of mechanoreceptors with the necessary properties, one in the skin and the other in deeper tissues. The rapidly adapting skin mechanoreceptors stimulated at 5–40 Hz produce a sensation of *'flutter'*. The deeper receptors stimulated at frequencies of 60–300 Hz produce a sensation of *'vibration'*. Though of no practical value to man, these forms of sensation have survival value to lower animals, particularly fish, as is known to every angler or huntsman, enabling the animal to detect vibratory stimuli in the environment. This primitive form of distance receptor is specialized in the lateral line organ of fish and in the organ of Corti in the ear.

The two groups of primary afferent fibres transmitting periodic bursts of impulses at the frequency of mechanical oscillation are apparently connected to two distinct populations of neurones in the thalamus and also in the somatosensory cortex. This phase-locking of cortical response to periodic peripheral stimulation is not unique to flutter–vibration sensation. It is also found in the visual cortex. Oddly enough, it is not apparent in the auditory system where frequency discrimination is based on spatial separation by receptors on tuned structures in the organ of Corti. The slower cutaneous 'flutter' sensation utilizes ventrolateral tracts as well as dorsal column, but 'vibration' only the latter.

The *receptors for flutter* are believed to be the quick adapting Meissner's corpuscles in glabrous skin, and hair follicle and field mechanoreceptors in hairy skin. The *receptors for (deep) vibration* include the Pacinian corpuscle. Joint receptors may also contribute but muscle stretch receptors probably do not.

The limitation of vibration sensation to fast conducting peripheral afferent fibres and the completely unilateral dorsal column–medial lemniscus pathway provides the neurologist with a unique method of testing the integrity of this pathway, but the perception requires that conduction velocity in the fibres concerned must be maintained. It is therefore very vulnerable to any factor such as age or disease which slows conduction asymmetrically in any part of the pathway.

Slowed conduction with increased temporal dispersion of impulses in adjacent fibres should not alter the perceived sensation provided that the impulse pattern reaching the next order neurone is adequate. This would be sufficient to account for dissociation between vibration and position sense in some patients with peripheral neuropathy or disease of the dorsal column, but there is no reason to assume that both sensations use the same afferent fibres.

POSITION SENSE

Conventional teaching in clinical neurology is that a sense of static position of limb segments and a sense of joint movement (*kinaesthesia*) depend on afferent impulses passing in rapidly conducting A fibres of sensory nerves to the dorsal column of the spinal cord with the first relay in the gracile and cuneate nuclei from which secondary neurones pass via the medial lemniscus to the contralateral thalamus, and that both first and second order neurones are either identical with those carrying the signals

perceived as vibration when stimulated appropriately or are intimately mixed with them and have similar conduction velocities. Occasional dissociation of vibration and position sense loss in disease would not be incompatible, as described above, if loss of vibration sense always preceded loss of position sense. The reverse situation could not be explained unless the neurones and receptors were independent and a number of clinical records indicate that this may occur. However, it is not clear that the distinction between flutter (cutaneous) and vibration (deep) sensation has always been made.

Swings of opinion regarding the putative role of receptors in the joint capsules, tendons, muscles and skin have arisen from conflicting reports of experimental work on animals and observations on the human. It is beginning to appear that some part of the anomaly may be due to differences between the large proximal joints and the small joints of the digits, and between upper and lower limbs.

Joint receptors, including the slowly adapting Ruffini endings, unquestionably discharge when a proximal joint is in certain positions (usually the extremes of flexion or extension) but it is not certain whether they respond to position or to torque in the joint capsule. *Position sense* in the digits requires slowly adapting mechanoreceptors in the skin overlying the joint. Muscle spindles and/or tendons may contribute to position sense as illusions of movement are generated by vibrating the tendons of various muscles but tension on exposed tendons is said not to produce a sensation of movement unless the distal structures are moved by the pulled tendons. All these methods of signalling static position and movement of joints may be used, the proportion differing from joint to joint as indicated above.

There is no question that the most important afferent fibres involved are A group fibres using the lemniscal pathway already described, but there is growing evidence that some fibres end in the dorsal horn and second order neurones ascend in the ventral quadrant of the cord (not necessarily the spinothalamic tract). These may be mainly (possibly exclusively) from the lower limbs except for the toes. It is not known which type of receptor is involved in this anterior pathway. It may be in part an explanation why posture is much more severely affected by sensory polyneuropathy and root entry zone lesions (eg tabes dorsalis) than by true dorsal column lesions.

THALAMUS

The medial lemniscus fibres, second order neurones, relay dorsal column signals from the gracile and cuneate nuclei and the spinocervico-thalamic signals from the cervical nucleus, to the *nucleus ventralis posterior lateralis* (VPL) of the contralateral thalamus in the same region as the termination of the spinothalamic fibres of the ventrolateral column of the spinal cord which have decussated in the cord.

Similar fibres of the contralateral trigeminal nerve terminate in the *nucleus ventralis posterior medialis* (VPM) of the thalamus, those of lemniscal type relaying in the principal nucleus and the nociceptive fibres in the descending nucleus of the Vth nerve.

The thalamus receives second order neurones from all peripheral receptive fields — interoceptive and exteroceptive, somato-sensory and 'special senses' alike with the important exceptions of taste and olfaction. Each afferent projection to the thalamus goes to discrete, modality-specific areas described by anatomists as separate nuclei. We will name some of them for convenience of referral to more detailed descriptions if required. Only anaesthetists involved in stereotaxic neuro-surgery need be concerned with the exact localization.

The principles described in this section apply to all sensory modalities relaying in the thalamus to the cerebral cortex. These thala-mic nuclei are sometimes termed the *specific relay nuclei* to distinguish them from less differentiated *intralaminar nuclei* which are the rostral part of the brain stem reticular forma-tion, important for pain sensation (p. 68). The latter system receives collateral branches from the sensory tracts projecting to the thalamus, with the possible exception of the medial lemniscus fibres. They are relayed to all parts of the cortex as a diffuse activating system (p. 49) and will not be discussed further at this point. An important projection of the intra-laminar nuclei and centromedian nucleus is to the striatum, possibly carrying integrated posi-tional data (Chapter 22).

It is possible that a 'crude' appreciation of afferent signals is possible at thalamic levels. If an 'interpreter' be required, it could be a thalamic relay to the amygdaloid–septal area of the diencephalon where there is a primitive mechanism for classifying sensory signals as desirable or dangerous (Chapters 6 and 10). For more discriminative analysis and cross-modality linkages there has been evolved a huge mantle of synaptic connections between thalamic neurones and the cerebral cortex of the neopallium, enfolding the archipallium, that is the analytic cortex of the diencephalon (p. 52). The possibility of separate 'pro-topathic' and 'epicritic' somatosensory systems is still debatable.

Some cross-modality linkage probably occurs within the thalamus but it must be minimal. There is little or no convergence on multi-input neurones. Most cell groups within the specific relay nuclei of the thalamus retain the topographic and functional characteristics of their afferent fibres.

DESCENDING CONTROL OF THALAMUS

There is indeed some dispersion of signals to a group of thalamic cells with some overlap, but inhibiting neurones and feedback from cortex to thalamus 'crispen' the signal by *surround inhibition* in the same way as in the dorsal horn and dorsal column nuclei.

AFFERENT CEREBRAL CORTEX

The same type of dispersal-overlap with surround inhibition is believed to occur in the cortex to which the ventral nuclei of the thalamus relay signals which still carry the local sign and 'modality' of the original peripheral receptor field. The apparent redundancy intro-duces a safety factor and also permits *integra-tion* of signals by convergence. At the cortex the third order somatosensory neurones end with large plexuses of terminal ramification in the IVth lamina (internal granular layer) of the cortex around a 'barrel' or *column of cells* orientated normal to the surface and associated with interneurones in other cortical layers, forming a cortical 'module' (p. 84). Each module retains the modality characteristics of its afferent neurone and its topographic sign (approximately a 'point-to-point' localization from receptive field to cortex), but of course the spatial distribution of cortical loci is different from that at the periphery.

The sharpened signals received by the large neurones of the thalamic VPL and VML nuclei are relayed by these third order neurones through the internal capsule and corona radiata to the somatosensory areas of the neocortex. (They are more correctly termed 'somatosensorimotor' as these areas have important efferent projections. Similarly the so-called motor cortex has some somatosensory functions.) Some authors recognize five or more somatosensory areas but only three are of known importance. The VML fibres project to areas for representation of the face but as there is no functional difference the rest of this discussion will refer only to VPL fibres. However, it should be noted that VML probably projects bilaterally (in parallel with the bilateral motor representation of the face).

FIRST SOMATOSENSORY AREA (SI)

The shortest third order sensory neurones project to cortical columns ('modules') in the *post-central gyrus*, spreading anteriorly into the pre-central gyrus (*Fig.* 8.1). Each contralateral dorsal root (and therefore each dermatome) is 'represented' in a narrow antero-posterior band across the gyrus. The body parts are therefore segregated from medial to lateral, but the serial order of nerve roots is changed so that the 'homunculus' illustrating the peripheral receptive fields shows an order of toes, foot, leg, trunk, head (but not face), arm, hand, fingers from medial surface of the hemisphere over the convexity to lateral surface, followed at the lower end of the post-central gyrus by the VPM projection from eye, face, lips, intraoral mucosa, tongue and pharynx in that order. Apparently out of sequence are the genitalia, bladder and rectum, lowest on the medial surface of the gyrus, and the intra-abdominal receptors, lowest on the lateral surface as it turns into the upper lip of the Rolandic fissure (*Fig.* 8.1). The odd proportions of the homunculus cartoon are intended to parallel the dimensions of cortex receiving afferents from the peripheral areas 'represented'. The cortical areas are roughly proportional to the *density* of receptors in the peripheral zones and to their *functional importance* as stimulus detectors.

Within the two-dimensional cortical 'map' which would be obtained if the first somatosensory area was spread out flat, there is a *mosaic of the columnar modules* described above. Each vertical column is modality-specific. Most are identified with the signals transmitted by the dorsal column–lemniscal pathway associated with 'discriminative' aspects of sensation–touch, position, flutter–vibration. There is still controversy about spinothalamic tract signals. With acute lesions of this area all sensory modalities may be lost contralaterally but there is gradual recovery of some aspects associated with spinothalamic signals. The first sensation to recover is pain, followed by touch, then thermal sensation. Vibration sensation, sense of joint position and discrimination of contact stimuli (*astereognosis*; loss of two-point discrimination) are permanently and severely impaired. The first to return are sensations from the face, larynx, pharynx and anogenital region, then neck and trunk. This is believed to indicate bilateral representation of these areas so it is possible that a similar explanation could account for the apparent sparing of pain and temperature sensation.

The cell modules for lemniscal sensation are to some extent segregated in vertical strips parallel to the axis of the post-central gyrus (orthogonal to the dermatomal strips). From front to back there are Broadman's areas 3, 1 and 2. Area 2 mainly receives from deep tissues, especially sensors of joint movements. Area 3 also receives from deep afferents, including muscle, area 3b from slowly adapting cutaneous mechanoreceptors, and area 1 from rapidly adapting cutaneous mechanoreceptors. The first somatosensory area is therefore well suited for the first stage of sensory discrimination by receiving an 'image' of the body in cortical space which is topological in that it preserves the connectivity of body parts and the specificity of detected stimuli. It is closely linked with efferent cortical neurones by intracortical axons, but its value as an organ of sensory discrimination depends on the further processing of the sensory signals in the parietal and other areas of the cortex as described in Chapter 12.

SECOND SOMATOSENSORY AREA (SII)

The VPL nucleus of thalamus also relays third order neurones to a more compact area at the lower end of the post-central gyrus in the upper bank of the Sylvian fissure adjacent to the insula. Somatotopic representation of all areas of the body is repeated here but the localization is less discrete and both sides are represented, though mainly contralateral. As many of the units in this area have large receptive fields it appears to be less specific for mode and locus of stimulation than the first somatosensory area.

The face area is rostral and the lower limb caudal. Electrical stimulation in conscious man evokes feelings of tingling, numbness and warmth in part of one or both sides of the body. (Note that a bilateral sensory aura in epilepsy does not exclude a unilateral focus.) No syndrome has been clearly associated with ablations of this area, but there is some evidence that its 'association cortex' (Chapter 12) in the left supramarginal gyrus is connected to the limbic system by way of the insular cortex, evoking the emotional response to pain. (Lesions of the left supramarginal gyrus occasionally cause 'asymbolia for pain'. Prefrontal lobotomy leaves intact the physical reactions to pain but removes the apprehension of its significance.)

Motor responses are also obtained by stimulation of this area (so it is sometimes labelled SmII) but the efferent pathway is unknown. The further processing of the sensory message is also obscure. Its relationships to the insula, claustrum and limbic system suggest a role for the second somatosensory area in affective responses to the environment. *Commissural connections* link SI with the opposite SII for axial areas of the body.

THIRD SOMATOSENSORY AREA (MsII)

Another projection of the VPL nucleus of thalamus is to the medial aspect of the cerebral hemisphere. This is a 'second motor area' but evoked cortical responses can be elicited by stimulating peripheral nerves or dorsal roots, and the stimulation of this cortical area causes sensations in the head and abdomen, and an unlocalized feeling of palpitation. The head area is anterior but localization is not well mapped. These sensory functions are presumably related to the motor functions of the anterior part of this area of cortex, whatever these may be, and sensory discrimination would be unlikely unless the signals are further processed in the superior parietal lobule.

CORTICOFUGAL CONNECTIONS

The signal traffic is not all one way, thalamus to cortex. Each somatosensory area sends efferent fibres to that part (VPL and VPM nuclei) of the thalamus from which its thalamo-cortical afferents arise (p. 83). In addition, the second somatosensory area projects in a somatotopical pattern to the dorsal column nuclei in the brain stem. It is virtually certain that these projections exert an inhibitory feedback control of signals passing to the sensory cortices. Why the latter should be multiple is unknown. It seems likely that some sorting occurs according to the further signal processing offered by the cortical association areas (Chapter 12).

Further reading

Burgess P.R. and Perl E.R. Cutaneous mechanoreceptors and nociceptors. In Iggo A. (ed.) *Somatosensory System: Handbook of Sensory Physiology*, vol. II. Berlin: Springer-Verlag, 1973, pp. 29–78.

Eccles J.C. *The Inhibitory Pathways of the Central Nervous System*. Liverpool: Liverpool University Press, 1969.

Granit R. *Receptors and Sensory Perception*. New Haven: Yale University Press, 1955.

Mountcastle V.B. and Powell T.P.S. Neural mechanisms subserving cutaneous sensibility, with special reference to the role of afferent inhibition in sensory perception and discrimination. *Bull. Johns Hopkins Hosp.* 1959; **105**: 201–32.

Sinclair D. *Mechanisms of Cutaneous Sensation*. Oxford: Oxford University Press, 1981.

Willis W.D. and Coggeshall R.E. *Sensory Mechanisms of the Spinal Cord*. New York: Plenum Press, 1978.

Chapter 9

Kinaesthesia: sensory signals from muscles, tendons and joints

The title of this section has been chosen because of some controversy about whether afferent signals arising in muscle, tendon or joint can be consciously 'perceived'. Since Sherrington's description of a 'muscular sense' — later termed 'kinaesthesia' to incorporate information derived from joint position receptors — the concept has undergone radical changes of view. In the 1960s it was denied that the muscle signals contributed to conscious perception, a view that few clinical neurologists could accept. In the past decade the Sherrington view has been adopted again as the result of observations on conscious human subjects, either by pulling upon a tendon exposed surgically under local anaesthesia or by selectively stimulating the primary afferent receptors of muscle spindles by a vibrator oscillating at 100 Hz which causes a sensation as if the vibrated muscle is being extended.

Conversely, the role assigned to joint position receptors is currently less defined. Whereas in the recent past it has appeared that appreciation of joint movement is due to information from receptors in the joint capsule (so that 'joint sensation' was to replace 'muscle-joint sensation' for the clinician), it is now beginning to appear that the role of joint receptors has been rehabilitated. Furthermore, the importance of signals from cutaneous receptors overlaying the joints is becoming increasingly clear. It is certain that many classic psychophysiological studies on 'proprioceptive sensation' must be re-evaluated.

JOINT RECEPTORS

At least two types of receptor have been identified in the *joint capsule* — one lamel-lated, like an elongated Pacinian corpuscle, with a rapidly adapting burst of action potentials to movement in any direction, and the other with a spray type of ending, like the Ruffini corpuscle, which is slowly adapting and so better suited for signalling static position since it has a characteristic frequency of discharge for any one position of the joint. It is convenient to include here two other types of receptors. One resembling Golgi organs does not occur in the joint capsule but is present in the extrinsic and intrinsic *ligaments*. It is of high threshold and adapts slowly, contributing to the signalling of joint position. The other, a plexus of fine unmyelinated fibres, is probably a type of pain receptor rather than a position/movement detector. It is found in all the soft tissues in and around joints.

Doubts about the validity of this interpretation have grown with the demonstration that joint receptors are apparently most active when the joint angle is at the extremes of its range. It seems to us that a possible reason for some discrepancies in the literature is that it has been assumed that all joints are the same in their afferent mechanism. Recent studies following intracapsular injection of local anaesthetic (knee) or replacement of a diseased joint by a prosthesis (hip, finger) indicate possible differences between proximal and distal joints. At the time of writing it may be postulated that muscle stretch receptors are important for signalling movement at all joints, and that joint capsule receptors are more important for proximal and less for distal (digital) joints. Conversely, cutaneous receptors in skin overlying the joints become progressively more important at distal joints for signalling joint movement.

RECEPTORS IN MUSCLES AND TENDONS

Pain nerve endings are also present in muscles and tendons. They are typical free nerve ending chemoreceptors. The appropriate stimulus has not been discovered but is presumed to be one or more metabolites of muscle, produced especially when muscle contracts under ischaemic conditions. Their slow conducting small fibred nerves follow the same central pathways as the pain fibres already discussed for cutaneous sensation.

Skeletal muscle and its tendon have specialized mechanoreceptors. The *muscle spindles* are present in all striated muscles though the relative density varies widely. As a general principle, muscles used in delicate controlled movements have a higher density of spindles compared to extrafusal 'power' fibres than do muscles used for coarse movements. Thus the spindle-poor muscles are those of the shoulders and thighs and the supply gets richer in more distal limb muscles and in the tongue and face muscles. On the other hand, the greatest density of spindles occurs in the neck muscles.

The muscle spindle is a compound transducer sensitive to various aspects of stretch applied to the organ. It is a spindle-shaped connective tissue capsule some millimetres long lying in parallel with the 'power' fibres of the muscle and connected at each pole to the tendinous origin and insertion of the muscle, either directly or through the perimysium of extrafusal fibres. The capsule contains fluid (the purpose is not yet identified) which surrounds a group of slender muscle fibres, hence called *intrafusal* fibres. (By derivation, the 'power' fibres which do not pass through the spindles are termed *extrafusal*.) The number of intrafusal fibres in one spindle is variable but averages ten in human muscle. These fibres differ in their contractile properties and morphology, the latter differences accounting for their description as nuclear bag fibres (of two types) and nuclear chain fibres. These differences are of considerable functional importance in regulating the sensitivity of the afferent receptors and so the description will be postponed until the basic functions have been described (p. 91). The stretch receptors are found on each of the intrafusal fibres.

PRIMARY SENSORY ENDING

Surrounding the equator of each intrafusal muscle fibre, a non-contractile part with many nuclei, is a spiral receptor which is the termination of a single group Ia (A alpha) sensory nerve fibre. (Occasionally one axon may branch to supply primary endings in two simple spindles.) The effective stimulus is passive stretch of the enclosed non-contractile part of the intrafusal fibre caused by stretching the whole muscle or by contraction of the striated pole(s) of the intrafusal fibres which have their own nerve supplies (p. 89). The former descriptive term 'annulospiral ending' has been discontinued as some secondary sensory endings may also have spiral form. The stem or parent nerve fibre (*group Ia*) enters the muscle nerve and passes centrally in a mixed peripheral nerve to its cell body in a dorsal root ganglion and then by a dorsal nerve root to the spinal cord, entering the dorsal column and rising to its first synapse in one of the dorsal column nuclei as described in Chapter 8. At the root entry zone a collateral branch travels anteromedially through the central grey matter of the spinal cord to end monosynaptically on a motoneurone supplying extrafusal muscle fibres in the area of muscle containing the original spindle, thus forming the mechanism for a very localized stretch reflex (*see Fig. 17.1*). Many spinal fibres relay in the nuclei of the dorsal column and decussate in the medial lemniscus to the ventroposterolateral nucleus (VPL) of the thalamus. Others relay to the cerebellum (*Fig. 9.1*).

The trigeminal nerve carries similar fibres from facial muscles. Some group Ia afferent fibres have their cell body in the semilunar or Gasserian ganglion and the central process relays in the main sensory nucleus of the trigeminal nerve instead of the dorsal column nuclei. There is, however, evidence in some animals that the spindle afferents pass into the medulla via the motor root of V. (The tendon organ afferents do not.) The second order neurone decussates in the trigeminothalamic tract and passes to the contralateral ventroposterior medial nucleus (VPM) of thalamus. Both thalamic nuclei send third order neurones to the sensori-motor cortices as already described (Chapter 8).

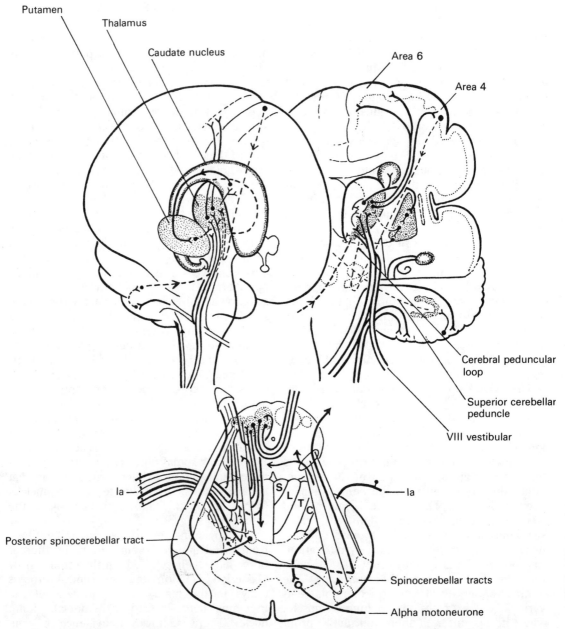

Putamen

Thalamus

Caudate nucleus

Area 6

Area 4

Cerebral peduncular loop

Superior cerebellar peduncle

VIII vestibular

Ia

S L T C

Ia

Posterior spinocerebellar tract

Spinocerebellar tracts

Alpha motoneurone

Fig. 9.1. Kinaesthetic afferents (mainly from muscles but also from joints and skin) are large myelinated A group fibres in the dorsal nerve root. Some Ia fibres (*right of cord diagram*) end monosynaptically on a motoneurone, the afferent pathway of the pluck reflex. (Polysynaptic stretch reflexes are shown in *Fig.* 17.1.) Some Ia and most of the Ib and II afferent fibres relay at the base of the dorsal horn or after ascending to its extensions in the medulla, the dorsal column nuclei and the arcuate and accessory cuneate nuclei to the cerebellum directly or via the inferior olive and lateral reticular nucleus of the medulla (*see Fig.* 23.1). The main spinocerebellar tracts are the ipsilateral posterior spinocerebellar tract (second order neurones from the dorsal nucleus of Clarke's column) and the contralateral anterior spinocerebellar tract (second order neurones from the lateral base of the dorsal horn).

A minority of the secondary neurones and primary fast conducting Ia fibres (which enter the dorsal column without synapse) ascend to the gracile and cuneate nuclei, grouped segmentally. Many of these send collaterals to the cerebellar afferent nuclei before relaying in the sensory decussation to the contralateral medial lemniscus to the VPL nucleus of the

The primary ending of the spindle provides signals of both the *degree and velocity of stretch* for kinaesthesia and for the stretch reflexes. It is also an important source of information to the cerebellum, presumably by collateral branching to second order neurones in Clarke's column and the nucleus dorsalis at the base of the dorsal horn (p. 78). Without this information, the central nervous system is unable to regulate the length of a muscle when it is passively stretched (hypotonia; absent jerks), to stabilize body posture when standing (sensory ataxia; Rombergism), or to appreciate the relative position in space of body parts (a form of agnosia characterized by 'pseudo-athetotic' wandering movements of the fingers).

SECONDARY SENSORY ENDINGS

A secondary sensory ending may be present on one or both sides of the primary ending. Formerly termed a 'flower-spray' or 'myotube ending', the newer term is preferred because the morphology varies in different muscles. It may be spiral and it is more common on the chain intrafusal fibres (which have a nuclear region resembling the myotubes of developing muscle). The secondary endings are now recognized by their situation and supply from group II afferent fibres rather than by morphology. They do not necessarily occur on each side of a primary ending (the ratio of secondary to primary endings is about 1·5:1). Some spindles ('simple' or type P) have no secondary endings, especially in muscles with rapid phasic rather than tonic contraction.

The zone of the intrafusal fibre bearing the secondary ending is less extensible than its equatorial region. The secondary ending is less sensitive to stretch of the muscle and functions mainly as a *tension receptor* since more tension is required to elongate the appropriate part of the fibre. It is supplied by the peripheral axon of a *group II afferent nerve fibre* which is more slowly conducting than the Ia fibre of the primary ending. Like other group II fibres, the central extension from the neurone in the dorsal root ganglion ends in the apparatus of the dorsal horn described on p. 78. Second order neurones supply the interneuronal system of the polysynaptic reflex system involved in the flexion withdrawal reflexes (p. 162), ie they are excitatory to flexor muscles and inhibitory to extensors, regardless of the nature of the muscle bearing the secondary spindle endings (*see Fig. 17.1*). They may, however, be important for the tonic stretch reflex (as distinct from the monosynaptic) which is so easily abolished by light anaesthesia when the monosynaptic response (tendon jerk) may be even brisker than before. The functions of the secondary endings have not been studied in the same detail as those of the primary endings. There is no incompatibility between a postural function with innocuous maintained stretch and a protective function when stretch becomes excessive. One of us has suggested an inhibitory role on local extrafusal fibres in the control of isometric tension.

TENDON RECEPTORS

These are of two types. Little is known about the functional significance of the *Pacinian corpuscles*. They appear to be vibration receptors with higher threshold to displacement than the primary endings of the spindles. They presumably contribute to proprioception and reflex control of movement as each has a single *group I* afferent nerve fibre and the receptors adapt rapidly. Thus, in clinical practice, it is common for both vibration sensibility and

---

Fig. 9.1. (contd)

thalamus. In the pons its fibres are mixed with the spinothalamic tract (*Fig. 6.1*) and the kinaesthetic afferents are joined by the lateral lemniscus carrying gravity-orientation second order neurones from the vestibular nerve which end nearby in the VL nucleus of thalamus.

A relatively small number of thalamo-cortical fibres are projected to the main somatosensory cortex and again to the superior parietal lobe. An important but not well-defined projection of the medial and lateral lemnisci is to the centrum medianum of the thalamus from which they are relayed to the neostriatum, the head ganglion for the righting reflexes. The centrum medianum also receives input from the contralateral cerebellum and ipsilateral pallidum and central cortex (by the 'cerebral peduncle loop'). These motor control fibres are indicated in dashed lines. The major outflow from the pallidum is omitted.

The large fibre input to the spinal cord and brain is predominantly for postural control. Perception of movement and position is a minor aspect of kinaesthesia.

'muscle-joint sensation' to be affected together by disease but as the receptors and nerve fibres involved are separate it is not surprising that only one or the other may be lost — position sense loss may occur through vibration sensation is retained. (The converse is common since appreciation of vibration requires retention of relative conduction velocities of afferent neurones, *see* p. 82.)

The better known tendon receptor is the *Golgi tendon organ*. A large *group Ib* myelinated nerve fibre branches and each branch terminates with a spray of fine endings between bundles of collagenous fibres in the tendon, usually near the insertion of the extrafusal muscle fibres. Unlike the spindles, this organ is in line ('in series') with the muscle fibres, a point of some importance since it senses the total tension generated by the muscle. It is generally agreed to be a *tension receptor* (as distinct from the length aspect of stretching). This is probably utilized in isotonic contraction of muscle and almost certainly in the inhibition of muscular contraction when the muscle is overloaded (*autogenetic inhibition*) and its antagonists are facilitated (both actions via interneurones) (*see* Fig. 17.1). The Golgi tendon organ may also be the receptor by which it is possible to judge the weight of an object held in the hand, but little is known about this aspect of perception. Discrimination of weights certainly requires integrity of the contralateral parietal lobe and probably of the dorsal column–lemniscal system projecting to it, but this function has not been studied in sufficient detail to discuss further. The peripheral afferent nerve fibre is certainly in the fast conducting type I group used by the nervous system for discriminative aspects of sensation.

Parallel and series endorgans

There are some important functional consequences of the anatomical situation of the muscle/tendon receptors. The primary and secondary endings stimulated by stretching the intrafusal fibres are in *spindle organs placed in parallel* with the extrafusal fibres. It is clear that they will signal passive extension of the muscle (or that part containing the spindle) and the primary ending will be exquisitely sensitive to very slight extensions, especially if applied rapidly ('velocity sensitive') whereas the secondary ending responds to maintained stretch such as will increase tension in the muscle. They are particularly appropriate as internal length-measuring devices. But the circumstance requiring immaculate measurement of muscle length is isotonic contraction. The spindle being in parallel with extrafusal fibres has less applied stretch as soon as the extrafusal fibres contract. To compensate for this, the nervous system drives the *intrafusal muscular fibres* to contract along with the extrafusal, thus resetting the spindle to the new length of the latter and so retaining its capacity to act as a measuring instrument. Nevertheless, during a rapid twitch of muscle, the spindle is briefly 'unloaded'. This is one example of the sensitivity of a peripheral receptor being regulated by impulses from the central nervous system. As the mechanism is then available for other motor control uses, it will be described further in Chapter 17.

Unlike the spindle, the *tendon organs are in series* with the extrafusal fibres and so they are stimulated whether the muscle contracts or is stretched passively, since in both cases the tension on the tendon is increased. The tendon integrates the tension produced by all the extrafusal fibres (the intrafusal fibres contribute a negligible amount). The autogenetic inhibitory reflex from this receptor is not only segmental but mainly (? exclusively) to the stretched muscle, via a single *inhibitory interneurone* in the cord grey matter. It protects the muscle from rupture due to excessive tension and probably plays an important role in allowing a muscle to relax under load during isotonic exercise. Examples of load-compensating responses are described on pp. 201 and 210. The inhibitory neurone is contacted by a collateral of the first sensory neurone in lamina V or VI of the dorsal horn at the level of the posterior root or one or two segments up or down the cord. Like the spindle afferents, some signals from the tendon reach the cerebellum.

Unloading of the spindle and the autogenetic inhibition from the Golgi tendon organ are two of the factors in the '*silent period*' (p. 245).

Central regulation of receptor sensitivity

The inhibitory role of the higher nervous system on incoming signals reaching the dorsal horn and higher nuclei is described in appropriate chapters. The availability of facilitatory and inhibitory interneurones makes this a relatively simple matter of feedback or feedforward control. In at least some situations a degree of control is exerted at the peripheral receptor.

MUSCLE SPINDLE

It is now necessary to amplify the description of the muscle spindles outlined on p. 87. These are now classified as two types of nuclear bag fibres (bag_1 and bag_2) and a nuclear chain fibre according to the nuclear structure of the equatorial region of the intrafusal fibre. The *central area* of each type of intrafusal fibre is devoid of contractile sarcomeres and so is readily stretched. The *extreme poles* of the intrafusal fibre (inserted into the perimysium and other connective tissue of the extrafusal fibres) have elastic tissue which is more abundant or more compliant in the bag_2 and nuclear chain fibres. Moving centrally from the elastic poles, one sees a *region of sarcomeres* with M lines (less well developed in bag_1 fibres). This is a site of local shortening in response to membrane depolarization by the action of a special efferent nervous system. This contractile region does not include the entire nuclear area of the intrafusal fibre. There is a *transitional zone* with myofilaments but instead of shortening occurring with membrane depolarization, as in extrafusal muscle fibres, the cross-bridges bind actin to myosin filaments to resist extension except for a slight 'creep' as the cross-bridges slowly detach. This gives the receptor a 'dynamic' action — ie an immediate and progressive though non-linear resistance to stretch. This is followed by gradual creep of the transitional zone, relaxing the stretch on the equatorial area (with consequent '*adaptation*' of the receptor). The overall contractile system can then be slow although the sarcomere mechanism is fast.

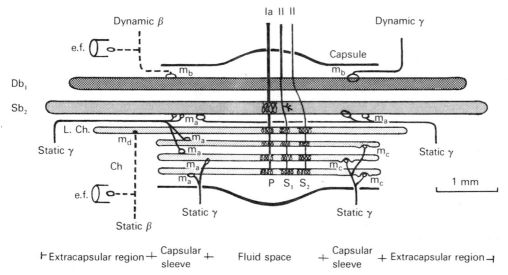

Fig. 9.2. Structure and innervation of a typical muscle spindle (cat) with one dynamic nuclear bag_1 intrafusal fibre (Db_1), one static nuclear bag_2 fibre (Sb_2) and four nuclear chain fibres (Ch), one longer than the others (L. Ch.). Primary sensory ending (P) has sensory spiral terminals of a group Ia axon around every intrafusal fibre. Secondary sensory ending in S_1 region has spirals around chain fibres and spray terminals on both nuclear bag fibres, more on Sb_2 fibre; secondary ending in S_2 region has sensory spirals on chain fibres only. The Db_1 fibre is innervated selectively by dynamic γ and β axons and Sb_2 and chain fibres are innervated both selectively and non-selectively by static γ axons. Static β axon innervates L.Ch. in some spindles only.

The intrafusal fibres receive motor nerve terminals at the two areas of localized cross-bridge binding. The local depolarization occurring under their terminals is a local junctional potential. It is not propagated in the bag fibres. In chain fibres action potentials may be generated but these do not seem to propagate throughout their lengths. These depolarizations occur at specialized nerve endings of two types described as 'plate' or 'trail' endings according to their structure. Both are believed to be cholinergic (but less readily blocked by D-tubocurarine than the endplates of extrafusal fibres). It is not known how they differ functionally — the original impression that each supplied a specific type of intrafusal fibre has not been confirmed.

However, a difference of function between the different intrafusal muscle fibre types has recently been identified.

INTRAFUSAL FIBRE TYPES

There are two types of nuclear bag fibres. The *bag$_1$ fibre* has a slow weak contraction followed by 'creep'. Its primary sensory receptor therefore transduces rapid stretch but adapts to sustained stretch. It is described as a 'dynamic' receptor.

The *bag$_2$ fibre* has more elastic tissue and a larger contraction. Its bag area is less sensitive to abrupt stretch but has less creep. Its primary sensory receptor is less dynamic and more 'static' in its response to stretch of the fibre.

The *nuclear chain fibre* has still faster contraction and little creep. It is a receptor of 'static stretch'.

EFFERENT NERVES TO INTRAFUSAL MUSCLE FIBRES

These properties of the muscle fibres within the spindle depend on activation of their sarcomere mechanisms by membrane depolarization at motor nerve endings, plate or trail. It is now clear that there are efferent nerves with corresponding 'dynamic' and 'static' functions.

The *gamma or fusimotor neurones* constitute a system of small motor neurones in the anterior horns (and motor cranial nerve nuclei) with small diameter myelinated axons conducting at only 21–25 m/s.

Dynamic fusimotor axons go exclusively to the dynamic bag$_1$ muscle fibres. When stimulated, there is no significant excitatory effect on the muscle unless the latter is being stretched in which case the primary afferent response from the bag$_1$ fibre is enhanced.

Static fusimotor axons go to bag$_2$ and chain intrafusal muscle fibres (either or both, *see Fig. 9.2*). The fusion frequency of the bag$_2$ fibres is rather low, but the chain fibres can follow static fusimotor stimuli up to 100 Hz. The functional significance of this difference is unknown but the dual mechanism may be related to an interesting and important functional attribute of the static stretch detection system. At very small stretches (around 1 mm) the transfer function (afferent nerve firing rate per increment of stretch) is remarkably high. With progressive increase in the magnitude of stretch the sensitivity of the system is reduced more or less abruptly. This enables the same system to function effectively for the small increments of stretch in postural control and for the large changes in voluntary movement. The explanation for this non-linearity is not known but the dual static stretch detection system is likely to be involved since the decoding apparatus of the central nervous system must be informed when the change of receptor setting has occurred.

BETA NEURONES

The gamma motoneurones do not innervate extrafusal muscle fibres. However, some motor fibres of alpha diameter innervate intrafusal as well as extrafusal fibres. They have been given the name 'beta' and have a conduction velocity at the lower end of the alpha range. They exert both static and dynamic effects on the spindle. As might be expected, 'dynamic' beta neurones end on bag$_1$ intrafusal fibres (dynamic) at a special plate ending. 'Static' beta axons end on chain fibres but have not yet been identified in the other (bag$_2$) static intrafusal fibres. Although the system has not yet been identified in man it is likely to be present as it seems to be a more 'primitive' system than the gamma motor system in so far as there is complete linkage between driving of extrafusal and intrafusal muscle fibres, whereas gamma driving has been demonstrated independent of alpha activity. An additional difference is that the beta neurones in the anterior horn probably receive monosynaptic Ia afferent input like pure alpha motoneurones, providing a mechanism to keep spindles functioning during shortening of the muscle.

An additional function of the gamma motoneurones may be to promote independent activation of the dynamic fibres which increase the sensitivity of the Ia afferents regardless of the passive value which depends on muscle length, whereas the balance of dynamic and static fibres may provide a continuous gain control of spindle responsiveness at all levels of stretch.

ROLE OF SPINDLES IN VOLUNTARY MOVEMENT

A hypothesis that alpha motoneurone activation of extrafusal muscle fibres driven reflexly by spindle afferent (Ia) firing induced in the first place by the gamma motoneurone could account for 'voluntary' muscle contraction (the *servo hypothesis*) has been abandoned because all research in this field has shown that gamma motoneurone and spindle activity never precede that of alpha neurones. Although the 'command' role for the fusimotor system has been abandoned it is undoubted that the system plays an important role during voluntary muscle contraction, both reflexly and as a route for supraspinal facilitation of length-regulation of the contracting muscle. In this sense, *co-activation of alpha, beta and gamma motoneurones* is probably the rule though not invariably. If the servo hypothesis were correct, it would be impossible to move after de-afferentation and this is not so. Motor control is still possible for 'pre-programmed' movements, but learning of new skills for the de-afferented muscles is impossible (p. 242). It could be said that the fusimotor system controls posture within movement under the higher control of the striatal complex (Chapter 22).

SUPRASPINAL CONTROL OF GAMMA MOTONEURONES

Efferent neurones projecting to the spinal interneurones connected with the gamma motoneurones have been identified in most of the descending pathways including the reticulospinal, rubrospinal, vestibulospinal and probably the corticospinal. They are believed to be coordinated and linked with alpha neurone activity by the anterior lobe of the cerebellum projecting via the fastigial and globose nuclei (p. 233). In the cat, the *alpha–gamma linkage* can be broken by freezing this area of the cerebellum and it has been postulated that similar absence of coactivation could account for some of the dysmetria and asynergia found in cerebellar disease in man. The areflexia of certain clinical disorders in man (Friedreich's ataxia, Holmes-Adie syndrome, phenytoin poisoning) has been attributed to failure of this supraspinal facilitatory system since the monosynaptic reflex arcs are intact. Conversely, overactivity of this system may play a role in some types of rigidity (p. 218).

Central control of receptor sensitivity in the ear

Another sensory system in which the intensity of stimulus reaching the receptor endorgan is under reflex control is the acoustic system. Reflex changes in the tone of the tensor tympani muscle alter the dampening qualities of the tympanum, and the stapedius muscle controls the position and tension of the ossicles which transmit the sound vibrations to the inner ear. Each of these muscles contracts reflexly in response to sounds of high intensity, thus dampening the pressure waves reaching the fluid of the inner ear and hence reducing the stimulus to the hair cells of the organ of Corti (p. 102). These reflexes are under control from the inferior colliculus of the mid-brain at which level central control is possible.

In addition, the cochlear nerve carries efferent fibres from the superior olivary nucleus (mainly contralateral) which pass to the cochlea and in some way inhibit its sensory outflow (appropriate nerve endings have been identified on the hair cells). The olivo-cochlear bundles are also believed to be under control from the acoustic cortex via the medial geniculate body and the inferior colliculus. Although most of this descending or centrifugal control of auditory pathways is likely to take place at synapses in the ascending pathways for hearing, it is clear that peripheral reflex control is also used in a manner reminiscent of the muscle spindles.

Central control of visual reception

It is unnecessary to elaborate the point that the intensity of light reaching the retina is controlled by the light reflexes varying the diameter of the pupils. This is more appropriately described in Chapter 10. With excessive illumination the eyelids are closed by a blink reflex (p. 164).

Active perception

These examples of 'central control' involve the use of muscle reflexes to adjust the stimulus intensity reaching the receptors. Previous suggestions that the reticular formation may interfere with peripheral sense organs have not been confirmed. By far the most common site of modification of the afferent bombardment is at the primary synapse. There is, however, another aspect of sensori-motor collaboration, which we have called, for want of an agreed term, 'active perception'. For some time it has been known that there are cortical neurones responsive to the orientation of an object in the visual field. Recently it has been shown that some neurones of layers III and IV of the somatic sensory cortex are differentially sensitive to the direction of a stimulus moving across their peripheral receptive fields, and still more commonly in area 5 of the superior parietal lobule to which the primary sensori-motor cortex projects (see Fig. 8.1). It seems unlikely that this has evolved to detect an insect walking over the skin — a more suitable project for lower level reflex action. It is strongly implied that palpation and manipulation are essential for discriminative sensation, a proposition self-evident to psychophysiologists. It need not therefore be surprising that a patient often describes a paralysed limb as 'numb', in full appreciation of the sensory significance of the adjective.

A related fact pointed out above is that so-called position sense is remarkably poor until a joint is abruptly displaced, be it ever so slightly. Skilled movements in extra-corporeal space would be impossible without accurate perception of limb position at the start of movement. A possible mechanism for maintaining the signalling function of muscle and joint receptors would be an imposed fine vibration. This could be the purpose, if such is needed, of *physiological tremor* but, strangely, the tremor vanishes when isometric contraction is maintained with the eyes closed. A possible clue may lie in the fact that an exaggerated form of physiological tremor occurs as a familial disorder and that it is reduced by β-adrenergic receptor blockers such as propranolol. The fluid-containing capsule of the muscle spindle receives an autonomic nerve supply which releases noradrenaline but its function is unknown. Alternatively, the adrenergic beta-2 receptors on extrafusal muscle fibres may alter the active state of these twitch fibres. Physiological tremor is modified by segmental stretch reflexes and central driving (in the Jendrassick manoeuvre) which synchronize the motoneurone pool, but it does not depend on afferent feedback for its initiation. Granit has commented that an oscillating muscular response may be a necessary consequence of the multiple biological operations contributing to the maintenance of a length setting. The spinal interneuronal pool certainly contains adrenergic receptors.

Further reading

Boyd I.A. Muscle spindles and stretch reflexes. In: Swash M. and Kennard C. (ed.) *Scientific Basis of Neurology*. Edinburgh: Churchill Livingstone, 1985; pp. 74–97.

Boyd I.A. and Gladden M.H.I. (ed.) *The Muscle Spindle*. London: Macmillan, 1985.

Gibson J.J. Observations on active touch. *Psychol. Rev.* 1962; **69**: 477–91.

Goodwin G.M., McCloskey D.I. and Matthews P.B.C. The contribution of muscle afferents to kinaesthesia shown by vibration-induced illusions of movement and by the effects of paralysing joint afferents. *Brain* 1972; **95**: 705–48.

Gordon G. (ed.) *Active Touch*. Oxford: Pergamon, 1978.

McCloskey D.I. Kinesthetic sensibility. *Physiol. Rev.* 1978; **58**: 763–820.

Matthews P.B.C. *Mammalian Muscle Receptors and Their Central Actions*. London: Arnold, 1972.

Matthews P.B.C. Review Lecture: Evolving views on the internal operation and functional role of the muscle spindle. *J. Physiol. (Lond.)* 1981; **320**: 1–30.

Mountcastle V.B. and Powell T.P.S. Central nervous mechanisms subserving position sense and kinesthesis. *Bull. Johns Hopkins Hosp.* 1959; **105**: 173–200.

Young R.R. and Hagbarth K.-E. Physiological tremor enhanced by manoeuvres affecting the segmental stretch reflex. *J. Neurol. Neurosurg. Psychiatry* 1980; **43**: 248–56.

Chapter 10
Vision

The somatosensory receptors for detecting stimuli at the surface or within the body are specialized endings of peripheral nerve fibres with their own satellite cell support system (Schwann cells). The receptor organ for light rays, detecting extracorporeal space, is radically different. The retina of the eye is an evagination of the cerebral hemisphere and its satellite cells are glial like the central nervous system (so that the retinae and optic nerves are vulnerable to a different range of diseases and noxae than the other peripheral nerves).

Encapsulated in a specialized globe with light transmission characteristics enabling light rays to be focused on the retina, the *retinal rods and cones* are not directly sensitive to electromagnetic energy. They are in fact chemoreceptors which light reaches after passing through the layers of nerve cells. Within the rods and cones are *visual pigments*, rhodopsin, porphyropsin and others, which are bleached by light and regenerate in darkness. It is still not certain how the photochemical process leads to the development of a receptor or generator potential but it is certain that the energy of a quantum of light is thereby amplified some 10 million times to produce the nerve impulse in tens of milliseconds. The reaction is extraordinarily resistant to low temperature, anoxia and ion concentration. The rod units are more sensitive than the cones but the latter generate a larger receptor potential. Not surprisingly, *rods* are the dominant receptor at the periphery of the retina and for night vision (to collect all available light) and *cones* at the fovea where maximum fidelity is required.

The receptor cells connect via *bipolar cells* to *ganglion cells* either directly or via interneurones (*amacrine cells* and *horizontal cells*)

(*Fig.* 10.1) in the eighth layer of the retina. Several rods converge on one ganglion cell, but the ratio of cones to ganglion cells is virtually 1:1, in accordance with the light gathering role

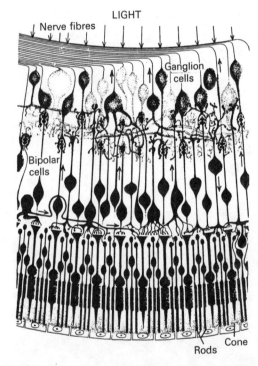

Fig. 10.1. *The retina.* Light, gathered and focused by the refractory media of the eye, travels through the layers of blood vessels, nerve fibres and supporting cells to the pigment epithelium of the outermost layer of the retina into which are inserted rod and cone cells which are depolarized by the photosensitive reaction. The receptor cells have synapses with bipolar cells which converge on the ganglion cells. These third order neurones have long axons which gather towards the optic nerve head. There they gain myelin (of central type) and pass without further relay to the lateral geniculate ganglia. In the bipolar cell layer there are lateral multibranched connections through interneurones, including the amacrine cells.

of the rods and the visual acuity role of the cones. (A price has to be paid for the cone insensitivity: they are easily saturated and so the intensity of light is modified by a rapid response reflex pupillary constriction. Remember that when the latter is tested for evidence of integrity of brain stem connections it is essential to shine the light towards the macula, not to the periphery of the retina as commonly practised.)

The rod is not only more sensitive to dim light, but as its photochemical cycle is faster than in the cone it is able to follow individual light flashes up to a higher rate of flicker before they are 'fused' than can the cone receptor. The cone is better for giving a constant picture of the environment, but the rod is a splendid *detector of movement* away from the direction of gaze. Indeed the more peripheral rods of the retina apparently detect movement (as the gaze fixation reflex is elicited) without any sensation of vision (p. 177).

The visual receptors in the pigmented layer of the retina furthest from the refractory media are in synaptic connection with dendrites of bipolar cells which in turn synapse with ganglion cells in the layer enclosing the vitreous humor of the eye. These are, in effect, third order neurones with long axons passing across the retinal surface to the optic disc where they turn centrally in the optic nerve and pass via the chiasma and optic tract to one or other *lateral geniculate body* (*see Fig. 19.4*). Those arising from the temporal side of the retina pass to the ipsilateral lateral geniculate body: those from the nasal side decussate in the optic chiasma to the contralateral lateral geniculate body. Note that the layers of the retina are homologous with dorsal horn grey matter, and the chiasma resembles the decussation of the lemniscal pathways but only those fibres transmitting impulses from the nasal half of the retinae are crossed. (Since light rays cross in the refractory media, the nasal retina 'sees' the temporal field of vision.) In this way fibres are sorted out so that left temporal and right nasal fibres pass to the left hemisphere, ie the left hemisphere receives stimuli arising from the right half of the visual field of each eye, and vice versa for the right hemisphere.

Since the retina is virtually 'explanted brain'

it processes the sensory signals in a way not seen with true peripheral nerves/receptors and many of the visual phenomena and illusions investigated by the experimental psychologist take place at retinal level. Already at this level there is convergence of several photoreceptors on each bipolar cell which in turn projects to more than one ganglion cell in both facilitatory and inhibitory modes. Thus the *lateral inhibition*, which we have already seen is a general principle for 'crispening' signals in the nervous system, is already present in the retina. It is so efficient that the most effective signal for onward transmission is a line between fields of different luminosity. The eye and brain 'see' the line and the cerebral cortex apparently interpolates between the lines an interpretation based on previous visual experience. (The brain has to 'learn' to see, cf. p. 100.)

Like most sensory transducers, a change in the environment is the most effective stimulus — some photoreceptors are excited by a light turning 'on', others perceive light 'off', and still others both 'on and off', but their firing rate drops significantly if the light flux is steady. These circumstances favour detection of moving line-borders.

COLOUR VISION

Cone receptors, mainly in the foveal region, do record continuous light, and furthermore they are specialized to respond to different wavelengths, a basis for colour (*photopic*) vision as distinct from the grey shadows (*scotopic*) of rod vision. It is generally agreed that there are three types of cone sensitive to wavelengths (long, medium and short wave) perceived as red, green and blue (violet) hues. The different colours are seen by a mixture of signals from the three systems. Many people are partially (rarely completely) lacking in one of the three kinds of cone systems. Presumably these receptors maintain separate connections through the retinal layers and at all synapses in the lateral geniculate and cortical relays since cortical cells have been identified which respond to one or other of these light wavelengths. Like somatic cutaneous sensation, the periphery and the cortex are linked in a point-to-point localization with retention of stimulus modality, and indeed the cortical cells have a columnar organization essentially the same as that described for somatosensory cortex.

BINOCULAR VISION

There is one important difference between skin and retinae. Both eyes see the same visual field and the signals from the temporal side of one retina must be linked with those crossing from the nasal side of the other retina (homonymous fields of vision). The crossed and uncrossed fibres (which are the axons of ganglion cells in the retinae) end in alternating layers of the lateral geniculate body with fibres from corresponding retinal areas ending in neighbouring parts of the different layers. They relay in the lateral geniculate body and the next neurones pass in the *optic radiation* to the striate area of the medial surface of the occipital cortex, maintaining such close topographic association that a lesion of the optic radiation causes virtually identical scotomas in the visual field of each eye (congruent homonymous defects).

The topographic arrangement from half-fields is maintained at the cortex. The upper retinal quadrants (lower field quadrants) are represented superior (dorsal) to the calcarine fissure and the lower retinal quadrants (upper field quadrants), inferior (ventral) to the fissure. However, like the cortical representation of cutaneous sensation, the area of cortex devoted to retinal areas is not in direct proportion to anatomical area but rather to functional importance. Thus, the macular (foveal) representation is much more extensive than that of the peripheral retina. It is situated posteriorly in the primary visual area. In keeping with its functional importance it has major blood supplies from middle cerebral and posterior cerebral arteries so that a hemianopia due to infarction of the visual area commonly 'spares the macula'.

Despite the topographic arrangement of cell layers in the lateral geniculate body which would suggest convergence of impulses from matching sites of both retinae, it appears that this is not the rule. Convergence is delayed until geniculo-striate fibres meet at the striate area of the cortex. The lateral geniculate body is interpolated into this point-to-point projection system as a rather complex interneuronal

organization at which *fibres from the cerebral cortex and the reticular formation gate the receptor to cortex flow* in a similar manner to that already described for somatic sensation.

VISUAL CORTEX

The fibres of the optic radiation end in contact with cells of the granular layers of the striate area (area 17) on the medial surface of the occipital lobe. It is a typical 'receptive' cortex but has prominent pyramidal cells in the (efferent) IIIrd and Vth layers which relay some processed data of the visual signals to the surrounding area 18. That area relays a further 'abstraction' to area 19, a large part of the convexity of the occipital lobe (*Fig. 10.2*). It is difficult to avoid such 'interpretative' terms since there is no language to describe in physiological terms the further data processing which goes on in this 'associative cortex'. Stimulation of the striate area produces sensations of simple optic events (sparks, flashes of light or scintillating scotomas) which are referred to the appropriate part of the visual fields. Stimulation of areas 18 and 19 also produces more complex visual sensations and movements of the eyes, not unlike the 'body image' hallucinations and commanded movements of parietal lobe stimulation (Chapter 12). Integration of visual impressions into a 'visual space image' related to eye movements may reasonably be postulated in analogy with the image of body and 'palpable' space associated with manipulation which characterizes the parietal lobe. Activity of neuronal circuits organized in columns where many visual impulses converge may be considered to represent visual 'symbols' linked to stored memories of previous events to give them significance in the behavioural pattern, a basis for *reading*.

A neuronal activity (or its stored version) could only acquire symbolic value if it could be linked with another modality of afferent input. The anterior extension of the visual association area is likely to be linked transcortically or subcortically with somatosensory influences via the parietal lobe. Perhaps more significant is an integration of visual impulses (via the superior colliculus) with auditory signals which are relayed by the *pulvinar nucleus* of the

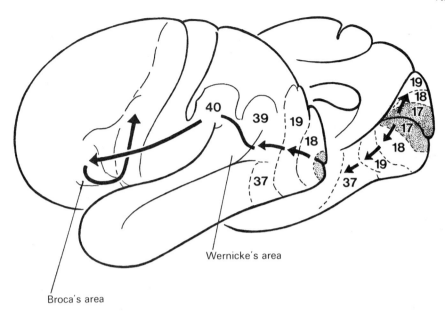

Fig. 10.2. The visual area of the cortex (striate area, 17) is around the calcarine sulcus. It is is connected radially to areas 18 and 19 (pre-striate area), a visual association cortex in which discrete zones process the information in parallel, according to wavelength of light and orientation of the optic stimulus, movement across the visual field etc. Further serial processing in area 19 and anteriorly uses the visual data for commanding movements of eyes and head and other aspects of visually guided behaviour. In the left hemisphere the forward projection from the angular gyrus (39) to Wernicke's area and then further forward to Broca's area (which is linked to the lower motor strip) is the substratum for speaking a written word. In the right hemisphere dominantly, projection to the parietal lobe adds a visual component to the body image, bilaterally. Connections with the inferotemporal cortex (37) are used for learning visual discrimination tasks including recognition of faces (mainly right hemisphere).

thalamus to area 18 as well as to the posterior sylvian receptive region (*supramarginal and angular gyri*) adjacent to the auditory projection area and the inferotemporal cortex. Thus lesions rarely cause 'pure' *alexia* or '*word deafness*' — usually both forms of speech reception are involved. The retina–colliculus–pulvinar–circumstriate cortex pathway may account for the unlocalized awareness of movements sometimes reported by patients with 'cortical blindness' after cardiac arrest.

In the reference to a physiological basis for the receptive aspects of speech (p. 107) we discuss the necessity for spatial and temporal sequential ordering of cutaneous afferent signals if they are to have symbolic value. Experiments on the visual cortex of the cat have been particularly instructive. Hubel and Wiesel (1977) have shown that some columns of cells in the visual cortex respond to a stripe of light and for each column it is most effective when the stripe has a particular orientation in the visual field. This property appears to be due to linkage at the lateral geniculate body of inputs from retinal receptors arranged in rows. The principle is similar to the direction-sensitive cortical neurones of the somatosensory cortex and the sequential order of activation may be equally important. There are '*complex*' cells which respond to appropriately orientated stimuli in all parts of the visual field — possibly integrating activity from many 'simple' *orientation-sensitive cells*. The elements for pattern recognition are there in the primary visual cortex (area 17).

It has recently been proved that (in the cat) there is a multiplicity of visual areas responsive to motion, form and colour individually which further project in parallel (not sequentially) to the different visual areas of the prestriate cortex. These analytic functions are in contrast with the synthetic function of visual activated neurones in the parietal cortex. These are particularly sensitive to stimulus movement and direction along the radii of the visual field, and relatively insensitive to stimulus, speed, orientation or colour according to Mountcastle. Anatomical evidence in monkeys points to direct geniculo-cortical projections to areas 18 and 19 as well as to area 17 which may therefore be receptive as well as associative cortices.

Interhemisphere connection by commissural fibres does not occur from area 17 but is considerable from area 18 (like the secondary somatosensory areas) (*see Fig.* 19.4). Cells in the cortex of area 18 are reciprocally connected to cells in the inferotemporal cortex of both sides. Some of the latter appear to respond to complicated visual patterns such as the shape of a hand. This area is important for *learning visual discrimination* tasks. A particular variety of visual agnosia in man concerns the non-identification of the human face (prosopagnosia) in lesions mainly of the right temporal lobe.

To recognize visual patterns they must be matched for similarity with 'remembered' engrams. This function appears to require linkage of visual areas with the *inferior temporal cortex*. When the latter is ablated bilaterally a '*psychic blindness*' occurs in which visual clues lose significance despite intact visual acuity. (Monkeys then identify objects by oral exploration as they are continually unfamiliar, part of the Kluver–Bucy syndrome, Chapter 13.) Experiments with kittens indicate that visual impressions only acquire significance when the developing animal actively explores and manipulates its environment. Note the similarity to 'active touch'.

It seems that the environmental influences in infancy affect neuronal connections which may persist throughout life and sensory deprivation may permanently prevent full development of potential.

DEPTH PERCEPTION

Instead of colour or movement, some cells of the visual cortex signal velocity of a light spot crossing the retina, or depth in the visual space. The psychophysiology of depth perception is a fascinating story but must be consigned to the bibliography (Gregory, 1966) as it is of little significance to the anaesthetist. The physiological mechanisms are not unique and depend on asymmetry of overlapping visual fields, direction and relative sizes of shadows, perspective and, perhaps most im-

portantly, a comparison of incoming positional signals from the retinae and extraocular muscles with the outgoing motor control systems which make the two visual axes converge at different depths in visual space. (The importance of corollary discharge is discussed on p. 242.)

STEREOSCOPIC VISION

The range-finder effect of monitoring eye *convergence* has a major limitation. It can only measure the distance of one object at a time. Stereoscopic vision, due to the disparity of the images received by the two eyes, is another method of judging depth. There are cells in the visual cortex which detect the disparity between the images on the two retinae, and *depth disparity* is detected by special cells in area 18, firing most briskly (or only) with binocular inputs. The difference in depth between two objects with disparate images depends on the distance of the objects: the scale of the disparity system is adjusted by the angle of convergence measuring system. But depth can still be assessed with only one eye. Most of the clues which enable this to be done are learned, eg perspective lines, parallax movements, distance haze and blueness, and size disparity of familiar objects. A comparison between a photograph (with suitable focal length of lens) and an artist's impression immediately demonstrates a psychophysical phenomenon of some importance. We tend to perceive familiar objects with a '*size constancy*' and geometrical perspective which makes distant objects seem to be larger than they must be in the retinal image. Observations on aboriginal people and young children indicate that the size constancy phenomenon is learned (and best learned by active manipulation of the environment), that is to say the true image is interpreted in terms of stored polymodality impressions — probably the same phenomenon as the comparison of afferent signals from the peripheral nerves with a stored 'body image'. It is difficult to escape the conclusion that this is a general principle of sensory perception. Inherent in it is the possibility of misinterpretation and of alternative interpretations of ambiguous patterns as in some well-known optical illusions.

A study of depth perception highlights some other important aspects of brain function.

Consider, for instance, the hemisphere representation of a point nearer or further than the object focused on by the two optic axes. Their image on each retina should be projected to different hemispheres (*see Fig*. 19.4) if each half retina is strictly homonymous. Electrophysiological experiments on animals show that this generalization is not absolutely true. The separate halves of the retinae do converge on single units in *both* hemispheres, at least so far as central vision is concerned. In the human, there is no evidence for projection of retinal ganglion cells into both optic tracts and a decussation in the corpus callosum seems probable (accounting for retention of depth perception from the temporal retinae/nasal fields after section of the optic chiasm). Depth perception by bilateral representation would be a poor biological development if it became impossible to decide whether an object near the fixation point in the same plane was to right or left of it. Confusion is eliminated by making one half retina-to-cortex projection *dominant* for any particular cortical cell.

This depth perception from bi-hemisphere stimulation is greatest for the centre of the visual field. The rangefinder–convergence method also requires accurate control of direction of gaze. Its further discussion is postponed until the control of gaze has been described (p. 185). Acute vision and perception of colour, and to a large extent form, are also central retinal functions. Clearly *visually guided behaviour* as distinct from detection of movements, depends on accurate direction of the axes of the two eyes and rotation of the globes to minimize disparities of images. It is not surprising to find (p. 185) that involuntary gaze is directed first by reflex response to movement of an object relative to others in the periphery of the visual field in such a way as to bring it into the central field, and then to that part of the central field at which disparity between the images of the two retinae is minimized, in the same way as the palpating hand is moved to bring the explored object to the most sensitive areas of the skin of the fingertips.

The control of head and eye movements is described in Chapter 19. They cannot be considered in isolation. At a primitive level, the identification of a stimulus and its localization in space are orienting reactions for prey-catching (slowly moving visual object) or avoidance behaviour (rapid movement). It will be shown later that visual attention elicits the EEG responses associated with alertness (Chapter 16) but that orientation responses are strongly influenced by motivation, which includes limbic lobe activity (Chapter 14). Both these cerebral functions are suppressed by light anaesthesia.

Threatening visual stimuli (rapid movement towards the eyes) evoke eye closure and evasive movements, turning the head away, sidestepping or compensating for tilting of the body. These are reflexes utilizing the thalamus (p. 164) and may use the optic relays at the pulvinar and superior colliculus rather than being cortex-commanded movements.

Some of the optic nerve fibres leave the medial side of the optic tract where it enters the lateral geniculate body and pass via the superior quadrigeminal brachium to the *superior colliculus* and pre-tectum of the mid-brain, bilaterally (*see Fig*. 19.3). These important centres for control of reflex eye movements and of the pupil diameter are not completely independent of the visual cortex. They send fibres via the pulvinar to areas 17, 18, 19 and inferotemporal cortex (*Fig*. 10.2), and receive corticofugal fibres from these areas. These connections may account for the reports of patients with cortical blindness who are able to distinguish sudden darkening or lightening of a room ('blind sight').

Further reading

Brindley G.S. *Physiology of the Retina and Visual Pathway*, 2nd ed. London: Arnold, 1970.
Gregory R.L. *Eye and Brain. The Psychology of Seeing*. London: Weidenfeld and Nicolson, 1966.
Hubel D.H. and Wiesel T.N. Functional architecture of macaque monkey cortex. *Proc. R. Soc. Lond.* 1977; **B198**: 1–59.
Zeki S. Looking and seeing. In: Swash M. and Kennard C. (ed.) *Scientific Basis of Clinical Neurology*. Edinburgh: Churchill Livingstone, 1985, pp. 172–87.

Chapter 11
Hearing

In the acoustic system mechanoreceptors have been developed as distance receptors by being placed on a membrane which is thrown into vibration by pressure vibration of the external air (or water) environment.

Fluctuations of air pressure are not transmitted directly to the membrane carrying the hair cell mechanoreceptors. They are linked by a mechanical impedance-matching device — tympanic membrane, chain of ossicles in the middle ear and cochlear fluid — which transfers sound energy from a gas to a liquid without significant loss of energy. The details of the external and middle ear are not relevant to this textbook except to note that the tensioning of the tympanum and dampening of the ossicular movements are due to two muscles (tensor tympani and stapedius respectively) both supplied by the VIIth cranial nerve and under reflex control to limit movement of the mechanical parts of the system in response to very intense sounds (signal limitation like that resulting from the pupil light reflex). Measurement of the mechanical impedance of the system to imposed pressure changes in the external meatus and the reflex response times are used clinically to measure the integrity of these reflex arcs.

Static pressure within the middle ear is maintained equal to that in the external meatus by allowing air to pass into it from the pharynx by the Eustachian tube. This tube has a soft pharyngeal orifice which opens only when the tensor palati pulls on it during swallowing, yawning and sneezing. If this muscle is paralysed or the Eustachian tube is blocked by inflammatory reaction in the intubated patient, the trapped air in the middle ear is absorbed, causing deafness and discomfort (like that experienced on landing after a long air flight).

Loudness is signalled by the amplitude of the longitudinal pressure wave transmitted to the cochlear fluid, and sound *pitch* by its frequency (approximately sinusoidal). *Timbre* and quality of sound are added by the relative amplitudes of harmonics of the vibrating pressure. '*Noise*' is caused by non-periodic vibrations.

COCHLEA

The coiled fluid-containing cochlear tube is divided into two canals by the transducer-carrying basilar membrane. The channel above the membrane (*scala vestibuli*) reproduces the pattern of pressure waves outside the tympanum. At the apical end of the coil (helocotrema) this channel leaks into a similar channel (*scala tympani*) under the membrane to equalize slow pressure differences. As fluid is incompressible, the scala tympani ends in a flexible membrane, the round window.

The ossicular movements are transmitted by the footplate of the stapes to the fluid in the scala vestibuli, causing the round window membrane to bulge and the basilar membrane to tilt towards the scala tympani on which lies a closed fluid-containing tube (*cochlear duct*) bathing the organ of Corti and its overlying tectorial membrane (*Fig. 11.1*).

Movement of the basilar membrane, imposed through this impedance-matched air-to-fluid interface, causes bending of minute hairs on the free surface of receptor cells of the *organ of Corti* (facing the tectorial membrane). There is still some uncertainty about the method by which different frequencies of sound induce selective deformation of the basilar membrane (there are resonance and standing-wave theories) but it is agreed that different frequencies of sound wave (pitch)

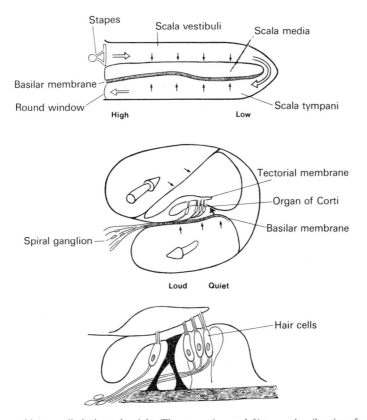

Fig. 11.1. *Upper*: the cochlea uncoiled, tip at the right. The stapes (*upper left*) transmits vibrations from the tympanum to fluid in the scala vestibuli which is continuous round the helicotrema (at the tip of the helix) with the scala tympani which ends at the round window, closed by a flexible membrane (*large arrows*). The fluid vibrations are transmitted (*small arrows*) to the closed scala media, setting up a standing wave in the basilar membrane (*grey*). *Middle*: represents a cross-section in larger scale. Movement of the basilar membrane pushes part of the organ of Corti against the tectorial membrane (a shelf-like structure) locally deflecting the stereocilia of hair cells. Pitch is represented along the length of the basilar membrane, loudness across its width. *Lower*: the organ of Corti. Inner and outer rows of hair cells are the receptor cells for acoustic nerve fibres with cell bodies in the spiral ganglion. These are bipolar cells, passing centrally in the auditory nerve (VIII).

evoke movement principally at discrete parts of the basilar membrane, high tones at the base of the coiled membrane, lower tones towards the apex. (More correctly, lower tones affect more and more of the length of the basilar membrane, spreading further to the apex as the pitch is lowered.)

The changes in electrical potential across the basilar lamina when the *hair cells* are distorted follow the amplitude and frequency of sound waves with remarkable fidelity. If suitably amplified and fed into a loudspeaker, words spoken into the ear are reproduced by the loudspeaker. For this reason these changes have been termed *microphonic potentials*. They are not action potentials of the acoustic

nerve, although they can be recorded from the nerve by simple electric conduction. Naturally they accompany the hair cell movement without latency. It is not known whether the microphonic potential is a derivative of the *transducer potential* of the deflected hair cell which inaugurates *action potentials* in a fibre of the acoustic nerve.

As the sound frequency is signalled by the *place* on the basilar membrane responding maximally, the intensity of sound can be signalled by both recruitment of fibres from this locus and by rate of firing (frequency) of the nerve fibres. The number of sensory units is greatest at that part of the membrane with the widest range of pitch discrimination, the middle range. The same principle of discrimination related to number of sensory units has already been encountered with touch sensation and visual acuity. As in these other sensory systems depending on topographic representation, some overlap is inevitable. That is, a hair cell unit will respond to a limited range of sound. *Fringe inhibition* (Chapter 4) is used to sharpen the signal.

There are two types of unit. An inner row of hair cells has several of them innervated by a single afferent fibre: an outer row has several neurones terminating on a single hair cell of different histological structure. The latter respond to low intensity sounds and the former to high intensity (like the difference between rods and cones in the retina) and it has been suggested that the high intensity responding units may account for the phenomenon of *loudness recruitment*. This term is applied to the ability of a partially deaf ear to hear intense sounds like a normal ear when the deafness is of the sensorineural type due to degeneration of the outer hair cells with advancing age or with disease. It has recently been suggested that only the inner hair cells are afferent to the auditory pathways. The outer cells may project nerve fibres to an efferent control mechanism modifying the micromechanics of deflection of the inner hair cells.

EFFERENT CONTROL OF HEARING

There are other mechanisms for increasing apparent loudness. One is paralysis of the stapedius reflex referred to above (p. 102), another is by loss of a cholinergic efferent system to the hair cells, presumably depolarizing them, as in pre-synaptic inhibition. The source of this efferent control of the receptor is the *olivocochlear bundle* (from the superior olive via the acoustic nerve). The superior olive and the cochlear nuclei receive fibres descending from the acoustic areas of the cortex. It is another example of corticofugal control of sensory input (p. 93) and its reduction by ageing may be another cause of presbyacusis and the difficulty of discriminating speech in a noisy environment ('cocktail party deafness'). It may be the efferent pathway which is responsible for an interesting phenomenon which may be used in sound

location — stimulation of one cochlea inhibits the input from the other.

LOCALIZATION OF SOUND IN SPACE

The source of a sound is assessed by comparing the loudness appreciated by each ear and by timing of the signals. Assuming normal hearing mechanisms and central pathways, a sound heard equally loud in both ears lies on the midsagittal meridian, provided that latencies are the same. Comparison of loudness and (more importantly) phase of sound waves is made at the *medial (accessory) superior olive* which receives afferent fibres from the *cochlear nuclei* on both sides of the brain stem, mainly for sounds of low frequency. Even at this level there may be diversity of function for different aspects of sound signals, with parallel processing similar to that identified for vision. The *inferior colliculus* and primary acoustic cortex are also important. They are linked to the motor system by unidentified paths to produce reflex movements designed to turn the head and eyes to look towards the sound source, ie to equalize the stimulus entering each ear. Some animals have an extremely sensitive location system, even for self-produced sounds reflected from the environment (sonar).

The auditory pathway

The hair cells of the organ of Corti are in synaptic connection with bipolar ganglion cells sending axons into the VIIIth nerve to the upper medulla oblongata. Each ganglion cell is related to a small number of hair cells (so the receptive fields of the afferent neurones overlap slightly). One branch is relayed in the anterior part of the nucleus and trapezoid body to the *superior olives* on both sides. The other branch continues posteriorly to the *dorsal cochlear nucleus* which relays to the contralateral *inferior colliculus*. From the superior olive of each side an ascending auditory pathway passes in the *lateral lemniscus* to the inferior colliculus of the mid-brain. (A study of *Fig.* 11.2 will show that the colliculus receives both second and third order afferent neurones.) It relays further to the medial geniculate body of the thalamus and thence to the auditory cortex. As it ascends, collateral

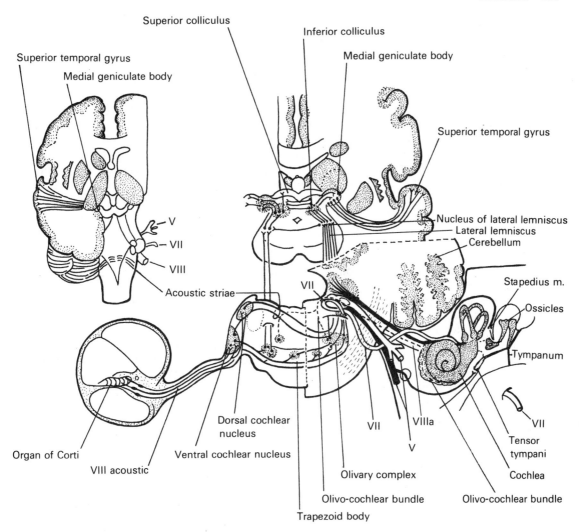

Fig. 11.2. *Hearing.* The organ of Corti lies on the basilar membrane of the cochlea and is stimulated by movement of the membrane transmitted in the scala vestibuli from the chain of ossicles linked to the tympanic membrane of the ear. The afferent fibres pass in the acoustic division of VIII close to the V, VI and VII nerves in the cerebellopontine angle. The V and VII nerves supply motor fibres to tensor tympani and stapedius muscles and inhibitory efferent VIII fibres pass to the organ of Corti from the superior olivary nuclei of both sides. These (and the nuclei of the trapezoid body) receive bilateral acoustic fibres, which join the mainly crossed fibres relaying in the dorsal cochlear nucleus to form the lateral lemniscus which ascends to the inferior colliculus. Further relay through the medial geniculate body passes to the superior temporal gyrus. Commissural connections occur at several levels and collateral fibres pass to the reticular formation (for arousal) and to the superior colliculus and cerebellum.

fibres are projected to the ascending reticular formation, cerebellar vermis and superior colliculus for functions involving arousal and orientation of head, eyes and body axis. The synaptic potentials generated at each of these relays and at the cortex give recognizable 'far field' responses which can be recorded by scalp electrodes as the 'brain stem auditory evoked responses'. Prolongation of their latencies there are of some localizing value in clinical disorders of the auditory pathways (p. 151).

The full connections are not described here but sufficient detail has been given to make it clear that signals detected in one ear are projected bilaterally but mainly contralaterally and that a synchronous volley entering the cochlear nerve from a transducer system capable of producing perfect microphony is nevertheless dispersed in time when it reaches the mid-brain and medial geniculate levels.

The medial geniculate body relays the ascending acoustic signals to the cortex of the temporal lobe in the most posterior part of the internal capsule. As with other sensory systems described in earlier chapters, there are at least two cortical acoustic or auditory areas.

The first acoustic area (AI) is on the first temporal gyrus (areas 41, 42) buried in the Sylvian fissure and the *second acoustic area* (AII) is in the frontal and parietal operculum. In these areas cells 'represent' receptive fields of primary cochlear nerve fibres from restricted areas of the cochlear basilar membrane and therefore 'represent' pitch of sound. (In fact, this tonotopical localization is not established beyond dispute in man.)

The problem of maintaining 'local sign' in a multi-synaptic afferent system has already been discussed. The principle of signal sharpening by surround inhibition applies to the acoustic system and it also has a *corticofugal control* of afferent impulses from acoustic cortex to superior olives and cochlear nuclei as well as the olivocochlear modulation of hair–ganglion cell input (p. 104) and reflex control of the peripheral impedance-matching device (p. 102). The latter protective reflexes (to tensor tympani and stapedius muscles) have relays in the inferior colliculi and efferent connections bilaterally to V and VII motor nerves respectively. Less well known but functionally important reflexes via the central grey matter and tectospinal pathways modify muscle tone of neck, trunk and limbs as part of a general alerting and orienting reaction to sudden noise.

Cortical analysis of sound

There is increasing evidence that (like somatic sensation and vision) some form of frequency discrimination is possible at medial geniculate level but the cortex is necessary for finer analysis including the acoustic equivalent of direction of movement of a stimulus over the receptive surface — in this case a *change in frequency* (rising or falling tone), and *temporal patterns of sound* — an essential substratum for receiving speech.

Intensity of sound (number of hair cells stimulated) is probably interpreted at quite a low level, even below the inferior colliculus. Some of the phase analysis necessary for localization of sound in space is believed to occur in the superior olives, but lesions at higher levels right up to the cortex do impair the capacity to localize the source of sound, especially in the vertical plane. Some cortical neurones respond to intensity differences between the two ears, others to phase differences. A few units have also been detected (in the cat) which are best excited by movement of the sound source in a specific direction in a certain sector of the auditory field. Analogies with the visual cortex are obvious and it is likely that a similar columnar organization of specialized cells exists in the auditory cortex. One similarity not yet clarified concerns the possibility of a highly discriminative area of each acoustic receptive field for each ear. Chapter 19 will describe how a 'foveation' reflex moves the eyes to bring a moving object detected peripherally into the foveal field for detailed analysis. The shape of the pinna and its reflex movement in respond to sound, coupled with appropriate head turning, suggest similar *orientation reflexes* to bring sound stimuli into the ears from a favoured direction — an 'acoustic fovea'. The reflex involves the *inferior colliculus*.

Motor commands are likely to arise in the acoustic as well as in the visual and somatosensory cortices. Some of these may involve the larynx and other bulbar motor mechanisms. In the bat these command neurones control bursts of high frequency sound for echo-location: the same connections are probably utilized in emotional responses and, in man, in *speech*. In the sonar function it is essential to have highly refined detection of the temporal pattern of sound, including identification of temporal order, and this capacity is fundamental to the development of speech reception, provided that the perceived pattern can be compared with engrams stored in a memory with other associates which give it symbolic value (Chapter 12).

The complex acoustic patterns of speech have no symbolic value unless the cortex is aroused by the reticular formation. In addition, observation shows that speech, even of threshold intensity, is by far the best arousal stimulus. The sleeper awakened by a whisper and the mother by her own baby's cry are part of received knowledge and give credence to the popular belief in the superior efficacy of a familiar voice in arousing a comatose patient. There is impressive evidence that the auditory system has evolved for the purpose of detecting and identifying those sounds that are significant for the adaptive behaviour of the species, including the rising and falling pitches (frequencies) for which the acoustic cortex is specially equipped. *Significance* is not a 'wired in' feature, eg the mating call of a male animal is only significant to the female when her brain is appropriately modulated by hormones, the general environmental situation and her previous experience of the particular male. Perception, or perhaps attention, of acoustic and visual signals also depends on psychological 'set' and on *expectation* based on previous experiences (stored in a memory). *Interpretation* of speech-mode acoustic patterns varies with the acoustic context that precedes and follows it. The brain hears what it expects to hear (cf. the importance of the title for a piece of programme music). Conversely, out-of-context or unfamiliar sounds have the characteristics of alarm signals — a psychoacoustic principle the anaesthetist should remember in the recovery room. (If space permitted, a discussion on the heard reassurance of familiar speech inflection and dialect and the authoritative implications of 'class' speech patterns would be highly relevant to management of the patient during induction and recovery from general anaesthesia.)

ASSOCIATION AREA FOR SOUND

The concept of significance of sound patterns implies that there is recognition by a central pattern detector. As well as recognizing innate or acquired templates, it could be used to modify self-generated vocal patterns by feedback control (monitoring either the sound or a corollary discharge, p. 242). Acquisition of vocal speech is notoriously impaired in the congenitally deaf. Conversely, it has been suggested that acoustic speech cues, ambiguous out of context, could be decoded by reference to articulatory motor command patterns, unlike perception of non-speech sounds. Experiments with dichotic listening indicate that, for right-handed persons, the sounds entering the right ear (delivered mainly to the left hemisphere) are better perceived for *speech sounds* either meaningful or nonsensical, and sounds entering the left ear for persons known to have language dominance in the right hemisphere. *Non-speech sounds*, including music, are heard better by the other hemisphere. Both hemispheres have the capacity to extract and analyse the acoustic patterns of speech sounds, but linguistic interpretation of them is only possible in the language-dominant hemisphere. This appears to be related to an inborn asymmetry of the temporal speech region: the *planum temporale* is larger on the left in 65 per cent of human brains, and on the right in only 11 per cent. The planum temporale, which contains the *auditory association cortex*, extends on to the lateral surface of the posterior portion of the first temporal gyrus (area 22) behind the *primary auditory cortex* in the transverse gyrus of Heschl (*Fig. 11.3*). Lesions in this area of the left hemisphere cause Wernicke's aphasia (fluent, incomprehensible speech).

Connections from and to other sensory modalities (vision and somaesthesis) are believed to reach Wernicke's area via the angular gyrus for the intermodality correlations necessary for speech, and for arousal of tactile and visual associations by auditory stimuli, especially speech. Damage to these connections causes severe disturbances of speech and behaviour. The *connections are interhemispheric* via the corpus callosum as well as transcortical. The very complexity of the acoustic and visual stimuli and the motor aspects of vocal, written and gestural speech have made it possible to trace connections uniquely in man. The subject is further discussed in Chapter 12.

Electrical stimulation of the primary acoustic cortex in man (during operations under local anaesthesia) does not produce sensations of recognizable pure tones. Stimulation of Wernicke's area may produce either vocalization or speech arrest. Some patients have stated that they 'heard' snatches of melody or of recognizable speech (reproducible on repeated stimulation) but such experiences cannot be dissociated from a memory function (*déjà vu*) which also utilizes the temporal lobes (Chapter 13).

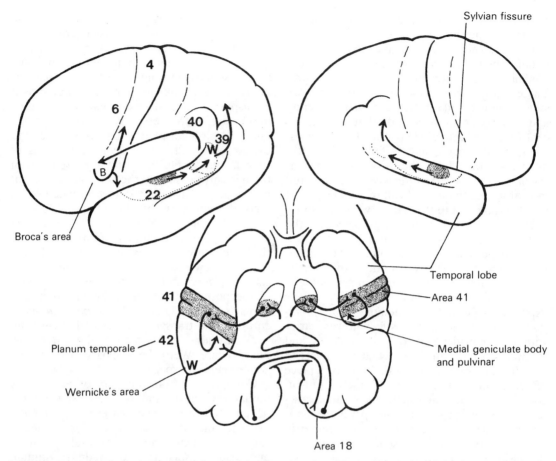

Fig. 11.3. *Hearing and speech*. The lower diagram is horizontal section of brain through the Sylvian fissures showing the temporal lobes from above. Fibres from the auditory nuclei ascending from the mid-brain terminate in the medial geniculate body and pulvinar. They relay across the internal capsule to the primary auditory cortex (Heschl's gyrus, 41) where aspects of sound are analysed in parallel. These aspects (e.g. pitch, timbre, loudness, change of pitch) are integrated in area 42, the planum temporale and in the surrounding area 22 which projects to the parietal lobe and insula. The planum temporale projects to the junction between the superior temporal gyrus (22) and the angular gyrus (39) at Wernicke's area (W). On the right there is untutored appreciation of music. On the left, Wernicke's area projects through the arcuate bundle to Broca's area (B) at the inferior end of the premotor area (6) which activates the movement synergies for speech (area 4). Note the asymmetry of the planum temporale, larger on the left in most humans, with left hemisphere 'dominance' for speech. The diagram also shows callosal connections of visual association areas (18) with each other and to the contralateral Wernicke's area.

Further reading

Celesia G.G. Organization of auditory cortical areas in man. *Brain* 1976; **99**: 403–14.
Rudge P. *Clinical Neuro-otology*. Edinburgh: Churchill Livingstone, 1983.

PART 3   Higher Nervous Functions

Chapter 12
Integrative functions of the cerebral cortex

In earlier chapters we have followed the input of sensory information into the cerebral cortex after relay in the thalamus (including its medial and lateral geniculate bodies) with retention of signs of modality and of locus of origin. Already in the primary afferent areas of cortex there has been evidence of synthesis of information derived from the spatial or temporal orientation of signals in overlapping or adjacent receptor fields, increasing the discriminatory capacity of the cortex with respect to intensity and significance of afferent signals. 'Significance' is here used in terms of a value judgement for the present and future welfare of the subject. This implies (i) integration of the whole contemporary sensory input, (ii) comparison with a stored template of previously experienced stimuli of a like kind, (iii) a decision on familiarity/novelty of the contemporary situation and (iv) emotional response of satisfaction or alarm. An appropriate motor response may then be made.

Present knowledge of the physiological basis of these functions is necessarily incomplete and based largely on interpretation of functional deficits seen in human subjects with discrete lesions of brain areas. It is usual to warn that a confident attribution of *normal* function cannot be made on the evidence of deficit when a part of the nervous system is damaged. Nevertheless, this proper reservation must not be allowed to conceal that the method has proved highly reliable in most circumstances if recognition is given to loss of inhibitory as well as of facilitatory control. Lesion studies indicate that spatiotemporal analysis of afferent area activity and also cross-modality linkage occur in specialized areas of cortex adjacent to the afferent areas and described as *association areas*. These are reciprocally connected to memory stores where a 'body image and diary' are constantly updated. The special, but not exclusive, role of the temporal lobes will be described. The memorized template is continuously matched against the contemporary input. Good matching ('familiarity') is apparently acknowledged by a limbic lobe response (p. 118) activating the parasympathetic autonomic system, appropriate hormonal and somatic motor response and diminishing the activity of the brain stem arousal system. Mismatching ('novelty'), on the other hand, evokes a limbic lobe response preparing for 'fight or flight' by activating the sympathetic autonomic system, appropriate hormonal and somatic motor response (gamma-motor) and maximal alerting by the arousal system.

Note that we are now entering an aspect of neurophysiology where *interaction* between a number of cortical and subcortical areas is of the essence and the following account of some aspects of individual areas must be read in this context. It should also be noted that a new and important element has just been introduced. Whereas a reflex is, by definition, an invariant response to a standardized input (modified only quantitatively by facilitatory and inhibitory controls), the new factor is the *choice* between alternative responses, a conservative choice which is determined by memory of previous experience but nevertheless a choice linked to efferent responses which, in turn, can be perceived (either peripherally or by corollary discharge, p. 242) as a 'feeling' of satisfaction, or of unrest requiring exploratory or interventional activity until the unrest is resolved. This elementary decision-making part of the brain with *emotional correlations* (afferent and efferent) is the *hippocampus*, developed during evolution in relation to an association area for the first of the distance receptors, olfactory/gustatory, and still the most evocative for feelings of familiarity and mood, being linked to the most primitive self- and species-protective drives, the appetites for water, food and sex (Chapter 14).

Association areas

In following the transmission of signals from peripheral receptors to primary sensory areas of cortex in previous chapters, we have seen modality-specific and topographic representation at thalamic and cortical levels but with additional development in the cortex of cells receiving convergent inputs from these neuronal channels so that they respond to spatiotemporal *orientation* of signals in the peripheral receptor field (retina or basilar membrane of the cochlea). For somatosensory signals to the post-central gyrus we have also hinted at integration of both spatial and modality information in the association cortex of the superior parietal lobule for matching with a stored 'body image' (p. 112). The same principle may be applied to the sensory data for vestibular sense, taste and smell.

A critical evolutionary development was the growth of neuronal circuits for convergence not only of same-type signals from different parts of the receptive field, but of modality-different signals, not just touch + nociceptive, but somatosensory + visual, visual + hearing, olfaction + hearing + vision etc., and linkage of these with a choice–decision mechanism based on judgement of *value* for the survival of the organism and species. *The association areas have been developed for this cross-modality linkage.* In addition, they have developed cross-hemisphere linkages which coordinate the responses of the two otherwise independent cerebral hemispheres.

The modality- and topological-specific projections from thalamus to primary sensory areas are entirely ipsilateral. Each thalamus is independent and few if any fibres cross in the massa intermedia (which is commonly absent in man). The primary sensory areas of one hemisphere do not communicate directly with their homologues of the other hemisphere via the corpus callosum (p. 53). There is, however, a massive interhemisphere linkage through the corpus callosum from the associa-

tion areas into which the primary sensory areas project (*see Figs* 11.3 and 19.4). *Callosal connections* from primary areas of sub-primate mammals are probably from 'association neurones' located within the primary areas. In the primates these cells are in overlapping perisensory areas and in man the separation is substantially complete. This evolutionary shift is associated with development of an additional thalamocortical projection from the posterior part of the thalamus (pulvinar) with identifiable fibre bundles to each of the association areas.

The obvious development of association cortices in the primate has diverted attention from the intricate synaptic connections in the thalamus. Some cross-modality linkage is probable at this level and the integrated message is then relayed via the pulvinar to the association areas (especially visual) and hippocampus. The *pulvinar* is linked especially with the medial and lateral geniculate bodies and perhaps the ventral posterior nucleus of the thalamus. It does not receive long ascending sensory fibres directly though some visual impulses may be received from the superior colliculus. The pulvinar also receives corticofugal fibres from the visual association area (areas 18 and 19), indicating *reciprocal thalamocortical and corticothalamic activity*, a possible mechanism for cross-modality linkage (*see Fig.* 19.4).

Cross-modality linkage also occurs reciprocally between association areas in one hemisphere. Some transcortical connections are by *subcortical bundles* of fibres. Short association fibres connect adjacent convolutions and long association fibres interconnect cortical regions in different lobes. Important transcortical bundles running longitudinally connect the association areas with the anterior (motor) part of the hemisphere. An important example is the arcuate fasciculus (*see Fig.* 11.3). A third level for cross-modality linkage is by *intracortical connections*. It is at this level (with the plasticity offered by multisynaptic connections) that man is more developed than other primates. Thus 'disconnection syndromes' due to breaking cross-modality linkages are most often related to cortical lesions but it should be noted that (*a*) disconnection syndromes, including speech disorders, may occur with subcortical or thalamic lesions, and (*b*) alternative linkage pathways exist and may permit very substantial recovery of function after an acute lesion, or minimizing of dysfunction with a slowly developing lesion. Even *transcallosal pathways* may be used (*see Fig.* 11.3), with some loss of speed and versatility. These alternatives apply only to association area functions. The thalamocortical projections to primary sensory areas do not have this built-in redundancy and functional plasticity. They can only communicate with the homologous areas of the other hemisphere through their own association area.

Higher cortical functions

Earlier chapters have described neuronal mechanisms for integration of convergent sensory signals to cells that respond to stimuli orientated in space and time, undoubtedly for vision, hearing and probably for skin contact and in principle for all sensory modalities. It has now been shown that an anatomical equipment exists for similar integration of signals of different modalities. That is to say, a cell, or group of cells, will fire in response to alternative or synchronous convergent inputs. It may have a unique output or, by divergence, a number of possible output pathways depending on facilitation/inhibition by the input signal and by the whole central excitatory state.

CONDITIONAL RESPONSES

By frequently repeating the two convergent signals either synchronously or within a limited time span the response appropriate to the first can be transferred to the second signal. This is the '*conditional reflex*' studied by Pavlov and his school. Clearly some 'memory' of the response to the first stimulus must be present, and repeated utilization of the convergent pathway facilitates one behavioural response. It is usually the response natural to the first of the paired stimuli, but not necessarily so. The dominant response is usually one involving an imprinted appetite response (hunger, thirst, aggression, flight, acceptance of another subject etc.). The *conditional responses* (they do not have the stereotypy of true reflexes) require regular reinforcement by reward and vary with states of alertness, alternative attractions or threats and many other factors. A full

account is unnecessary but enough has been presented to indicate some important features — (i) convergence of afferent signals, (ii) divergence of motor responses, (iii) modification of 'preferred' response by linkage with limbic system behaviour, (iv) memory, (v) motivation or reinforcement by the limbic connection, (vi) modification by state of arousal and total environmental pattern. Although conditional responses are given a lower place than Pavlov might have wished, they do indicate important properties of the higher nervous system including elementary forms of memory and of learning based on cross-modality linkage. A not inconsiderable part of human behaviour is at this level and the higher functions now to be described differ in complexity and precision rather than in principle.

SYMBOLS

Consider the famous experiments of Pavlov. A bell is sounded every time a hungry but domesticated dog is given food in a familiar environment. After a number of repetitions, the sound of the bell evokes the somatomotor and autonomic behavioural pattern normally evoked by the sight or smell of food. (Note that smell itself was originally 'conditioned'. A chain of conditional responses can be built up.) It could be said that the bell sound has become a 'symbol' for food: they have become equipotent stimuli with the same significance. In the same way a pattern of lines on paper or of varying pitch sounds, or palpable surface discontinuities can become a 'symbol' of another sensory input. The written or spoken 'CAT' is immediately related to a small furry animal if the appropriate *symbol code* has been learned by repetition of the paired stimuli (in the first instance). Studies on acquisition of human speech and its dissolution by disease indicate the necessity for cross-modality linkage in the association areas (or parts of them) and the reinforcing effect of the limbic system.

Somatosensory perception and discrimination

The somatosensory areas of the cortex discussed hitherto are related topographically and in modality to discrete receptor fields at the periphery, a rather fixed type of organization.

But reaction-time studies and the better sensory discrimination achieved with 'active touch' (p. 94), including, apparently, discounting of the component of movement of receptors with respect to object palpated, both indicate that perception occurs after a further process of sensory analysis in which the 'perceived' stimulus pattern is integrated with information about body posture and movement, and also visual and acoustic information. The further processing is believed to require relay from the somatosensory receiving areas to areas 5 and 7 of the parietal cortex (*superior parietal lobule*) which is an area of convergence for somatic sensory, visual and acoustic signals, formerly described as an *association area*. Stimulation studies suggest that the input is bilateral and not topical, indicating major connections through commissural systems such as the *corpus callosum*.

Convergence of axons on to a common neurone or neuronal system is a fundamental feature of the structure of a polysynaptic nervous system. Indeed, if signal intensity could be preserved, there would be no need for an arrangement more complicated than a nerve net unless there were operational requirements for convergence and divergence contingent on activity at other inputs or outputs of the system. A second or third order neurone may indeed fail to pass on the signal unless facilitated by other neurones. It is in fact a coincidence detector (p. 45). (The concept of 'gate control', p. 45, is essentially the same.) If some response to a previous afferent input ('memory') can be stored, scanned and matched with novel afferent signals, the convergent neurones become a recognition system. The temporal and frontal lobes have this capacity particularly well developed but there is little doubt that 'memory', 'recognition' and 'coincidence detection' are general attributes of all grey matter. So far as the parietal lobe is concerned, the stored information appears to be concerned mainly with somatosensory information which is continuously updated (with a time lag) as a '*body image*'. The right parietal lobe is particularly implicated in this, as indicated by functional disturbance associated with disease of this part of the brain.

At this point is it unnecessary to review possible mechanisms for memory storage. The psychological term '*engram*' will serve for discussing the stored memory. If coincidence detectors recognize that current afferent input (from the periphery and from the emotional system) is 'familiar' they can activate a previous motor response ('*conditional reflex*'), as described so well by Pavlov and his followers. This is clearly an economical system if linked with an alternative output so that a novel stimulus pattern is directed to the alerting system (Chapter 15) and to the motor system for active exploration of extracorporeal space.

Failure to recognize similarity of old and new patterns of afferent signals is described by the neurologist as *agnosia* and the resulting failure to activate appropriate motor programmes is *apraxia*. The failure of pattern recognition is the essence of agnosia. Primary stimuli (touch, pain, movement etc.) are detected and localized, but they are not integrated conceptually. Similarly, the fragments of movement are not lost (there is no paralysis) but they are not assembled and used appropriately in apraxia. These disturbances may be quite localized — eg apraxia for the movements of dressing only, or agnosia for one part of the body such as the fingers (in Gerstmann's syndrome from a lesion of the angular gyrus).

It is helpful to consider receptive neuronal firing patterns as symbols for the object in the external world, and the motor neuronal firing patterns similarly as symbols for particular complex movements. Thus the parietal neurones can store and compare sound, visual and touch 'symbols' linked by conditioning and training to patterns of peripheral stimulation — the receptive aspects of speech (auditory, written and Braille). In the same way the motor responses of the respiratory system, vocal cords, lips, tongue and fingers used in vocal and written speech are pre-programmed in certain areas of cortex linked with these symbols for receptive speech (Chapters 10 and 11). These specialized groups for recognition and reproduction of speech are mainly in the left hemisphere. *Receptive and expressive aphasia* are special forms of agnosia and apraxia.

The economy provided by a convergent system with storage and recognition of symbols for recurrent sensory patterns useful for personal survival and interpersonal communication (survival of family and tribe) has some limitations. It would be useless and cumbersome if only able to recognize an exact replication of the stored symbol. Storage of essential features only, with coincidence detectors able to recognize similarity rather than identity, would be adequate and more economical. This may well have been the most important development in the evolution of the brain, especially if the coincidence detection system is not too rigidly coupled, since it allows storage of vast amounts of symbolic representation of abstractions, and of 'association of ideas', the essential components for logical thought. It cannot be accidental that thought and speech have evolved together and are so intimately linked. Eccles and others have doubted whether thinking is possible in the absence of speech.

The contribution of the *medial temporal lobe* to speech functions is sufficiently great as to indicate that many of the transcortical connections between sensory association areas must be relayed through the hippocampus and it is possible that at this level long term memory stores are implicated. In lower animals there is indeed evidence that the major part of cross-modality linkage is via the gustatory and olfactory (rhinencephalic) association area — ie convergence of visual–olfactory/gustatory and auditory–olfactory/gustatory connections link vision with hearing. Stable non-limbic sensory modality linkages only occur in man, using the transcortical and intracortical connections described above. Geschwind believed that the development of propositional speech (as distinct from emotional ejaculations) depends on this, but the limbic linkage is apparent in oratory and the entertainment industry. Constant effort is required to remove it from juristic and scientific communication, the most precise form of speech involving brain circuits developed late in evolution and in ontogeny.

Before we examine this, it is necessary to point out that the concepts just developed have an application wider than for speech. It has been suggested that the corticolimbic connections are less important for man than for the monkey because of the development of a connection between association areas through the *inferior parietal lobule*, particularly of the left hemisphere. A lesion of the *left supramarginal gyrus* may cause asymbolia for pain. The subject can feel pain and correctly identify pain stimuli at normal threshold but it does not evoke an emotional response, suggesting that a link between the upper parietal lobule and the limbic system has been cut.

Multimodal linkage

THE INFERIOR PARIETAL LOBULE (angular and supramarginal gyri; approximately areas 39 and 40)

This is an extremely important structure, appearing in the human for the first time in the evolutionary series. Not only is it phylogenetically new, its fibre connections myelinate late and it forms dendrites late (adolescence). It is clearly different from the primary sensory and the association areas in having few thalamic afferent fibres. It is not essentially concentric with the primary projection areas but is at the junction of the somatosensory, visual and auditory association areas to all of which it is reciprocally connected. It is an 'association area of association areas', allowing powerful intermodality association, a body image incorporating visual and auditory data. It has been said that the inferior parietal lobule frees man to some extent from the limbic system except for learning.

FRONTAL LOBE IN HIGHER CEREBRAL FUNCTIONS

The posterior (pre-motor) part of the frontal lobe is part of the thalamocortical development of association cortices which is responsible for some aspects of motor programming, and these will be discussed in Chapter 24. The orbital surface is part of the limbic system. This chapter will consider the unique contributions of the frontal pole. Like the inferior parietal lobule, the most anterior part is phylogenetically new, late to mature in young people and not connected directly with the thalamus. It does not project directly to the brain stem. A large bundle of fibres (*superior longitudinal fasciculus*) connects it with the parietal and occipital lobe, and the *cingulum* connects it with the medial temporal limbic structures. The frontal lobe does not receive primary sensory data directly. It processes signals generated in association areas, and some would claim that it can inject signals into the limbic circuits to modify the contemporary *v*. template matching (Chapter 13).

The ability to sort and assess environmental cues by deriving transmodality symbols or *models* enormously increases the computing power of the brain. Furthermore, so long as there are memory stores it becomes possible to manipulate the models when the subject has moved away from the environmental input. It is this consideration that has made many writers comment that the development of thinking is inseparable from that of speech. (Of course in this formulation 'speech' implies symbolic transforms from the most primitive to the most sophisticated.)

It is not surprising, then, that the parietal lobes (particularly the left) play such a major role in higher nervous functions, provided that they are linked with certain receptive and motor areas of cortex on both sides of the brain and with those areas specialized for *memory and coincidence detection* (temporal lobes) and for the taking of decisions based on reviewing the options derived from remembered previous experience (frontal lobes) (Chapter 13).

The afferent and efferent engrams for speech and logical thought require more than association by convergence. It is necessary to preserve *serial order* in a time dimension that is polarized. Whatever may be the basis of that aspect of memory in which the temporal lobes are involved, if an epileptic discharge or an electrical stimulus evokes a hallucination of a tune or words, it is always in the correct serial order. It is not different in principle from the neuronal organization required to detect the direction of a visual or moving cutaneous stimulus, a property of some thalamic VPL neurones as well as in the cortex. (Indeed the necessity to move a noxious stimulus at a particular velocity and in a special direction over the plantar skin to elicit the plantar reflex suggests that a similar mechanism is present in the dorsal horn grey matter.) A possible mechanism could be that synapses sequentially excited by a moving stimulus could be spatially arranged on one dendrite so that each has a different potency, requiring them to be activated in the correct order to provide sufficient temporal and spatial summation to depolarize the spike trigger zone of the cell (*see Fig.* 4.2). Some direction-sensitive neurones in area 5 of the parietal lobe are excited by joint movements, particularly when the movement is initiated by the animal (they have been found in the monkey) rather than by passive manipulation, a property which is probably used in 'active touch' (p. 94).

Some cells in areas 5 and 7 are thought by Mountcastle (1978) to be part of an apparatus for initiating and driving to completion a behavioural act under a specific motivational drive. According to this concept they are *'command neurones'* directing attention to a selected object within the immediate extrapersonal space within reach of the hand, driving the contralateral hand and both eyes to examine the object visually and by manipulation. The pattern of activity of these cells is independent of the *particular sensory cues* and the motor response is not stereotyped; the average patterns of their activity are not influenced by the specific spatial trajectory of the arm. The movement commanded is goal directed rather than reflex, a property of cortically controlled movement always emphasized by Sherrington. This will be discussed further in Chapter 24, but before doing so it is necessary to examine the contributions of temporal and frontal areas of the cerebral cortex and the sources of the motivational drives necessary to activate the command neurones.

Goal-directed movements beyond the immediate extrapersonal space require input from the 'distance receptors', the so-called special senses. An animal which uses its hand as the principal examining organ to bring an object close to its eyes and peer at it has taken a major evolutionary step. It has an arboreal existence with limbs which are to some extent prehensile, unlike the lower animals which examine with the snout, sniffing and nuzzling with their whiskers. The highest functions of its brain are no longer associated with olfaction and trigeminotactile areas. A neopallium is becoming dominant over the paleopallium. When the parietal lobe is damaged in man, the defects are gnosic, ie disorders of corporeal awareness, of visuo-spatial conceptions and of interdimensional manipulations. The part played by the hand as a tool connecting the personal space of the body with extrapersonal space has been suggested to account for the *finger agnosia* and *agraphia* which are such prominent features of a lesion of the left angular gyrus (with right–left disorientation and dyscalculia: Gerstmann's syndrome).

HEMISPHERE DOMINANCE

The striking relationship of aphasia, finger agnosia and hand preference with the left parietal lobe has led to the concept that the human brain has a 'dominant' left hemisphere. There is considerable truth in this (even with many left-handed people, speech functions are largely controlled by the left hemisphere) but it is less well known that other functions are better 'represented' in the right hemisphere, eg unsophisticated aspects of music, manipulation of mathematical symbols and recognition of faces (*see Figs* 10.2 and 11.3). It is common experience that 'eye dominance' does not necessarily match 'hand dominance'. There is increasing evidence that these lateralized *specializations* (rather than unique functions) correlate with differences in cortical dimensions, but it is impossible to be more specific until more is known about cortico-cortical connections and their disruption in the causation of deficiency syndromes. They may be blocked temporarily by drugs. For instance, if the left hemisphere is dominant for speech, that function is briefly abolished in the conscious subject by injecting sodium amylobarbitone into the left internal carotid artery, but not the right. Normal speech returns in about 10 minutes.

Allowing for specialization of some aspects of symbolization on one or other side, it is increasingly clear that no absolute distinction can be made between a dominant and a non-dominant hemisphere. Interhemisphere (and particularly inter-parietal) collaboration is probably essential for higher mental functions.

In the model presented up to this point we have stressed the importance of the limbic lobe in cross-modality linkage as a pathway connecting association areas and for reinforcement of linkage establishment by introducing *memory* and *emotion*, both important in *learning* of primitive type. This reinforcement is essentially immediate and highly suitable for modifying behaviour in such a way as to maximize pleasure and minimize discomfort. Some animals can apparently anticipate and avoid a potentially harmful situation. It would clearly be of evolutionary survival value if it could choose to forego immediate advantage in favour of a predictable delayed advantage. Once a conceptual system can be handled by 'speech models' it would be a major step forward if the models could be assembled in different ways to predict probable outcomes of behavioural responses in the light of previous remembered experience, especially if the immediate limbic reinforcement could be inhibited. This is preferred as a model of frontal lobe function. From the continuous model processing of the inferior parietal lobule (which appears to continue during sleep and to play a role in dreams) a derivative is transferred forwards to the frontal pole which (free from immediate thalamic input) suppresses the limbic choice based on expediency and extrapolates the data into future time, calculating probable consequences of different behavioural responses based on previous experience (testing hypotheses) *and on the possibility of actively manipulating the environment*.

To the subject, interpersonal relationships are important, his action on others, and vice versa. (There is a price to pay. Pain and hardship may continue until a chosen goal is reached. Choice of behaviour may be removed from the limbic system, but emotional response is not.) The anticipation of the future is 'intelligent' according to the ingenuity with which models are constructed. Cross-linkage of concepts ('association of ideas'; lateral thinking) is in principle the same as the linkage necessary for speech symbols. To some extent we all use both limbic-reinforced thinking (artistic, based on belief, faith, herd experience) and frontal-reinforced thinking (juristic, scientific, 'rational'). The wonderful versatility and variability of the human mind depends on these differences. But progress depends on the frontal lobes. Their function will be studied further after an account of the mechanisms of memory and learning without which the frontal lobes cannot function.

Further reading

Critchley M. *The Parietal Lobes*. London: Arnold 1953.
Mountcastle V.B. Brain mechanisms for directed attention. The Sherrington Memorial Lecture. *Proc. R. Soc. Med.* 1978; **71**: 14–28.

Chapter 13
Memory and learning

For an animal to learn from experience or to develop elaborate but non-random behavioural responses to similar or novel environments it must 'learn by experience' and this implies that it retain a 'memory' of important aspects of significant environmental signals. Much of the confusion regarding a physiological basis for memory functions lies in the many attempts to define a single mechanism. Even the simplest synaptic nervous system exhibits some properties of memory. A reflex pathway facilitated by repeated stimulation 'remembers' that it has received the appropriate afferent signals previously, presumably by growth of terminal boutons, dendrites etc., and perhaps ultimately by modifying the receptor structure and DNA of one or more neurones in a chain. A single-modality memory of this type is likely to be sited at each stage in the central processing of afferent signals (eg dorsal horn, lemniscal nuclei, thalamus, primary afferent cortex) and particularly in its analyser in the appropriate association area. There is evidence for this statement in simpler brains, such as that of octopus.

In principle, there is no difficulty in extending this concept to a hierarchy of feedback arcs, both facilitatory and inhibitory, with possibility of integration of signals from neurones coverging on to cells which only respond (*a*) to appropriate simultaneous or serial inputs ('coincidence detectors') or (*b*) to signals accompanied by suitable 'gating' messages. Thus a response laid down by embryological development can be cued by a secondary stimulus of different modality as in the *imprinting* response of the neonate to its mother or surrogate parent and in the conditional responses of Pavlovian type (Chapter 12). The elaboration of an interconnected higher nervous system increases the possibilities of linkages of this type in the association areas.

At an early evolutionary stage there is strong survival value in the development of conditioned responses for acquisition of food and a mate and for avoidance of potential danger, so it is not surprising that in lower animals cross-modality linkage most commonly involves the appetite receptor and effector areas of the brain in the limbic system and hypothalamus. Even in man the memory evocative powers of smell and taste are well known, and the importance of linkage with sexual experience and territory-establishing behaviour in all 'higher' behavioural patterns is a well-established psychiatric principle. *Rewards and punishments* are effective aids to conditioning of the laboratory animal and the young child but as the human subject matures the *satisfaction can be postponed* indefinitely and this is related to (i) the development of more and more elaborate cross-modality linkages, (ii) superior memory storage and recall, (iii) suppression of primitive survival responses, (iv) ability to use mental models (p. 114) and (v) to compute possible consequences of a modelled scenario. The roles of the frontal lobes in functions (iv) and (v) and of the 'association cortices' in cross-modality linkages have already been discussed. It is now necessary to look at the superior memory storage and recall of man and the higher primates overlaid on a limbic system by the development of a neocortex which is able to *suppress* primitive response patterns.

PRIMITIVE SURVIVAL RESPONSES

In this section we use the term 'response' rather than 'reflex' to indicate a general pattern of behavioural and autonomic reaction modulated according to a variable input, rather than the invariant response of a simple reflex. Indeed we do not know what is the effective stimulus for hunger, thirst and sexual desire, though these can be increased in the non-satisfied alert animal by a display of food, water and an appropriate mate, indicating potentiation by olfactory, gustatory and visual stimuli. Thus at an early stage of central processing the cortex of the rhinencephalic area on the medial surface of the anterior temporal lobe, and the visual association cortex of the medial and inferior surface of the posterior temporal-occipital cortex, are involved and perhaps cross-linked in the hippocampal formation.

The olfactory and gustatory cortices project to a subcortical nucleus, the *amygdala*, which is at the termination of the caudate nucleus (p. 216). Its high concentration of dopamine suggests a close relation to the neostriatum. It probably also receives signals from the viscera. The efferent projections from the amygdala pass via the stria terminalis and substantia innominata to a wide area of the hypothalamus, septal region, brain stem reticular formation and dorsomedial nucleus of thalamus where they evoke the endocrine, autonomic and somatic responses for flight and defensive reactions, with the associated emotional experiences (Chapter 14). At the same time the appetitive responses are arrested.

THE HIPPOCAMPAL FORMATION

The rhinencephalon–amygdala–hypothalamus response is activated by novel (unfamiliar) sensory experiences of all types, but is inhibited by environmental stimuli recognized as familiar (and hence stored in some component of memory). This appears to depend on a transcortical linkage of rhinencephalon to hypothalamus via the hippocampal formation which may be regarded as an association cortex linking olfactory–gustatory influences with the association areas for all other afferent inputs to the cerebral cortex. O'Keefe and Nadel (1978) have described the hippocampus as a 'cognitive map' storing *models*, but not details, of experienced extrapersonal space, the model being 'verbal' in the left hippocampus. It also

receives information from the cingulate gyrus, superior temporal gyrus, insula and septal region, linking environmental information with the system controlling the emotional state, *the limbic lobe*. Hippocampal activation promotes behavioural responses to remote associations of primary afferent stimuli by actively inhibiting the prepotent defensive reactions of the amygdala circuit. This allows flexibility of reactions to changing circumstances.

The corticofugal connections from hippocampus to hypothalamus, thalamus and reticular formation are complex (*see Fig. 14.1*). An *alvear pathway* crosses to the contralateral hippocampus and it appears that either hippocampus alone or together can activate central structures by the main outflow through the fornix. A secondary olfactory cortical area, the prepyriform cortex, sends fibres by a '*perforant*' pathway into the hippocampal formation, relaying from its pyramidal cell layer to the fornix, a large bundle arching upwards, forwards under the corpus callosum and then downwards to the *mammillary body* posterior to the hypophysis (with some fibres diverging to the amygdaloid nucleus and tegmentum of the midbrain). The mammillary fibres again relay to the *anterior nuclear group of the thalamus* and to the central grey matter of the *tegmentum*, which in turn projects forwards to the *septal region*. Thus the hippocampal outflow brings a limbic-influenced cortical control to important centres for endocrine and autonomic (hypothalamus) and somatic behavioural responses (thalamus) and to the alerting mechanisms (tegmental grey matter and septal region). The integrative function of these connections must be important.

MEMORY

We still have no satisfactory model for the special features of human memory as distinct from conditioned learning. It is certain that some aspects of memory are disturbed by lesions of the hippocampus, mammillary bodies, dorsomedial thalamus and amygdala. Resulting amnesia is practically never complete and shows a marked tendency to recover. Single modality *recognition* (eg vision, hearing, tactile patterns) is rarely lost. It is mainly the cross-modality linked 'models' to which access cannot be gained unless an adequate clue is provided (eg the initial letters). A clue may give access to stored models of extrapersonal space (the subject is disorientated in space and time) and in particular those models stored as language symbols. Much of the confusion regarding research on memory is caused by the necessity to instruct or test the amnesic person by means of speech. Clinical evidence suggests that the *dorsomedial nucleus* of the left *thalamus* is involved in recording of verbal memory, and that on the right with spatial memory.

With most lesions the problem is one of *recall*, ie the amnesia is *retrograde*, especially for memory of recent events and less so for long-established memories. Lesions of the mammillary bodies and medial thalamus tend to cause islands of retrograde amnesia which can subsequently be recalled. The 'permanent' memory stores, be they hippocampal, in other association cortices or at lower levels, are not eliminated by brief arrest of cortical function, electroshock or by general anaesthesia. This supports the concept of a structural basis in synaptic connections or DNA templates in a distributed system (p. 47).

An acute injury to the head (the physical basis of concussion is still unknown) commonly causes *anterograde* amnesia. For a period of time no experiences are recorded. This period of amnesia is permanent, suggesting interference with a *storage* function, in contradistinction to the recall function impairment of retrograde amnesia. Neuropsychological studies suggest that there is a *short term memory* before memoranda are 'consolidated' into the permanent storage and that, unlike the latter, it is extremely vulnerable to brief interruption of neuronal activity. The ability of certain drugs such as benzodiazepines and scopolamine to block this storage system is used in premedication before surgical operations. An obvious mechanism would be a reverberating circuit in which some derivative of the original signals (from sensory receptors plus contributions from the permanent stores) would circulate within a closed chain of neurones which would thereby acquire the facilitation necessary for permanent storage. A similar facilitatory-imprinting mechanism of neurones repeatedly stimulated by epileptic discharges is known as *kindling*.

As there must be some limit to the storage capacity, priority would be given to those patterns given the imprimatur by the limbic system as 'satisfying' or 'dangerous'. Clinical experience points to the *hippocampus* as an *area for consolidation of memory*. The substantial preservation of memory storage and recall after unilateral ablation of a hippocampal formation indicates that there is access to the entire store from either side. This could be due to the commissural nature of the fornix, or to convergence at mammillothalamic level. We postulate that one reverberating circuit could be hippocampus–mammillary body–anterior nucleus of thalamus–cingulate gyrus–hippocampus, coupled with inhibition of the rhinencephalon–amygdala–hypothalamus response. It would be inconsistent with the cortical functions previously described to suppose that this would be the sole memory reinforcing circuit. Obviously the signals returning through the thalamus could be routed through appropriate primary afferent association cortices and a major integration could occur by corticothalamic and transcortical connections as already described, reinforcing 'local' memory stores. Indeed the circulating signals could be deposited in the hypothalamic and upper brain stem grey matter as proposed by Penfield and others. Stores of intrapersonal or skin-contact data may indeed be stored in a more primitive area than those of extrapersonal data and of the linguistic models which are the building bricks of conceptual thought. These stores are more likely to be cortical and to involve the hippocampus and frontal lobes. As judged by the effects of brain damage, the right temporal lobe is associated with establishment of new visuo-spatial material into long term memory, whereas the left frontotemporal region is involved in the retrieval from long term memory of old verbally encoded material. Observation indicates that memory for events is consolidated as a verbal model. It is aided by a diary or by regular rehearsing. The fixity and gradual conviction of 'an oft told tale' is legendary; it is remembered in preference to a trace of the true environmental signals.

An experiential record is only useful to an animal if it can be compared with contemporary experience for the latter to be judged as familiar or novel. Neurones connected as coincidence detectors are common, even in quite simple nervous systems, gating novel signals to the 'fight–flight–alertness' behavioural pattern and familiar ones to the 'rest–recuperation–sleep' pattern with appropriate autonomic–hormonal responses and affect (Chapter 14).

With electrical stimulation or a focal epileptic discharge there may be amnesia for a previously experienced environmental pattern which is interpreted as novel ('*jamais vu*') or a truly new one may trigger the coincidence detector and be experienced as familiar ('*déjà vu*'). These judgements are commonly associated with hallucinatory experiences (possibly memory recall) from the uncal and posterior temporal association cortices, an appropriate motor pantomime, and affective experiences (pleasure, religious experience, terror, demonic possession etc.). There is simultaneous disturbance of the *content of consciousness* but no loss of consciousness unless a generalized epileptic seizure follows. (It should be noted that the hippocampus, amygdala, thalamus and tegmental grey matter are implicated in many theories of 'idiopathic' epilepsy.)

The experiential record is also useless unless the brain is alert to detect novelty, and its value would be immeasurably greater if the nervous system could then *concentrate attention* on the unfamiliar aspects until the limbic system had made its choice. The brain cannot lay down new memory stores until consciousness is restored, but *conscious awareness* returns long before memory storage is resumed after concussion. The excitatory pathway through the amygdaloid nucleus to upper brain stem (p. 131) and its inhibitory partner from hippocampus via the fornix could provide a mechanism for the conscious brain to attend to selected items of the thalamocortical bombardment. In addition to contemporary inputs, this bombardment includes signals from some, perhaps all, memory stores. If the currently appropriate signals could not be isolated for attention the resulting interference would be as effective in causing functional amnesia as would faulty consolidation or retrieval (Warrington and Weiskrantz). Mountcastle stresses the conditional nature of behavioural responses to signals from the environment. In addition to

being matched against 'memory' for novelty, the signals must be assessed according to motivational drives.

Having selected part of the environment *or of the verbal model of possible environments* with possible long term consequences computed by the frontal lobes, the hippocampal formation can then gate one of alternative motor patterns to satisfy its limbic partner either now or at some postponed time. This is as near as one can get to the choice factor implied by the term '*voluntary behaviour*'.

We have now dealt with the reception, analysis, storage and recall of sensory data reaching the two cerebral hemispheres and have noted separate systems with bilateral access due to commissural and intracortical connections. An extensive literature on 'split brain syndromes' cannot be reviewed, but it will be necessary to consider whether each hemisphere 'has its own consciousness'. Fascinating speculations will occur to the reader. Since the ability to recognize that one event has occurred before another provides a method for appreciating a vectorial time dimension, can the two hemispheres have independent clocks and, if so, which is the master? What maintains serial and temporal order in remembered events? Is that imposed by the verbal model or is it intrinsic? Ability to learn improves with increasing literacy (capacity to use verbal models) but memory for events and future appointments does not. Is learning therefore different from memory? Ability to recall a scene like a mental photograph (*eidetic memory*) is exceedingly rare. Is the 'effort' to memorize and to recall evidence of a corollary discharge, and if so where does it originate and what structure perceives it? Despite growing understanding of higher nervous functions 'the will' still eludes us.

Contrary to popular conceptions, no memory storage or learning occurs during sleep, though recall seems to be possible (perhaps even facilitated). Learning and memorizing require (i) attention, (ii) motivation. Motivation will be discussed in Chapter 14. Learning and recall in hypnotic states are only apparent exceptions to this statement. The importance of these aspects should be remembered in assessing claims for improvement of memory storage with adrenergic arousal drugs (caffeine, amphetamine) or of memory recall with drugs that block inhibitory adrenergic effects (strychnine, picrotoxin) or with cholinomimetics (physostigmine). Recent interest in hypophyseal peptides (pitressin) cannot be assessed until more is known about the effects of neuromodulators on distributed neuronal systems.

DOMINANCE

The dominance of the left cerebral hemisphere with respect to speech is associated with asymmetry of an important area of association cortex (*see Fig.* 11.3). Clinical experience with brain-damaged children suggests that the two hemispheres are more equal for signal processing in the young. So far as non-speech modes of learning activity are concerned, there is increasing evidence for bilateral representation with some 'dominance' of one hemisphere, not always the left hemisphere even in strongly right-handed people. It is difficult to sort out different aspects of some activities. For instance, experiential responses of music are more often evoked by electrical stimulation of the right superolateral temporal cortex, and temporal lobectomy on that side disturbs comparison of tonal patterns and judgements of tone quality. But after sophisticated musical education both hemispheres participate equally or the left becomes dominant. Clearly it is not a general category 'music' that is 'represented' but a data processing system. There is no 'musical faculty' as there is no 'speech faculty' as such, and there are as many aspects of amusia as there are of aphasia. Both hemispheres have visual association areas but the right hemisphere is of primary importance for complex visuo-spatial functions, including recognition of a face (Chapter 10).

LATERALIZATION OF LEARNING

Observations on man and animals with severed corpus callosum ('split-brain') show a capacity for learning by each hemisphere. Capacity to store information seems to be symmetrical but complex learning tasks are best performed by the *left hemisphere*, regardless of handedness, possibly involving arrangement and acquisition of *serial ordering*. Numeracy is predominantly a right hemisphere function though the speech mechanisms involving the left supramarginal gyrus may be necessary to test it. The *right hemisphere* tends to use *parallel processing* rather than sequential processing — better for perception of visual space but inferior for handling the symbolic aspects of vision and hearing. Each method of handling signals has its advantage: in the human brain there is access to both processing systems via the callosal connections of the association areas, not directly from primary sensory areas.

Interhemisphere transfer of skills is well established (skill trained on one side later evident in untrained unexercised muscles of the other side). The *corpus callosum* is the main route for signal transfer but subcallosal pathways are used for transmitting high order tactile information. *Anterior and hippocampal commissures* are accepted but it may be that the possibility of communication through the thalamic massa intermedia should be re-evaluated.

Frontal lobe

In previous sections we have followed inputs into the cerebral cortex via the thalamus for relating body position and movements to extrapersonal space, both contactual (parietal) and extracorporeal (occipital and temporal) and noted the consequences of cross-modality linkage for interpretation of cues, resulting in conditional responses, association, symbolic representation and processing of derived data which at its highest evolution is the basis of speech and verbal programming, a substrate of thought. In the hippocampal structures and other parts of the temporal lobes the integration is highly complex and linked with the greatest development of a generalized memory function for identification of novelty or familiarity of environmental situations even though no identical stimulus pattern has been experienced. Unfamiliar patterns evoke an orienting response, familiar ones a satiety response, with appropriate cortical alerting/sleeping, muscular tension/relaxation set and autonomic fight–flight/recuperation responses due to limbic output via amygdala and caudate nucleus to the brain stem alerting system, the striatal

122

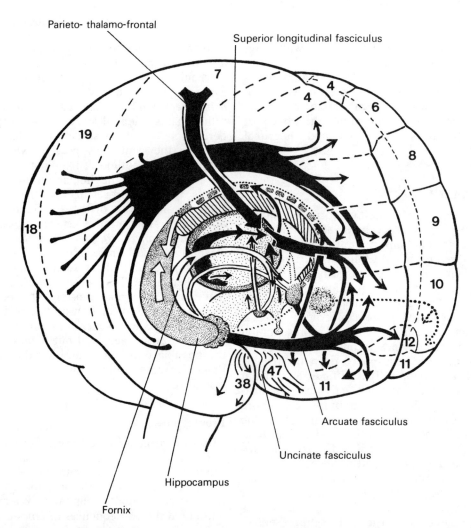

Parieto- thalamo-frontal

Superior longitudinal fasciculus

7

4

4

6

19

8

9

18

10

12

11

38

47

11

Arcuate fasciculus

Uncinate fasciculus

Hippocampus

Fornix

Fig. 13.1. *Frontal lobe: afferent connections.* Looking into the right cerebral hemisphere from above the right forehead, the brain stem and right thalamus are seen (*light shading*) (deeper structures including the left thalamus and fornix are dotted). There are four major inflow pathways, the largest being the superior longitudinal fasciculus conveying fast conducting fibres from the visual and auditory association areas to the dorsal (lateral and medial) part of the frontal lobe (areas 6–8) and also to the ventrolateral (9, 10, 11) which receives the second main projection from the dorsomedial thalamic nucleus (DmTN).

Somatosensory association cortex (7) projects to areas 9 and 10 by relay from DmTN which also receives fibres from the ventrolateral thalamus (termination of the lemniscal pathways) and from the hypothalamus. The third main bundle to the orbitofrontal complex is from the amygdalo-septal area (which are closer together than would appear from the diagram where they are dark shaded) at the forward end of the brain stem (septum) and the anteromedial end of the hippocampus. The hippocampus (*shaded area left with white arrows*) passes medially upwards and over the thalamus to the indusium griseum, an archipallial cortex projecting to the cingulate gyrus ('limbic lobe'). It receives inhibitory retrograde fibres from the anterior thalamus but the indusium also projects anteriorly to the orbital area (47). The hippocampus outflow to the hypothalamus (by the fornix to mammillary body) and thence to the anterior nucleus of thalamus (*unshaded paths, thin black arrows*) joins the DmTN projection but also goes to the septal nuclei. The septum also receives short and long (stria terminalis) connections from the amygdala and these two nuclei project to the orbital area. Thus the limbic and hypothalamic inputs to this area are closely linked at several points.

One outflow is shown, from the orbital area 47 to 38 of the anterior temporal lobe (uncinate fasciculus). It is inhibitory to the limbic controlled ('emotional') motor behaviour, a target for leucotomy. Area 8 ('pre-central cortex') projects back to visual association area 18 and to the caudate nucleus for control of eye and head posture. The frontal polar cortex (9–12) exerts inhibitory control on the dorsomedial thalamus, hypothalamus, tegmentum and by the frontopontine tract to the cerebellum (*see Fig.* 23.3). The most important crossed connections are through the corpus callosum and anterior commissure. The frontal poles function as a single organ. Anterior callosal lesions severely disrupt mental functions.

motor system and the hypothalamus (Chapters 15, 22, 25).

The animal with this system is well equipped to survive in a familiar or predictable environment. The primate frontal lobe, most highly developed in man, adds a new dimension, though not different in kind. The temporal lobe memory system is essentially a coincidence detector (p. 45). It is adequate for learning difficult discrimination tasks but is poor for response tasks involving delays of more than a few seconds and it gives priority to processing of novel stimuli (distractability). *Delayed response tasks* require storage of data in correct temporal sequence. With the acquisition of the ability to manipulate verbal models (p. 114), this type of cortical processing enables the brain to work out the possible consequences of various response strategies to a given environmental situation and to *inhibit the hippocampal choice-making system* in order to achieve delayed reward, even at the price of immediate discomfort or appetitive deprivation, in fact, 'cold-blooded' calculation.

Delayed responses and *anticipation of future consequences* are functions of the *frontal polar cortex* (area 10), in front of the agranular areas of the *pre-motor strip* which controls goal-directed movements of eyes, head and limbs (areas 6 and 8). The pre-motor strip receives thalamic input from the N. ventralis lateralis. It projects via pyramidal pathways and also to the centromedian and parafascicular nuclei of the thalamus (and thence to the neostriatum, *Fig.* 9.1). It will be considered with other aspects of the motor system (Chapter 22). Immediately anterior is the granular cortex of the *ventrolateral frontal lobe* (particularly areas 9 and 10), which has an input from the dorsomedial nucleus of the thalamus (*Fig. 13.1*). This is an association nucleus and is not a direct relay from the primary afferent pathways. It derives its connections from other thalamic structures and the sensory association areas so that integration, or cross-modality linkage, has already occurred before projection to the ventrolateral frontal cortex. Modality and accurate localization are of less interest to the frontal granular cortex than the total body image and its relationship to extracorporeal space. Most of the pre-frontal cortex projects fibres back to the rostral intralaminar nuclei of the thalamus. The *orbitofrontal cortex* (areas 9, 10, 11, 12) is in reciprocal connection with the amygdala and also receives fibres from the dorsomedial nucleus of thalamus (believed to originate in the piriform cortex, amygdala and hypothalamus) and from the memory systems of the temporal lobes. This is an important connection because the delayed responses permitted by the frontal lobe processing system demand that otherwise prepotent behavioural and emotional sets should be inhibited in favour of behavioural responses computed as being of superior ultimate advantage despite contemporary autonomic responses experienced as anxiety, relationships which are the basis of *personality*. It is the so-called limbic connections from the amygdala/septal area to the orbitofrontal cortex and from there back to the hypothalamus and temporal lobe, which are the targets for various leucotomy procedures designed to limit emotional responses and obsessional behavioural patterns. These represent the unacceptable face of forward prediction, unreal expectation of distressful or harmful results from harmless experiences.

The inhibitory role of the frontal cortex is extremely important. It appears to be concerned mainly with the granular cortex of the *dorsolateral and dorsomedial frontal lobe*. This resembles and is reciprocally connected with the infraparietal lobule (39), previously described (p. 113) as an area for highest integration of afferent signals, in that it has no direct input from the thalamus, receiving only transcortical connections. This makes it difficult to identify the full complexity of the connections and functions of the granular cortex. The frontal granular cortex is the only region of the neocortex to project directly to the hypothalamus and it has been suggested that it inhibits 'ingestive' behavioural patterns. No motor responses result from electrical stimulation of the dorsolateral frontal cortex.

The effects of lesions in man point to an important role in the inhibition of hippocampus–amygdala–hypothalamus sets. They are well described by Milner (1982). Inability to overcome a previously established response set causes a *perseverative tendency*. Preferred modes of response are not suppressed (eg the contactual grasp reflex, p. 166). *Inertia* results from failure to shift from one motor programme to another, especially if it is verbally programmed (despite persisting memory of the verbal command). Serial organization of actions is reduced or abolished (eg a patient may know a match and be able to strike it and know a candle, yet be unable to light the candle with the match). Goal-orientated behaviour is grossly impaired. The subject is unable to evaluate the adequacy of his own actions. His *mood* alternates between euphoria and depression or irritability. Inappropriate jocularity is common. Most importantly, especially with left frontal lesions, there is disturbance of the directive role of speech in the organization of appropriate movements. Even the vegetative components of the orientating reflex (Chapter 14) are disturbed.

These features, along with the disturbance of the highest forms of attention and of the most complicated control of memory processes when the prefrontal area is damaged, point to the controlling role of the frontal lobe over the limbic system on the one hand and over the goal-directed motor systems on the other. Nauta (1971) has described appropriate connections in monkey brain. With the frontal lobe, consequences of actions can be computed from contemporary input and previous experience or even entirely from verbal models. It can deal with *abstractions* instead of first derivatives of sensory data. This ability to process verbal symbols, coupled with a capacity for cross-linkage with actual, memorized, or previously constructed (imagined) symbols gives an outstanding versatility since other observers' abstracted data can be fed in — ie true *education* as distinct from conditioning. With the ability to communicate by speech, this is the critical evolutionary development for civilization since each generation can start with a stock of verbal symbols and relations laboriously discovered by earlier generations. The unique associations and logical inferences of a single exceptional brain are not lost but become the common heritage of all humans with developed frontal lobes. The average artist depends on the temporal lobes, the jurist on the ability of the frontal lobes to derive systematic relationships between classes, but the scientist especially uses the model building and testing functions of the frontal poles. Gifted people in each of these categories use all three. Insight demands the frontal lobes.

Goal-directed movements and alterations of postural sets reacting to verbal models generated from memory stores cannot be discriminated from 'volition' and the distinction seems unnecessary. The most baffling voluntary activities are introspection and concentration. The 'effort' experienced strongly suggests a corollary discharge (p. 242).

Further reading

Clark W.E. Le G. Connexions of the frontal lobes of the brain. *Lancet* 1948; **i**: 353–6.
Milner B. Some cognitive effects of frontal-lobe lesions in man. *Phil. Trans. R. Soc.* 1982; **B298**: 211–26.
Nauta W.J.H. The problem of the frontal lobe: a reinterpretation. *J. Psychiatr. Rev.* 1971; **8**: 167–87.
O'Keefe J. and Nadel L. *The Hippocampus as a Cognitive Map.* Oxford: Oxford University Press, 1978.
Pribram K.H. and McGuiness D. Arousal, activation and effort in the control of attention. *Psychol. Rev.* 1975; **52**: 116–49.
Sperry R.W. Mental unity following surgical disconnection of the cerebral hemispheres. In: *The Harvey Lectures.* New York: Academic Press, 1968, pp. 293–323.
Warren J.M. and Akert K. *The Frontal Granular Cortex and Behaviour.* New York: McGraw-Hill, 1964.

Chapter 14

Appetites and motivation: the limbic system

It is not surprising that the most primitive sensing system for detection of food or toxic substances in the environment (originally aqueous) should be highly sensitive chemoreceptors and that the central processing of these signals in evolving nervous systems should be used for *appetitive behavioural patterns*.

Gustatory sensation

The taste receptor cells of mammals are collected in taste buds. Most of these are in the papillae on the tongue, but taste buds are also found in the mucous membrane of the posterior buccal cavity and upper pharynx. The *taste cells* have chemoreceptors for numerous chemicals but four main classes are recognized by the subjective interpretation of their effects as sweet, salt, bitter and sour. The taste buds have mixed receptor cells but one type predominates in different papillae. In man the different classes of taste sensation are best appreciated at the tip of the tongue (sweet and salt), base of the tongue (bitter) and along its edge (sour). The sensitivity of the receptors is increased by movement of the tongue and by application of saliva.

Appropriate chemicals on the receptor sites depolarize the taste cells and the generator potential fires repetitive action potentials in a peripheral fibre of a gustatory nerve — the lingual nerve for the anterior two-thirds of the tongue and the glossopharyngeal (IX) nerve for the posterior third. The terminal fibres form a plexus beneath each taste bud and there are also chemosensitive free nerve endings between receptor cells. Thus the receptive area for each neurone is large, overlapping is profuse and the sensory signal has little local sign.

The taste fibres in the *lingual nerve* pass into the chorda tympani which enters the middle ear cavity (where it may be damaged in mastoidectomy), crosses the tympanic membrane and joins the *facial nerve (VII)*. Each fibre is the peripheral part of a bipolar ganglion cell in the *geniculate ganglion* of that nerve. Central processes from the ganglion cells pass by the *nervus intermedius* of Wrisberg into the medulla oblongata and terminate ipsilaterally in the *nucleus solitarius*.

The lingual fibres of the *glossopharyngeal nerve* from the posterior tongue taste buds have their cell bodies in the *petrosal ganglion* and their central processes run in the trunk of the glossopharyngeal nerve to an adjacent part of the *nucleus solitarius* of the same side. Some taste fibres probably pass centrally in the vagus (X) and trigeminal (V) nerves and may account for 'anomolous' retention of taste sensation. More important is a '*common chemical sense*' transmitted by the trigeminal nerve (V) which is not specific for any particular taste sensation.

Second order gustatory neurones from the solitary nucleus decussate almost immediately within the reticular formation and pass by the tractus solitarius to medial and ventral nuclei of the thalamus for perception of taste. Less well known but functionally important fibres terminate in the mammillary body and hypothalamus.

The ventromedial thalamus relays third order neurones to the *cerebral cortex*. There is some uncertainty as to the exact destination in man — hippocampal formation, or the operculum, or the insula at the lower end of the pre- and post-central gyri, the anterior portion of the second sensorimotor area (Chapter 8). Efferent fibres from the same cortical areas have been traced to the striatum and globus pallidum and also back to the thalamus, doubtless involved in motor responses to taste sensation (p. 220).

There are also *efferent neurones* in the lingual nerve which inhibit the afferent response from the taste receptors (reminiscent of similar efferent control of acoustic and vestibular inputs to the brain). They are activated through the vagus and solitary nucleus by gastric distension or by osmotic pressure in the stomach and intestine, and by sympathetic activity. It appears that the functional level of the taste receptors can vary to a level suitable for changing combinations of internal and external conditions. Within the central nervous system, the gustatory signals are further inhibited by afferent signals from the stretch receptors of the body wall.

The nervus intermedius branch of the facial nerve and the glossopharyngeal and vagus nerves also transmit *visceral afferent fibres* relaying in the contralateral solitary tract nucleus to the superior and inferior salivatory nuclei respectively which send efferent parasympathetic neurones through the VII and IX nerves to the *salivary glands*.

Olfactory sensation

Olfactory sensation is a related sensory function. The savour of food depends on simultaneous activation of smell sensation along with the true taste sensation which only appreciates the four basic types described above. Molecules of numerous substances landing on the moist mucous membrane of the nose stimulate a wide variety of chemoreceptors on the peripheral axons of bipolar neurones in microvilli within the nasal mucosa. Bundles of their central processes passing through the cribriform plate of the ethmoid bone into the cranial cavity are readily damaged by accelerative forces to the head. They terminate in the olfactory bulb which, with the olfactory nerve, is a protrusion of brain tissue, not a true cranial nerve.

In the *olfactory bulb* complex connections of olfactory fibres (glomeruli) surround the mitral cells of the secondary olfactory neurones, an area similar in function to the dorsal root entry zone of the spinal grey matter. The mitral and

tufted cells are the most prominent of a number of neurones in a highly ordered structure for editing afferent signals, not unlike the retina of the eye. They project centrally in the secondary olfactory pathway to the cerebral hemisphere and receive centrifugal inhibitory neurones. This structure is of some importance in clinical neurology as it is compressed by expanding tumours of the frontal lobe. Unilateral anosmia may be the only detectable clinical sign.

The *olfactory tract* contains discrete bundles of axons and their collaterals which separate on reaching the undersurface of the cerebral hemisphere into distinct medial and lateral tracts to the *rhinencephalon*. With this important evolutionary development the thalamus was bypassed and an integrative cortex, the paleopallium, developed. In the same way as the head ganglion of the proprioceptive system (the cerebellum) had its cross-modality linkage system exploited in later evolution (Chapter 23), so the cerebral cortex was progressively exploited for sensorimotor processing in the neopallium, but the later sensory inputs were all relayed from the thalamus.

The medial olfactory tract (or stria) extends towards the subcallosal area on the medial surface of the frontal lobe (*see* Fig. 14.1). The lateral olfactory stria passes laterally and bends around the limen of the insula to enter the anteromedial part of the temporal lobe. Some intermediary fibres enter the anterior perforated substance between the tracts. In many animals there are complicated connections to an extensive area of the basal frontal and medial temporal cortex but in man the primary olfactory cortex is probably restricted to the *uncus and anterior end of the hippocampal gyrus*. They reach this agranular cortex without relay in the thalamus. The major inputs from the olfactory tracts go to the surrounding *entorhinal area* (area 28) or pyriform lobe, from which they are relayed to the hippocampus in the perforant and alvear pathways (p. 118), constituting its main input. Other fibres enter the septal region and amygdala. They are related to important behavioural responses concerned with the major appetites and with motivation. The motor outflow of the olfactory cortex, via the parahippocampal gyrus, hippocampus, hypothalamus and habenular nucleus to the mid-brain motor systems (Chapter 20) has been incorporated, in the course of evolution, into 'conditional' behavioural responses.

A complex undifferentiated input would be useless for such a refined analyser and it seems likely that the function of the inhibitory efferents to the olfactory bulb glomerular system is to use inhibitory 'sharpening' (Chapter 4) by way of interneurones (granule cells) to discriminate different olfactory stimuli, lateralize them, and probably in lower animals to derive directional localization data. The amazingly precise and sensitive identification of odours by carnivores has been all but lost in man, but the cerebral substratum is put to further use.

Motivation

At a very early stage of the evolution of species the development of a neuromuscular system increased survival potential for self and for species by allowing the animal to move towards food or sexual mate and away from harmful stimuli detected by the chemoreceptors of the leading segment (olfaction) and monitored by similar receptors at the food intake stoma (taste). It is not surprising that memory and behavioural patterns should have evolved round these two sensory modalities and that they are linked with afferent feedback from the viscera and internal monitors of the body's biochemical state. The smell of a hospital, especially the operation suite, terrifies many people, though the regular inhabitants have become so habituated that they no longer notice it.

Hunger and sexual drives have supreme survival value and their primacy is well recognized by psychologists and, since Freud, accepted without question by laymen. Drives such as power-seeking, stressed by some schools of psychology, are readily derived from the *survival drives* and clearly their linkage in association cortex permits many other secondary motivations to initiate behavioural patterns. Similarly, the *satiety signals* relevant to the hunger and sexual drives become linked to alternative *symbols* (in the sense used previously for that word — p. 111).

It will be convenient to postpone a brief description of the elementary forebrain and hindbrain reflexes based on olfaction and taste to the chapters on control of skeletal muscle (Chapter 20) and the efferent mechanisms of the hypothalamus will also be described separately (Chapter 25). Here we examine the cortical superstructure which evolved on top of this input–output system. It was the first development of a cerebral hemisphere in relation to the first distance receptor of the leading segment of the organism and is sometimes termed the 'paleocortex' on this account. With the later evolution of the neopallium superimposed on the thalamus, this primitive cortex with the even earlier hippocampus (archipallium) now circles the foramen of Monro, the thalamic stalk and the corpus callosum. Because of its obvious anatomical relationship to the olfactory system it was formerly named the *rhinenecephalon* ('smell brain'). With recognition that only the antero-inferior part of the old cortex is directly involved in olfaction (the pyriform lobe) the descriptive term *'limbic lobe'* was given to the ring of grey matter surrounding the stalk of the cerebral hemisphere — hippocampus, cingulum, cingulate gyrus and related structures. Recognition of the importance of this area in emotional reactivity led to concepts such as the Papez circuit which regarded the hippocampal formation and its principal projection system, the fornix, as an efferent pathway between the neocortex and the hypothalamus and so to the brain stem for exteriorizing the somatic and visceral responses which we regard as emotional. At the same time, 'impulses concerned with emotion' were regarded as being relayed transcortically from the hippocampal formation to the cingulate gyrus and from there to other cortical regions, to add emotional colouring to their analyses of afferent signals.

Paul D. McLean's model was a great step forward, incorporating the nuclei of the amygdala and septal area into a *limbic system*, a descriptive term adopted from Broca. When we use the term in this book it is for its convenience, but the term is passing out of favour as seeming to imply restriction to the archipallium. Throughout this book we have stressed that most functions are distributed anatomically and the same mass of grey matter (not necessarily the same synaptic connections) may be used in more than one distributed system.

The neural substratum for *motivation*, and its related subjective experience of *emotion*, is best understood by looking at the distributed functions separately. It will become clear that there is considerable overlap with the circuits for memory, olfaction, taste and the association cortex derivatives of hearing and vision. This has caused a problem for clinical neurology since disease, including epileptic activity, commonly involves several of these distributed functions and this does not necessarily imply that they are normally integrated. Thus terms such as 'temporal lobe epilepsy', 'psychomotor epilepsy' and 'limbic epilepsy' are being discarded in favour of such uncommitted terms as 'complex partial seizures'.

Consider now the behaviour required of the primitive animal. It has detected smell signals, investigated them by the sniffing responses described in Chapter 20, and tentatively sampled the same chemical soup with its taste receptors, nibbling with its oral and lingual apparatus. It must now decide whether to swallow it or spit it out with reflexes centred on the nucleus of the solitary tract (Chapter 20). At that level the taste signals are integrated with afferent signals from trigeminal receptors in the mouth and with vagal receptors in the intestinal tract and projected to the cortex at the lower end of the contralateral *post-central gyrus* via the medial part of the ventral posteromedial nucleus of the thalamus (ie medial to the thalamic relay nucleus for facial sensation). The solitary nucleus is also linked to a specialized area of the trigeminal nucleus, the *locus coeruleus*. Although we are not aware of evidence for an anatomical connection, it may be considered that the taste centres also project to the *raphe nuclei* at the midline of the reticular formation since this complex of reticular formation nuclei, extending from the pons to the dorsal tegmental nucleus of the mid-brain, forms a reciprocal pair with the locus coeruleus for arousing and suppressing the amygdaloid and septal areas among others. Hunger or an *interesting* (appetizing or unpleasant) smell/taste stimulus would activate appropriate behaviour responses; satiety or an uninteresting stimulus would cause it to be abandoned and the animal to return to a resting/sleeping state with inhibition of the lower olfactory and taste synapses by the efferent neurones previously mentioned. These decisions depend on the uniqueness or familiarity of the stimulation. The connections of the hippocampal formation which make it suitable for orientating responses, memory and recognition have been discussed in Chapter 13. It is now necessary to add the special contribution of taste and smell, and of any other influences acting on the locus coeruleus and raphe nuclei.

LOCUS COERULEUS: AN ADRENERGIC ACTIVATOR

The locus coeruleus is a large structure near the central grey matter of the upper pons. It has cells containing granules of melanin-pigment and catecholamines, mainly noradrenaline and dopamine, both of which have levodopa as precursor. It is related in some way to dopaminergic neurones in the substantia nigra and nucleus accumbens, but also to a dopaminergic system in the parolfactory gyrus. The exact role of this *mesolimbic dopaminergic system* (Chapter 3) is unknown but deficiency of this system has been related to the pathophysiology of affective and psychic disturbances in Parkinson's disease.

The *noradrenergic neurones* are considered to be more important. They ascend in dorsal parts of the midbrain and enter the diencephalon by the *medial forebrain bundle* (MFB) passing forwards to the septal regions (*see Fig. 3.1*). In addition, the noradrenergic fibres are widely distributed to cerebral and cerebellar cortex and directly to the hippocampal formation and medial hypothalamus. It is generally accepted that this is part of a general activating system along with the reticular activating system. There is pharmacological evidence of a reciprocally acting *cholinergic system*. Its neuronal basis has not been identified but the basal nucleus of Meynert is certainly involved (*see Fig. 3.4*).

Stimulation of the limbic system with α-adrenergic chemicals elicits feeding responses in rats and cholinergic stimulation elicits drinking. On the other hand β-adrenergic agonists inhibit eating, even in food-deprived animals (a possible basis for the appetite-suppressant effect of amphetamines).

This eating-regulating mechanism has been incorporated by the limbic system into an important mechanism of behavioural suppression. The coeruleus–MFB–septal route bombards the septal area nuclei with noradrenaline when an animal is 'rewarded' with food. It has been proposed that the noradrenergic neural systems of the basal forebrain subserve a 'pleasure system' which suppresses aversive reactions mediated by a cholinergic 'punishment system'. It is important, however, to recognize that most of the experimental work has been done with food-rewarded animals.

RAPHE NUCLEI: A SEROTONIN ACTIVATOR

Stimulation of the raphe nuclei leads to a widespread release of *serotonin* (5-hydroxytryptamine) throughout the forebrain (*see* Fig. 3.2). This potentiates a marked increase in the startle response which does not habituate. There is no general hyper-reactivity or somnolence. Inhibition of serotonin synthesis causes prolonged insomnia, and serotonin blocking agents such as the hallucinogenic drugs inhibit the serotonin responses and disrupt behaviour. Monoamine oxidase inhibitors and tryptophan, which elevate brain serotonin levels, slow raphe discharge. Tricyclic antidepressants also slow the raphe neurones and locally elevate serotonin levels by inhibiting their pre-synaptic uptake.

The ascending serotoninergic fibres enter the ventral part of the medial forebrain bundle and are distributed to the septal region and onwards through the cingulate cortex to the hippocampus. Some fibres pass to the hypothalamus via the mammillary body and by the stria terminalis. A bundle ending in the caudate nucleus may be important in the abolition of antigravity muscle tone during sleep. It is well known that involuntary movements 'released' by basal ganglia lesions are absent during sleep.

This important system, which has been revealed by a fluorescence technique and an immunohistological method, may indeed be distributed throughout the neocortex where serotonin is considered to be an inhibitory neurotransmitter or modulator. It is postulated that it is concerned with the active production of sleep (Chapter 15) and with the behavioural and autonomic changes associated with recuperation of the body. Rather surprisingly this is not a phase for metabolic recovery of the 'exhausted' waking brain. Neuronal discharge may actually be increased, and cerebral circulation and oxygen consumption increased.

The primitive drive associated with the basic appetites is incorporated into other behavioural patterns in higher animals. The elaborate association cortex of the limbic system and the integrative relays of amygdaloid and septal areas have absorbed these important modulatory systems for the control of the activity of the entire cortex and hypothalamus by *forebrain commands*. The incompletely identified cholinergic system promises to be particularly important for intellectual functions, especially memory.

THE AMYGDALAR CIRCUIT

The *amygdaloid nuclear complex* is the tip of the caudate nucleus which has rotated with the developing cerebral hemisphere so that this structure, starting inferior to the body of the lateral ventricle, comes to lie on the roof of the temporal horn. It is located internal to the uncus in the temporal lobe and receives olfactory fibres from the lateral olfactory tract and pre-pyriform cortex. Thus it receives both direct and indirect olfactory inputs (*Figs* 14.1, 14.2). The amygdala is, however, a complex of nuclei and the basolateral division is strongly associated with the thalamus and pre-frontal cortex. It is the most pronounced nuclear group of the human amygdala and its high density of acetylcholinesterase suggests that it may be a target organ for the cholinergic system projecting from the brain stem or from the substantia innominata (*see* Fig. 3.4). It is under inhibitory control by the noradrenergic brain stem fibres passing through the MFB. Many of its neurones are dopaminergic.

The amygdaloid complex has two major outflow pathways, all leading directly or indirectly to the *hypothalamus*.

The stria terminalis relaying most of the olfactory input is the most prominent outflow path from the amygdala. Its fibres arch along

130

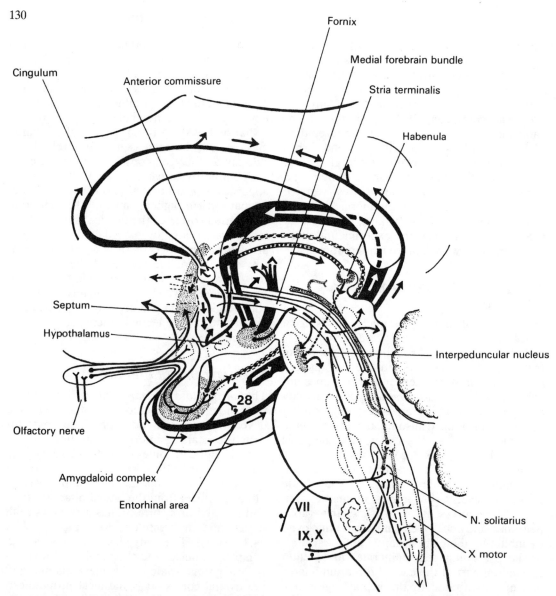

Fig. 14.1. *The limbic system: taste and olfaction.* Gustatory neurones of cranial nerves VII, IX and X relay in the nucleus solitarius and thalamus to the insular area of cortex, to salivatory nuclei and hypothalamus. The olfactory nerve (I) relays in the olfactory bulb by olfactory tracts to the rhinencephalon. Shown are the additional projections to the entorhinal area (area 28), orbitofrontal area and amygdaloid complex (*see text*). The medial olfactory tract passes to the septal area and into the cingulum anteriorly. The lateral olfactory tract fibres project to the preoptic region and anterior hypothalamus after relay in the amygdaloid complex, either directly (*black arrows*) or via the stria terminalis. (Some fibres cross in the anterior commissure.) A large component of the lateral tract (*solid black line*) bypasses the amygdala and divides in the temporal lobe into two major components, one passing posteriorly to enter the cingulate gyrus, the other relaying in the hippocampus (*white arrows*) and projecting in the fornix to the mammillary bodies and anterior hypothalamus. The mammillary nuclei relay to the anterior thalamus by the bundle of Vicq d'Azyr and by the mammillo-tegmental bundle to the tegmentum.

The septal and pre-optic areas direct olfactory and gustatory stimuli by the medial forebrain bundle to the tegmentum and tectum of the mesencephalon and by the stria medullaris (*dotted line*) to the habenula and interpeduncular nucleus.

The brain stem projections control orientation of head and eyes with respect to olfactory and gustatory stimuli. The amygdaloid, septal, hippocampal, diencephalic and cingulate areas constitute a 'limbic system' important for motivational and conditional responses and for memory. The hypothalamus regulates hormonal and autonomic responses associated with appetitive activity.

the medial border of the caudate nucleus near its junction with the thalamus to its bed nucleus dorsal to the anterior commissure where they are relayed into the pre-optic area and ventromedial hypothalamic nucleus. The bed nuclei of the right and left striae terminales are linked through the *anterior commissure* (*Fig.* 14.1).

THE VENTRAL AMYGDALOFUGAL BUNDLE

Relaying some of the olfactory and probably most of the important non-olfactory input of the amygdaloid complex, the anterior commissure spreads medially and rostrally beneath the lentiform nucleus, through the substantia innominata to the hypothalamus (*Fig.* 14.2). Especially in higher mammals, an important projection bypasses the preoptic region and hypothalamus and enters the inferior thalamic peduncle to the dorsomedial nucleus of the thalamus, linking the motivation part of the brain with the cerebrum. Ventral fibres from the amygdaloid complex also reach the hypothalamus and thalamus via the hippocampal formation — fornix–mammillary body–mammillothalamic tract described in Chapter 13. It is a major input of amygdaloid function to the limbic system and the most prominent re-entrant pathway through the hippocampus.

From both of these amygdalofugal arching pathways and by direct connections, the amygdaloid complex is linked with the septal area. It also contributes directly to the main outflow path of the latter, the *medial forebrain bundle*, for projection to the tegmental area (Chapter 22). Thus the amygdaloid nucleus complex fires into the hypothalamus and the central core motor system, the substratum for *emotionally determined autonomic and motor responses*, as well as into the most highly integrated areas of cortex (to which it is reciprocally connected) and the mid-brain reticular 'arousal' system.

Stimulation of the amygdala causes an 'arrest' reaction in which the experimental animal stops all ongoing activities, including feeding behaviour, and assumes an attitude of aroused attention with desynchronization of the EEG indistinguishable from reticular activation. This '*orientating reflex*' is followed by flight and defensive reactions. From different regions of the complex are evoked either withdrawal behaviour with the somatic manifestations of fear, or rage and aggression reactions, both with pupillary dilatation, piloerection and appropriate vocalization. Stimulation in man produces feelings of fear, confusional states, disturbances of awareness and amnesia for events occurring during the stimulation, but rage is rare. The manifestations are very similar to certain 'complex partial seizures' formerly termed 'temporal lobe epilepsy'. The autonomic and endocrine responses accompanying the behaviour will be discussed in Chapter 25. After-discharges following repetitive brief stimulation of the amygdala spread to remote brain regions and eventually produce generalized epileptic seizures ('*kindling*' see p. 119).

The amygdala appears to be important with the hippocampus in the establishment of *conditional emotional responses*. A basic conditional response is the affective component of pain. The spinal cord bundle known as the spinothalamic tract has relatively few fibres that terminate in the thalamus and an extremely small thalamocortical projection (Chapter 6). The bulk of the fibres terminate in the reticulum of the medulla and the central grey matter of the mid-brain. This area is closely linked with the small fibre pain system (*Fig.* 6.1) and with the frontotemporal portion of the limbic system for the *psychological appreciation of pain* (p. 135). This has important implications for treatment.

Destruction of the amygdaloid complex removes these 'emotional' reactions and releases sexual responses ('hypersexuality') and feeding behaviour (hyperphagia) suggesting that the amygdaloid complex inhibits the lateral hypothalamic area which is driven by the septal nuclei (*Fig.* 14.1). The animal can still orientate towards new stimuli but requires the motivation of a 'reward' to do so repeatedly. Bilateral amygdaloid lesions are usually associated with destruction of the hippocampal formation and of neighbouring association areas for vision and also the cross-modality linkages and 'coincidence detection circuits' necessary for memory (Chapter 13). With this combination the animal is docile, hypersexual, obsessed with feeding, unable to identify

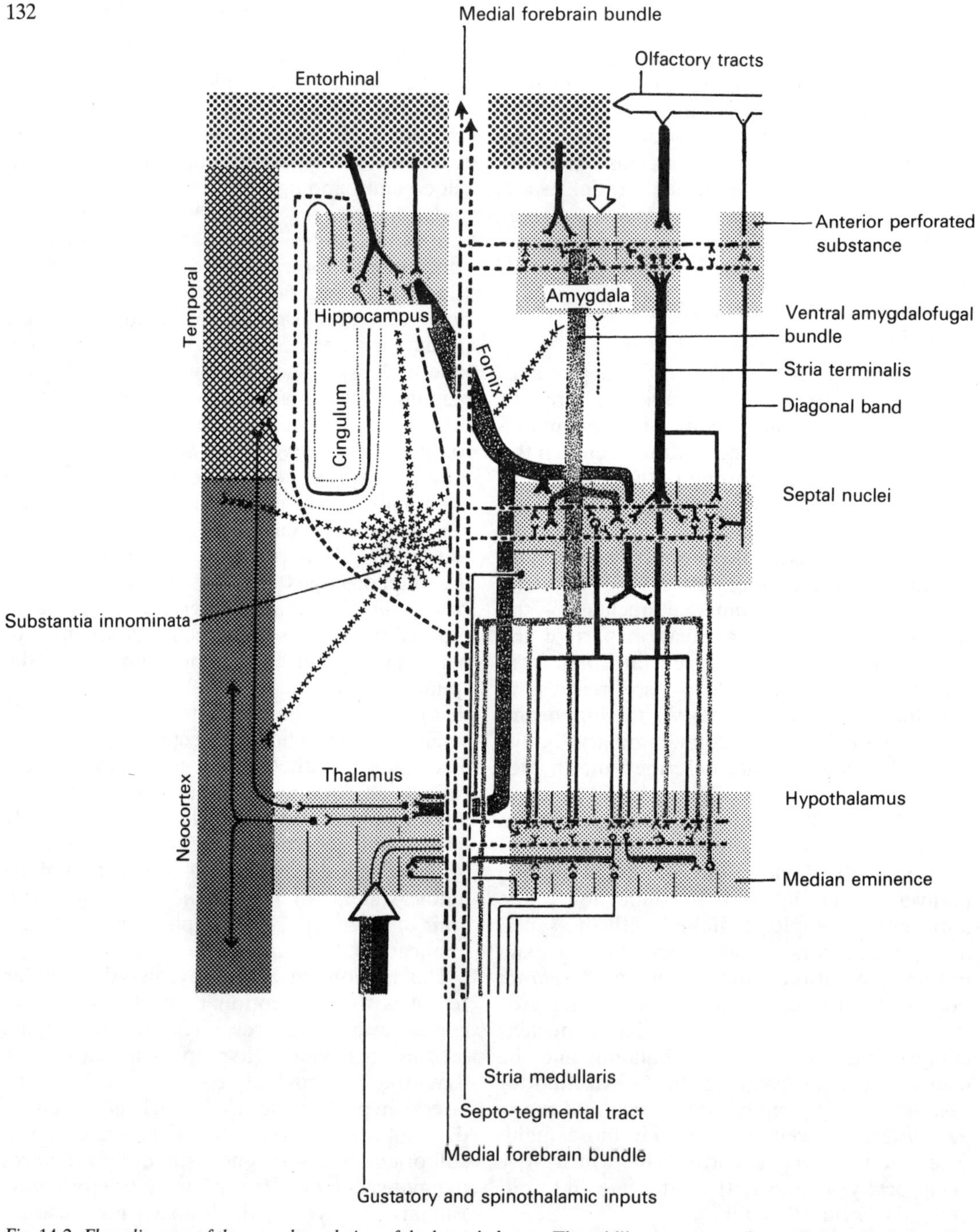

132

Fig. 14.2. *Flow diagram of the neural regulation of the hypothalamus.* The midline represents the medial forebrain bundle. The right border is the wall of the IIIrd ventricle. The unshaded block (*top right*) represents olfactory input which goes directly or after relay into several nuclear masses. These are (*from left*) (*a*) the hippocampus projecting by the fornix to the septal and mammillary areas and by re-entrant circuits through the cingulate gyrus; (*b*) the amygdaloid complex. The basolateral division of the amygdala projects a ventral amygdalofugal bundle to septal nuclei, hypothalamus and mammillary nuclei at the base of the inferior thalamic peduncle (*lower left*) where it is interconnected with the neocortex. The corticomedial division projects by the stria terminalis, to its bed nucleus and to the preoptic area and ventromedial hypothalamus (*lower right*), with connections to the septal area (*right centre*); (*c*) the anterior perforated substance and olfactory tubercle are connected to the midline septal area by the diagonal band of Broca.

whether an object is edible or not until it is smelled and mouthed, and immediately forgets the decision so that the same object is repeatedly re-examined. Conditional emotional responses such as *social reactions* with other animals in a colony are reduced, the animals become social isolates. This *syndrome of Kluver and Bucy*, first described in the Rhesus monkey after complete bilateral temporal lobectomy, is occasionally seen in man with bilateral temporal lobe disease. The human also develops religiosity, a compulsion to write and may be sexually impotent. The full syndrome is not produced by lesions confined to the amygdaloid complexes, and certainly not with unilateral ablation, so deliberate stereotaxic amygdalotomy has been used for the treatment of certain psychiatric and epileptic disorders associated with paroxysmal aggression. The hypothalamus remains under the regulatory control of the septal area. It can still respond aggressively, but the threshold to do so is raised by amygdalotomy. Regrettably, the major neurotransmitter of the amygdala is unknown for pharmacological blockade. The profound sleep-promoting serotonin effect on the hypothalamus is released.

THE SEPTAL AREA

In some respects acting reciprocally to the amygdaloid complex is the septal area at the anterior pole of the diencephalon. It is a complicated system of nuclei with an unpaired medial part and right and left lateral parts. In man it lies below the septum pellucidum and in front of a commissure joining the hippocampal formations of each side. It receives convergence of fibres from the hypothalamus, preoptic area, hippocampus and the amygdaloid complex. As already described, it receives important olfactory tract and brain stem inputs from food/sex exploration systems. In preference to eating behaviour, it is responsible for initiating, maintaining and completing the *intake of water* in response to a detector of the volume of body fluid.

All these converging signals are strongly modulated by the massive reciprocal chemical systems ascending via the medial forebrain bundle (Chapter 3). Some authors consider that these regulate two reciprocal output systems. A dorsal efferent system arising in the dorsal and lateral nuclei of the septal area enters the hippocampal fornix pathway to the hypothalamus which it *facilitates*. A ventral efferent system enters the stria terminalis pathway to the hypothalamus which it *inhibits*. Antagonistic actions of these two outflows could account for apparent disagreement of various experiments on ablation and stimulation of the septal area. It is certainly not a single function nucleus. In addition to the outputs to the hypothalamus, the septal nuclei project to the mid-brain motor control systems for head movement and feeding behaviour by two large pathways, the medial forebrain bundle and the stria medullaris.

The medial forebrain bundle, already described as an important afferent route from mesencephalon to septal area, is also a very important efferent tract from the ventral septal nuclei to the interpeduncular nucleus of the mid-brain. The *stria medullaris*, a smaller bundle of efferent fibres, projects from lateral and ventral septal nuclei along the dorsomedial margin of the thalamus (near the roof of the IIIrd ventricle) to the *habenula* where the fibres are relayed to the tegmentum and the interpeduncular nucleus. The role of the habenula, tegmentum and interpeduncular nuclei in movements of the head and in feeding

---

Fig. 14.2 *(contd)*

The lateral part of the septal area (*right centre*) has dorsal (facilitatory) and ventral (inhibitory) efferent systems to the hypothalamus, running with the fornix and stria terminalis respectively. A septal-tegmental outflow enters the medial forebrain bundle and stria medullaris.

The amygdaloid and septal inputs to the hypothalamic nuclei are regulated by a branch of the fornix. The median eminence is chemosensitive and linked by neurones and a portal vascular system to adjacent neuroendocrine areas including the pituitary body. Posterior hypothalamic nuclei at the base of the thalamic peduncle project autonomic control fibres in or near the stria medullaris and to the mammillary body. The ventral thalamus also relays gustatory, thermal and pain stimuli to the hypothalamus.

All of the deep nuclei shown receive serotoninergic (-----) and noradrenergic (–·–·–) fibres from the brain stem via the medial forebrain bundle. The substantia innominata (including the basal nucleus of Meynert and the diagonal band) have cholinergic neurones (∗∗∗). Their distribution is uncertain in man but includes the neocortex (*Fig. 3.4.*).

is described in Chapter 20. Some fibres go to the superior and inferior colliculi to direct eyes and ears towards a target.

SEPTAL-CORTICAL CONNECTIONS

The outflows just described constitute pathways for septal control over the basic autonomic and somatomotor systems involved in feeding, drinking and probably sexual behaviour. Though they are less well defined by anatomical and physiological studies, it seems highly probable that, like many of the neural systems already described in this book, evolutionary development has superimposed cortical functions which are more important in man, and there are only hints at their complexity from animal studies (*Fig.* 14.2).

Like the amygdala, the septal nuclei also project to the mediodorsal nucleus of the *thalamus* and so to the cortex, mostly to the *orbital-frontal cortex*. Most of the septal connections with the hippocampus are afferent, but some efferent fibres do pass through the hippocampal gyrus to the cingulate cortex. Thus the *'limbic' cortex* (orbitofrontal, hippocampal, indusium griseum and cingulate) may be considered to bear a relationship to the amygdaloid-septal area comparable with that of the neocortex to the thalamus. Its outflow through the hypothalamus and medial forebrain bundle is fundamental for the *appetitive responses* of the living animal and it is difficult to sort out the contributions of different parts.

ELEMENTARY FUNCTIONS OF THE SEPTAL AREA

The regulatory role of the amygdaloid complex with respect to eating appears to be paralleled in the septal area with respect to drinking water. In experimental animals ablation of this area causes hyperdipsia. Nevertheless, when water is offered as a reward of a conditional operant task the animal is less responsive, apparently because it is *less motivated* to win the reward regardless of its body's fluid balance. Drinking is increased by cholinergic stimulation. Ablation and stimulation studies are difficult to interpret or to generalize from different species but it appears that the septal nuclei are involved in a *pleasure-rewarding*

system with the fornix system positively reinforcing the hypothalamus and the stria terminalis system inhibiting it. In response to an environment producing pleasure and lacking threat, the septum potentiates the predominant behavioural tendencies of the animal, both genetic and acquired. The hypothalamo-autonomic system is inhibited by septal stimulation except for the responses preliminary to copulation and reproduction, including penile erection in the males. The behavioural response is, contrary to that evoked from the amygdala, manifestations of pleasure, friendliness and social behaviour, with grooming reactions. *In contrast to the amygdaloid circuit which promotes behaviour conducive to self-preservation, the septal circuit promotes activity for preservation of the species.*

Whereas the amygdala stimulates release of ACTH during stress, the septal circuit stimulates the infundibular portion of the hypothalamus to secrete sex hormones, androgenic and follicle stimulating.

SEXUAL BEHAVIOUR

Interestingly, the behavioural response is similar to, if not identical with, anger and defensive behaviour which can be stimulated from the same area. McLean has drawn attention to the close neural organization of oral (amygdaloid) and genital (septal) functions in relation to the olfactory sense and comments that even in mammals excitation in one sector readily spills over into the other, so that sexual excitation may result in reflex mouthing and biting, and vice versa. In later evolution vision and manipulation become progressively more important in guiding sociosexual behaviour. The olfactory apparatus is bypassed by inputs from the anterior thalamus and the cingulate cortex. Stimuli that would normally cause pain may be sexually arousing. Visual signals are transmitted to the hippocampus and thence by the medial thalamus to the hypothalamus. The love play of the higher cortex is less aggressive than that of the rhinencephalon but the septal circuit produces the necessary emotional, muscular, and neuroendocrine 'set'.

In rodents, experimental lesions of the septal area cause a 'septal syndrome' with increased rage reactions described as hyperemotionality, with enhanced social contacts, overreaction to pain and photophobia. The startle reaction is increased. This syndrome has never been adequately explained. On the analogy of the post-labyrinthectomy syndrome, one wonders if the lesions were asymmetrical in a system balanced across the midline or balanced against the amygdala. A differential emotional drive to the two hemispheres would hardly be conducive to survival. At any rate, the septal syndrome soon subsides and leaves the animal apparently less motivated to respond to thirst, rewards and pleasurable stimuli. The animal can still fight but it appears to be less motivated to do so. Its instincts for race preservation may be said to be reduced. Learning responses are retained but it is difficult to motivate the animal, even to avoid punishment. Animals with septal ablation will 'perseverate' in behavioural responses though unrewarded or positively punished. Indeed they show a heightened tendency to initiate responses and will not wait for appropriate cues. One hypothesis about septal function is that it exerts inhibitory control of the sensory input, motivation mechanisms and evaluation of reinforcement contingencies, or inhibition of responses in collaboration with the hippocampus.

Clearly the behavioural responses evoked by stimulation of the amygdaloid and septal circuits are exteriorized through the hypothalamus and mid-brain. They are under feedback control from the hippocampal formation where these appetitive drives are integrated with *satiety* responses from the ventromedial nucleus of the hypothalamus (p. 248) and with the total association function of the hippocampus in the formation of *conditional responses*, memory and reasoning (Chapter 13). The whole 'limbic system', with its alerting and sleep provoking mechanism, constitutes a 'gate control' for alerted attention. As shown earlier, this involves inhibition of unwanted sensory signals. Painful signals are of no further necessity when they have caused an orientating reaction and been assessed as dangerous or not dangerous by the limbic system. If not further suppressed, pain sensation is linked with an unpleasant emotional tone which gradually dominates.

THE 'AFFECT' OF PAIN PERCEPTION

Some spinothalamic fibres are relayed to the amygdala from the posterior complex of the thalamus and can thus enter the hippocampal formation and the orbitofrontal cortex, in addition to the spinoreticular and mesencephalic relays to limbic cortex (p. 68). This suprathalamic spread may account for pain which persists after all surgical procedures at or below the thalamus but which can be dissociated from its affective component by prefrontal leucotomy. This *'mental pain'* as it has been called is scarcely alleviated by conventional analgesics but may be relieved by a combination of an analgesic drug with one that suppresses limbic system responses such as a phenothiazine. Unfortunately, this pathway is specially suited for incorporation of pain signals into conditional responses so that a non-pain stimulus or its central 'symbol' (Chapter 12) may suffice to reactivate the sensation interpreted as pain.

It is not difficult to suggest a role for the above mechanisms in *motivation*. Primitive feeding and sexual drives are seen to involve the area of the brain most intimately concerned with conditional responses and learning, with outflow to the ergotropic and trophotropic functions of the hypothalamus and to the brain stem control for vocalization and axial movements (best seen in facial expression in man who does not have a tail to wag). An anencephalic infant with intact diencephalon, mid-brain and parts of the thalamus had apparently spontaneous whining and smiling and its face puckered after salty and bitter flavours. Sleep–wakefulness rhythm and brain stem and spinal reflexes were retained. The syndrome resembles the so-called *apallic syndrome* of decortication, with wakefulness but no consciousness. The EEG slowly but progressively returns to normal, including sleep–wake cycles (p. 144), but conscious awareness does not.

The *septal arousal system* is greater for the hippocampal and cingulate gyrus than for the neocortex, but all areas of cortex, including the motor areas, are facilitated by septal discharges. We can describe the somatomotor and autonomic results as the expressions of *emotion* but, perhaps by definition, this term should be restricted to man's introspective nervous system. We leave it to the philosophers to decide whether emotional feeling triggers this outflow or is the result of its experience in the context of remembered circumstances which evoked the same sensations. The neural apparatus is available for both views.

The role of the hippocampal formation in higher nervous functions is described in Chapter 13. The hypothalamic mechanism for sleep and arousal is reviewed in Chapter 15. They are driven by the amygdaloid and septal circuits, and it may be that the latter are involved in *sleep* and other *circadian rhythms*.

Lesions of the septal region in humans produce a form of coma described as *akinetic mutism*, a syndrome in which a patient lies motionless, speechless but with open eyes moving in all directions, apparently at random. They sometimes follow a target though without recognition. Protective reflexes are retained and may be exaggerated. Sphincter control is lost. Consciousness is disturbed, varying from deep coma, through coma vigile, somnolent coma, to an akinetic state with preservation of simple intellectual faculties. As recovery takes place, there is return of voice and facial expression and eventually spontaneous movements. Other limbic lesions (cingulate gyrus, fornix, mammillary bodies) may produce a similar syndrome. Clearly this is not a disconnection syndrome but rather a withdrawal of a diffuse activation system. It may be related to a marked depression of cortical and hippocampal acetylcholine, a deficiency which may also explain hyperdipsia. Cholinergic blockade in the medial and ventral aspects of the septal area mimics the effects of septal lesions. Interestingly, the major psychotropic drugs are anticholinergic as well as anti-adrenergic and anti-dopaminergic. The cholinergic output of the septum activates the neocortex and hippocampus, inhibits the hypothalamus except for the drinking response to corporeal fluid balance, and it activates the habenula. The other pathway to the mid-brain central grey matter through the medial forebrain bundle is possibly dopaminergic. (The upward flow of noradrenaline and serotonin in the bundle dominates chemical analysis.)

It may be speculated whether certain anaesthetic agents, such as the steroid anaesthetics, block the septal arousal system rather than the mesencephalic–thalamic reticular system. For light anaesthesia with block of contemporary memory and retention of vital reflexes the septum would seem to be an ideal target for the pharmacologist. Meanwhile, the amnesic effect of the centrally acting anticholinergics, atropine and scopolamine is a bonus for the anaesthetist.

Further reading

Kimmel H.D., Van Olst E.H. and Orlebeke J.F. (ed.) *The Orienting Reflex in Humans*. New York: Wiley, 1979.

Chapter 15
Arousal, attention and consciousness

Throughout this book it has been obvious that the central nervous system is a conglomerate of interconnected but relatively discrete functional systems each of which is dispersed anatomically. It has been necessary to ascend, descend and traverse the neuraxis many times in the presentation and a simple regional approach to function would have been grossly misleading. The same is true of 'the ascending arousal system' to which attention was drawn by the 1949 paper of Moruzzi and Magoun. It is misleading to consider that cortical arousal is the sole function of the upper reticular formation of brain stem and thalamus, or that only the reticular structures are involved in arousal (and the related desynchronization of cortical electrical activity as recorded in the EEG). In a book of this nature it is impossible to pursue all the ramifications of the reticular formation and its connections. The following section deals only with the distributed system, which is commonly known as the *diffuse activating system*. It activates both the cerebral cortex and the anterior horns of the spinal cord. Some cells project only caudally (reticulospinal), others only rostrally (reticulocortical) but they are commonly linked synaptically and many cells have branching axons passing both up and down. Nevertheless, it is too simplistic to regard the system as acting either diffusely or not at all. Discrete connections are well recognized and provide a mechanism for selective activation as well as diffuse arousal.

Believed to be a 'primitive' neural system appearing early in evolution, it would be surprising if the reticular formation depended only on collateral branches from the axons carrying sensory data into the brain. This early concept of its anatomy has now been abandoned. Sensory impulses entering the spinal cord by dorsal nerve roots are relayed in the dorsal horn to the *spinoreticular tract* (which is intermingled with the spinothalamic tract) running to the *lateral part of the reticular formation* of the medulla, pons and mid-brain. These are relayed onwards by long ascending fibres, including the *central tegmental tract*, and by short chains of neurones to the 'non-specific' nuclei of the thalamus. The trigeminal sensory nucleus sends an important contribution of primary sensory fibres (*Fig.* 15.1). The anaesthetist should be aware that cutaneous stimulation is most effective for arousal when applied to the trigeminal area. It probably has particular significance in activating the central nervous system and the reticular control of respiration at the time of birth. Primary sensory fibres can also be traced from the glossopharyngeal and vagal nerves.

On the other hand, the special senses (receptors for distance detection) contribute generalized arousal stimuli only through collateral branches or relays in the mid-brain (eg superior colliculus for light stimulation). The observation that visual, auditory and olfactory stimuli are more effective promoters of arousal if the stimulus is 'meaningful' may indicate that corticoreticular or limbic connections (or both together) are important. They descend with the corticospinal fibres and in the central tegmental bundle (p. 52). Nevertheless, convergence of spinoreticular and corticoreticular fibres on the lateral part of the upper brain stem reticular formation suggests that it is an 'association' area, in the same sense as we have used that term for certain areas of the cortex and so some possibility of 'conditional' arousal is implied.

From the cells of the lateral reticular formation of the medulla and pons, dendrites

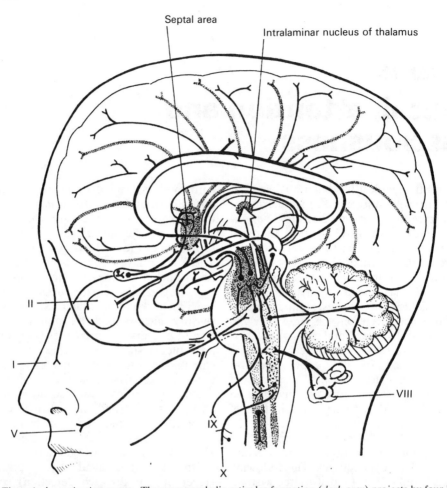

Fig. 15.1. *The reticular activating system.* The mesencephalic reticular formation (*dark grey*) projects by four bundles to the intralaminar nucleus of thalamus, the septal area, and secondarily to limbic lobe and neocortex. It also projects to cerebellum and spinal cord. The system is stimulated by ascending spinoreticular impulses and by collaterals from cranial nerves I, II, V, VIII, IX and X. The mesencephalic reticular formation and septal areas are linked but separate 'arousal' areas for the cortex.

pass transversely to synapse with cells in the *medial reticular formation* for upward and downward relay. The functional significance of the reticulospinal projection is discussed on p. 220. The rostral projection is important for activation of higher centres. This does not exclude more restricted localized functions although early writers found it difficult to see how any specificity of input could be maintained in a virtual network. Later research showed that the reticular net is more apparent than real. Discrete input–output connections can certainly be identified for some parts of the complex (*Fig.* 15.1). Furthermore, it has

become clear that the reticular grey matter is not the only connection between afferent signals and arousal behaviour. Fibres from the medullary, pontine and mesencephalic reticular formation project directly or via interneurones to (i) 'non-specific' nuclei of thalamus, (ii) septal area, (iii) hypothalamus, (iv) neostriatum.

The so-called '*non-specific*' *nuclei of thalamus* include the intralaminar nuclei, midline nuclei and the reticular thalamic nucleus. Unlike the 'specific' nuclei they do not project to primary sensory areas of the cortex. A prominent one is the *centromedian nucleus* and it certainly does not project diffusely to the whole cortex as formerly believed but almost exclusively to the claustrum and striatum. We have suggested that it relays kinaesthetic and vestibular influences to the striatum (Chapter 7). The *intralaminar and midline nuclei* project to the entorhinal and limbic areas. Other localized parts project to the orbitofrontal or parieto-occipital cortex, but apparently none to the cortex as a whole. Even the *reticular thalamic nucleus*, which surrounds the thalamus, is no longer believed by anatomists to project to the cerebral cortex. It is now considered to integrate signals passing from thalamus to cortex and back again and then to give feedback control to the lower 'non-specific' ascending projections, possibly acting as a 'gate' for selective alerting (p. 137).

Some authorities still regard a 'non-specific' thalamocortical relay as important and advocate the *ventral anterior nucleus* of the thalamus as the relay centre, but clearly the original model of a non-specific alerting system relaying in the thalamus is fighting for survival. This pathway does seem to be involved in certain recruiting EEG responses to rhythmical peripheral stimulation but not to the EEG desynchronization of arousal which was the original observation. That response can be evoked by high-frequency thalamic stimulation as well as by peripheral stimulation but it now seems that the thalamus projects down to the mesencephalic reticular formation which then desynchronizes cortical electrical activity by an ascending pathway bypassing the thalamus ventrally to reach the subthalamus, hypothalamus and septum (*Fig.* 15.1).

The nuclei of the *septal area* (in front of the anterior commissure at the base of the brain above the olfactory tubercle), receive fibres from the posterior hippocampus and feed back to an adjacent hippocampal area and also downwards to the lateral hypothalamus. An interplay of two reciprocal connections, septal-hypothalamic and amygdaloid-hypothalamic, appears to be involved in some form of attention response or *orientating reflex* which is at least as important as the mesencephalic reticular formation system in arousal but which is coupled with behavioural reactions for flight or defence, suppression of ongoing behaviour and with emotional and autonomic reactions.

Bilateral destruction of the amygdala in experimental animals reduces the flight response whereas bilateral destruction of the septal area is said to produce aggressive behaviour, with manifestations of rage, but responses to stimulation are contingent on concurrent activity elsewhere in the brain. The subject is discussed further in the chapter on 'the limbic system' (Chapter 14). The septal and amygdaloid nuclei, along with the fornix–mammillothalamic–hypothalamic path previously described (p. 118), form alternative connections from hippocampus to hypothalamus and reticular formation involved in arousal and probably in selective attention of the cortex while novelty and significance are being assessed, and no doubt they provide connections for alerting the brain in response to the conceptualizing processes involving memory and verbal modelling which are designated as 'thought'. When they are out of action, the subject can still be wakened by the mesencephalic system but he is *akinetic and mute*.

The behavioural responses to forebrain-induced arousal are predominantly septal to the *hypothalamus* (for regulation of the internal organs) or amygdaloid to the reticular formation and *neostriatum* (to prepare the 'set' for somatic motor responses). They are complementary, not alternative outflows from the hippocampal system, and are strongly interconnected by catecholamine- and serotonin-containing fibres. The *medial forebrain bundle*, one of the important connecting systems between septal and tegmental grey matter, also carries an upward-directed polysynaptic system of neurones which has been postulated to govern the synthesis of catecholamine transmitters in the forebrain.

Pribram has emphasized three neurally distinct and separate attentional systems — arousal, activation and effort—all integrated in the hippocampus. According to this model, there is a simple stereotyped stimulus–response relationship using upper brain stem connections to produce 'automatic' behaviour (as seen during epileptic fits involving the medial surface of the temporal lobe). If a sensory input is not 'recognized' as a match for stored memory signals, the median raphe and associated mesencephalic reticular formation transmit by serotoninergic neurones to the hippocampus, as an *'orientating arousal'* or 'stop' signal which inhibits the reticular formation via the amygdala. Electrical activity of the amygdala becomes synchronized and the hippocampal cortex desynchronized. A parallel ascending system from the more laterally situated periaqueductal grey matter, including the locus coeruleus, sends dopaminergic and adrenergic fibres to the hippocampus as an *'activating arousal'* or 'go' signal which relays to somatomotor mechanisms via the basal ganglia, initiating a tonic motor 'set' preparatory to movement — a 'what is to be done?' response. Electrical activity of the hippocampal cortex assumes a 4–8 Hz theta rhythm: the posterior cortical alpha rhythm is desynchronized, and the motor area of the cortex shows a DC negative shift ('contingent negative variation') which goes sharply positive when a motor decision is taken (Chapter 16). A third system is a hippocampal coordination of amygdala and basal ganglion activity, uncoupling the lower level stimulus–response reflex and delaying the response until central computation (parietal and frontal), and fairly described as *'reasoning'*, takes place. The attention involved is *voluntary*, therefore, in the sense that it is initiated by the organism rather than by some input event.

Pribram considers that what he terms *'effort'* is used to maintain efficiency by reducing equivocation between sensory channels. The sensation of effort may be related to isometric contraction of the musculature which commonly accompanies concentration and problem-solving. (It cannot be an afferent feedback from proprioceptors but may be an awareness of corollary discharge, p. 242. Even the layman refers to cognitive effort as work.) Recent studies show local differences of cerebral blood flow and metabolism associated with 'cerebral work'.

The effort to reduce afferent equivocation by concentration is not always desirable. Free association in a relaxed state or even during light sleep may be more profitable for problem-solving as well as for artistic pursuits. Serial associations, delayed in time, require the distributed memory systems already discussed and the additional circuitry of the frontal lobes.

Consciousness

It is notorious that consciousness is not amenable to definition in terms of simpler concepts. Nevertheless some of its homonyms, awareness, concentration, voluntary activity, alertness, indicate an integration of sensory associations with higher motor controls and arousal. The temptation to localize this 'function' at a convergent area such as the pre-frontal lobes must be resisted. The single lesson from our analysis of sensory processing, and to be confirmed in the motor system, is that the central nervous system uses distributed systems sharpened by feedback controls. There is no reason to suppose that consciousness is different and it is not unreasonable to seek various attributes of the conscious state in local circuits, concentration and volition anteriorly, awareness post-centrally with interpretation based on limbic memory and emotion circuits, and alertness on a dispersed arousal system.

Clinical experience does not indicate a single 'centre of consciousness'. In metabolic brain disease there is progressive loss of higher integrative functions in a remarkably regular sequence:

1. Loss of concentration and volition ('apathy') with defective appreciation of concepts (symbols) and of temporal factors including short term memory.
2. Loss of appreciation of extracorporeal space and recent memory while self data and long term memory are retained. Disorientation in time, and then for space and for persons.
3. Confusion, delirium, loss of access to all memory and failure to store new memories, so that serial subtraction is impossible. Defective perceptions and illusions may cause violent behaviour. Decreasing awareness is accompanied by drowsiness, sometimes alternating with agitation in delirium.
4. Stupor, no awareness, still responsive to stimulation but unable to form new associations.
5. Coma, with motor response only to maximal stimulation.
6. Coma with progressive loss of brain stem reflex functions in a rostral–caudal sequence (ocular motility, pupil reflexes,

respiration, cardiovascular control). Unexplained 'release' phenomena include irregular tremor, asterixis and multifocal myoclonus.

In slowly progressive disease states, this sequence is very suggestive of progressive synaptic block from higher associative cortices through hippocampal circuits to the mid-brain and pontine reticular formation.

Waking, sleep and coma

The term 'waking state' is to be preferred to consciousness to avoid semantic confusion between the 'level' of consciousness and its 'content'. Levels of the waking state range from directed attention through alertness, relaxed mood, drowsiness to sleep, stupor and coma. Various 'coma scales' such as that advocated by our neurosurgical colleagues in Glasgow (*Table* 15.1) do not grade the level of awareness, but rather the degree of stimulation required to evoke a range of motor responses (EMV = Eye opening; best Motor response; best Verbal response). They are given a numerical value and the items are chosen because low EMV scores have been shown to correlate with poor prognosis for recovery from coma after head injury and a number of other cerebral disorders.

SLEEP

The gradations from drowsiness, with vagal visceromotor dominance, to alertness and directed attention with sympathetic and somatomotor activation have been described above. The questions now arising are (*a*) is sleep merely an inhibition of arousal mechanisms, and (*b*) does it differ in kind from coma?

When interest was first directed to the possibility of a general arousal system projecting from reticular formation to cortex, with possible relay from non-specific areas of the thalamus, it seemed plausible that sleep and coma were essentially the same and due to withdrawal of sensory stimulated activation. It soon appeared that 'deactivation' is also an active function involving specific parts of the reticular formation.

ANTERIOR HYPOTHALAMIC ACTIVATION

The classical studies of Hess showed that (in cat) apparently natural sleep could be induced by low frequency stimulation of points in the medial thalamus, caudate nucleus and hypothalamus (preoptic and supraoptic). Further experiments on animals, and clinical studies on man, indicate a 'sleep centre' in the *anterior hypothalamus* which has a reciprocal

Table 15.1. Glasgow Coma Scale

Motor response		Score
Eye opening	Spontaneous	E 4
	To speech	3
	To standardized pain	2
	None	1
Best motor response	Obeying command	M 6
	Localizing	5
	Withdrawing	4
	Abnormal flexion ⎫ to standardized pain	3
	Extension ⎭	2
	None	1
Best verbal response	Orientated in time and space (aware of self and environment)	V 5
	Confused conversation	4
	Inappropriate speech, exclamatory, expletive	3
	Incomprehensible (not recognizable words)	2
	None	1

functional relationship with the general activation and arousal system. Natural sleep is an active process of the anterior hypothalamic system which is believed to entrain recuperative autonomic and metabolic processes. Coma and general anaesthesia are due to interruption or synaptic blockade of the arousal system, clearly different from natural sleep.

In sleep the cerebral blood flow and metabolism are increased and pituitary secretion of human growth hormone is increased. In coma, including general anaesthesia, these functions are decreased. Exceptions are ketamine and diazepam which cause loss of consciousness without any reduction in cerebral metabolic rate. Demonstrably, sleep differs from coma in being associated with *metabolic changes for growth and conservation of energy*. These features are not, however, continuous throughout the sleeping state, indicating that the hormonal secretion does not have an independent circadian rhythm. The rise in human growth hormone (HGH) is loosely associated with a phase of sleep characterized by slow wave activity in the scalp EEG, especially during the life stage of sexual maturation. Although circadian and other rhythms may be dominant, it has been clearly established that secretory activities of growth hormone, prolactin and pubertal luteinizing hormone secretory activities are closely linked to the sleep–wake cycle. Other hormones (ACTH and thyrotropin-releasing hormone) that have more complex cycles tend to be suppressed by sleep. Nitrogen retaining, anabolic effects are dominant and form a basis for the traditional belief in the recuperative effects of sleep and its special requirement in the growth period. Serotoninergic neurones play an important but complicated role and endorphins may have a role in controlling the secretion of growth hormone and prolactin.

POSTERIOR HYPOTHALAMIC RELEASE

From an early stage of sleep there is water retention associated with augmented secretion of antidiuretic hormone (ADH) (a cause of morning oedema though beneficial for bladder comfort). The pupils constrict, heart rate slows, the blood pressure falls and gut activity is reduced. Skin blood vessels dilate and muscle tone is reduced, a combination leading to a fall in body temperature which is terminated by the arousal effect of coldness of the skin. All these features point to a degree of posterior hypothalamic release (Chapter 25) during natural sleep, rather than to withdrawal of reticular formation arousal alone. The ease with which the sleeper can be aroused by a range of stimuli, especially conditional ones ('meaningful'), points to the continuing activity of the reticular formation. Withdrawal of light and noise *permits* sleep, but warmth, satiety (for food or sex) and fluid intake along with injection of ADH will actively *induce* sleep. Best of all is a quiet mind, from a hippocampus not aroused by the septal area. Stimulation of the anterior hypothalamus in man produces behavioural unresponsiveness, and excitation of the posterior hypothalamus (in animals) evokes arousal. Changing dominance of these functions causes recognizable 'sleep phases'.

The possibility that endogenous ligands for opioid receptors in the brain have an active role in sleep is an intriguing variant on the old concept of a hypnotoxin as the 'cause' of sleep but it is without convincing evidence. Sleep-associated HGH secretion is reduced by somatostatin which is widespread in the nervous system, including the hypothalamus. At this time, monoaminergic *neuronal* control of sleep–wake behaviour involving related hypothalamic neurones seems more probable than a humoral mechanism conveyed by the blood.

Phases of sleep

It is necessary to guard against swinging from one extreme to the other. To recognize the primary importance of the hypothalamus in 'going to sleep' is not to deny any role to the reticular activating system. Two distinct forms of sleep have been identified. As both occur in most sleep cycles they are described as phases of sleep rather than types.

SLOW WAVE SLEEP

Slow wave sleep, or the 'orthodox phase', is so called because of its EEG correlates: others refer to it as non-rapid eye movement (NREM) sleep because of absence of a feature characteristic of the other phase. Some muscle tone is retained. Tendon jerks are depressed, plantar responses dorsiflexor ('extensor') and pupils constricted. The eyelids close and the eyes roll slowly. Breathing and heart rate are regular. Parasympathetic tone is dominant. Dreaming is virtually absent. The various stages are more conveniently described with the EEG phenomena (p. 148). This phase of sleep is due to the active influence, probably serotoninergic, of the posterior hypothalamus, released by the amygdaloid-septal controls (Chapter 14). It is becoming acceptable to describe it as 'the forebrain phase of sleep'.

RAPID EYE MOVEMENT SLEEP

Light sleep associated with low voltage, faster (2–6 Hz) EEG activity, dreaming and rapid eye movements (REM) is different in character. Rapid eye movements and fine twitching of face and limbs are associated with dreams that have an emotional content. In man muscle tone is reduced between the movements. Respiration, heart rate and blood pressure fluctuate quite sharply. Body metabolic rate is increased, gastric acid output is raised, urine volume decreases and osmolarity increases. Very characteristically there is penile erection in the male or increased vaginal blood flow in the female unless the concomitant dream has a high anxiety content. All these phenomena make it difficult to accept that this is a 'hindbrain phase of sleep', as it is often called. That rubric is more appropriate for another type of sleep with which REM sleep is often homologated.

PARADOXICAL SLEEP

In the cat, the slow wave phase of sleep is followed by a phase of *deep* sleep with low voltage EEG activity identical to that of wakefulness in both neocortex and hippocampal formation. There is good experimental evidence that it is associated with suppression of the reticular arousal system of the mid-brain coupled with activity of the mesencephalo-mammillo-hypothalamic fibres in the mammillary peduncle (*see Fig. 14.1*), a chain of neurones starting in the pontine reticular formation. It is possibly the ascending limb of hippocampal mid-brain circuits which shows considerable species differences. In some respects it is different from REM sleep in man and it may be premature to accept that REM sleep and 'paradoxical' sleep are interchangeable terms. After total sleep deprivation the cat has more frequent stages of REM sleep: the human has more stage IV of non-REM sleep and relative absence of stages I, II and III (*see below*). In the cat, 'paradoxical' (EEG desynchronized) sleep is deep sleep. In man REM sleep occurs while emerging from deep sleep. Bearing these reservations in mind, the contemporary view is that human REM sleep is the homologue of cat 'paradoxical' sleep. Paradoxical or REM sleep is not activated until the subject has first experienced slow wave sleep except in certain pathological states such as narcolepsy in man, or after withdrawal of hypnotic drugs from a person who has been adapted to regular drug administration.

The rapid cortical EEG of REM sleep activity is activated by ponto-cortical ascending fibres (to mammillary and hypothalamic nuclei, transmitter unknown but possibly acetylcholine) additional to the ascending reticular system responsible for cortical arousal. The latter are considered to be *noradrenergic* neurones from the *locus coeruleus* (Chapter 3) ascending in the ventral part of the mid-brain and relaying in the hypothalamus to be distributed widely to all areas of the cerebral cortex bilaterally and to the cerebellum and via the central tegmental bundle, to the spinal cord where they inhibit muscular tonus. The locus coeruleus innervates the entire neuraxis. In the waking state, stimulation of the same area causes agitation with increased muscular tone. As noradrenaline is inhibitory to cortex, Purkinje cells and motoneurones, it is likely that arousal is through disinhibition of interneurones. A current simplification that reticular formation serotonin induces sleep and noradrenaline causes arousal is certainly too naive. The ventilatory response to CO_2 is much decreased during REM sleep and it is at this time that the risk for *sleep apnoea* is greatest (p. 192).

SLEEP STAGES

Normal nocturnal sleep has characteristic sleep stages. These are recognized by the associated EEG phenomena and will be described later. The EEG characteristics are used to define drowsiness and four stages of slow wave sleep of increasing depth. The REM type of sleep is recognized as a separate sleep stage by the muscular and autonomic responses described above as well as by the EEG features.

SLEEP CYCLES

Normal sleep shows a cyclical sequence of sleep stages. As the drowsy person 'falls asleep' the first cycle begins with stage I of non-REM sleep, deepens to stages II–IV and then, after about 60 minutes, sleep lightens but to a REM stage unless roused by a meaningful stimulus. This is followed by further cycles of longer duration (80–120 minutes), usually five to seven cycles but varying with age and other factors. Some 20–25 per cent of sleep time is in REM sleep, proportionately more in young people.

It is difficult to give a definition of sleep which will subsume all these variables. It is certainly a loss of wakefulness but it is not a complete loss of consciousness. By certain criteria of responsiveness it can be shown that a degree of consciousness (awareness of significance of stimuli) continues until stage II begins, and cortical vigilance (as shown by evoked responses or K-complexes) continues into stage IV. It may be that *wakefulness* is controlled by the noradrenergic system of the locus coeruleus and *awareness* by the cortex, especially the hippocampus. On the contrary, with coma awareness is lost earlier than wakefulness.

Stupor and coma

Stupor and coma are pathological disturbances of consciousness/wakefulness. *Stupor* is unresponsiveness from which a person can only be roused by strong repeated stimulation. *Coma* is a more advanced stage of the same disorder in which the unresponsive subject is unrousable (p. 141). Unlike sleep, which is an active physiological process, coma is due to loss of function of both the cerebral cortex and the ascending reticular activating system.

GENERAL ANAESTHESIA

Both of these grey areas with multisynaptic connections are very vulnerable to abnormal metabolic states, including hypoxia and drugs. Pharmaceuticals used for sedation and general anaesthesia are important examples of the latter. The clinical signs of coma, whether from disease or drugs, are due to loss of synaptic functions at all levels of the central nervous system. As this is a progressive impairment, it is possible to construct a series from alert wakefulness, through lethargy/drowsiness, obtundation, stupor, *coma vigile*/akinetic mutism, to coma. The unrousable state of coma cannot be further subdivided: so-called 'coma scales' (p. 141) record associated losses of cerebral functions. The wakefulness to coma series indicates progressive loss of higher (cortical) functions followed by depression of the brain stem arousal system or its disconnection from the integrative cortex. It is a loss of diencephalic and pontomesencephalic arousal systems rather than imposition of an active process as in sleep.

General anaesthesia produces coma, not sleep. The same is true with most hypnotic drugs used to induce sleep but it is the intention of pharmacologists to produce true sleep promoting drugs. That the difference is a genuine one is shown by the fact that sleep cycles can often be identified in the comatose patient, though the wakeful behaviour is rudimentary and without self-awareness.

Stages of anaesthesia

STAGE 1: ANALGESIA

Before consciousness is lost the subject can reply to questions and has normal reflexes but no pain is felt from tissue damaging stimulation. Respiration is quiet and regular.

STAGE 2: EXCITEMENT OR DELIRIUM

Awareness is lost. The subject is unable to respond to commands but may talk, move his limbs or show aggressive behaviour. The motor behavioural pattern is not a rational response to the environment. Reflexes remain active, including pharyngeal and autonomic. They may be disinhibited. (The cardiovascular risks of premature surgical stimulation are well known.) Respiration is irregular and breath holding may occur, a supranuclear response. Vomiting may occur.

STAGE 3: SURGICAL ANAESTHESIA

There are four phases of stage 3:

Phase 1 Breathing becomes regular ('automatic') and limb movements cease, though tone is not completely destroyed. Pharyngeal reflexes begin to disappear but laryngeal and peritoneal reflexes remain. There are marked eyeball movements.

Phase 2 Respiration continues regularly but it is shallower. Muscle tone is less and laryngeal and peritoneal reflexes disappear. The eyes are now fixed centrally.

Phase 3 Intercostal muscles become paralysed and the limb and trunk muscles relax.

Phase 4 With progressive paralysis of the diaphragm the respiratory volume becomes very small. There is full muscular relaxation. Autonomic reflexes are progressively reduced.

STAGE 4: MEDULLARY PARALYSIS

Respiration is gasping and finally ceases. Vasomotor reflexes are depressed. Vasoconstriction causes coldness and pallor of the skin but it is insufficient to maintain blood pressure and the pulse is feeble. The pupils are widely dilated.

The drug affects all levels of the neuraxis simultaneously and it must not be assumed that lower levels are normal in the early stages of anaesthesia. With this proviso, it is clear that stages 1 and 2 indicate major hemisphere depression followed in stages 3 and 4 by progressive arrest of function from the midbrain down to the medulla. As their function is not required by the comatose subject it is less evident that the cerebellum and spinal cord are

also depressed but not sufficiently to block reflex responses to painful stimuli, or sphincter continence.

As in many other conditions of neural damage (synaptic or axonal) loss of function may be preceded by brief hyperexcitability. Hypoxia causes decreased accommodation (p. 8), lowered stimulation threshold and withdrawal of higher level inhibition over lower levels of the nervous system. Vomiting, myoclonus, laryngeal spasm and autonomic overreaction including salivation, bronchorrhoea, bronchospasm and tachycardia are transient if stage 2 is not prolonged. Epileptic fits of generalized type are probably caused by withdrawal of inhibition but the site of the de-repression is unknown. Every coma-producing drug has the same potential but there are important differences in the concentrations required to produce stages 1 and 4. This difference, the 'safety margin', is important in the selection of a chemical as an anaesthetic agent.

Brain stem death

The discussion on coma has concentrated on (i) alertness, (ii) awareness of environment and self, (iii) appropriateness of behavioural responses with speech function as an index of highest awareness. The so-called coma scales do not attempt to evaluate the degree of facilitatory-drive from the central reticular formation or the amygdaloid-septal complex. Damage at brain stem level is potentially lethal. Whereas signs of brain stem damage are not included in the coma scales, the situation is entirely different with regard to survivability. It is now generally accepted that no meaningful life can persist if the lower brain stem is grossly damaged by a lesion known to be irremediable and causing failure of CO_2 responsiveness of respiration (Chapter 20).

The criteria for 'brain stem death' vary from one country to another. The following summary is of the British criteria which are being increasingly accepted. Provided that a human subject is in apnoeic coma due to irremediable structural brain damage caused by a 'disorder which can lead to brain death' (defined to clinicians), the subject may be considered to be dead if certain brain stem reflexes are absent and if there is no respiratory response to a standard CO_2 challenge. (If oculocephalic responses, p. 170, are present it is unnecessary to test the following reflexes as surviving brain stem function is thus demonstrated.)

Given the above preconditions, there should be:

1. No pupillary response to light (p. 181).
2. No corneal reflex (p. 164).
3. No vestibulo-ocular reflexes (p. 172). (In coma the response is tonic deviation of eyes. The nystagmus quick phase may be absent.)
4. No motor responses within the cranial nerves' distribution in response to adequate stimulation of any somatic area (head, trunk or limbs).
5. No gag reflex response (p. 165) to bronchial stimulation by suction catheter passed down to the carina.

Failure of the apnoea response must be demonstrated after disconnection from a ventilator. The important defect is loss of the CO_2 response, not failure of anoxic driving. For this reason the subject should be pre-oxygenated with 100 per cent oxygen for 10 minutes before disconnection, then given 5 per cent CO_2 in 95 per cent oxygen for a further 5 minutes to ensure a starting $Paco_2$ of $5 \cdot 3$ kPa (40 mmHg). The patient is then disconnected from the ventilator and 100 per cent oxygen (at 6 l/min) should be insufflated into the trachea to maintain diffusion oxygenation. (The intra-tracheal catheter should be passed to the carina. Disconnection from the ventilator should be maintained for 10 minutes.) Failure to evoke an inspiration response indicates complete apnoea since the $Paco_2$ of the blood will certainly exceed the necessary level. (It should be checked if possible at the end of the test.)

Further reading

Parkes J.D. *Sleep and its Disorders*. London: Saunders, 1985.

Routtenberg A. The two arousal hypotheses. Reticular formation and limbic system. *Psychol. Rev.* 1968; **75**: 51–80.

Chapter 16

The electroencephalogram

The electroencephalogram (EEG) (*Fig.* 16.1) is the electrical activity recorded by conventionally placed electrodes over the scalp. It is an attenuated and smoothed form of the *electrocorticogram*. In the waking but relaxed state rhythmical sinusoidal potentials wax and wane. A characteristic of the human EEG is the 8–12 Hz *alpha rhythm* in areas posterior to the central sulcus, occurring independently in both hemispheres but with similar frequency on each side. Children have a prominent 4–7 Hz *theta rhythm* over temporal areas, decreasing in amplitude and distribution as the brain matures, but tending to recur transiently in response to emotional disturbance. Some persons have a non-sinusoidal 14–16 Hz *mu rhythm* (*rythme en arceau*) over the motor cortex, near the vertex or more commonly over the hand motor area. It is usually bilateral but asynchronous. Anterior to this the potential changes may be of considerable amplitude but are not rhythmical except in persons with frontal lobe disease.

The waves are not action potentials but are believed to 'represent synchronized *dendritic potentials* superimposed on slowly varying potential differences across the cortex (DC shifts). Arousal, and especially fixation of attention on a visual pattern or performance of mental activity such as calculation, desynchronizes the alpha rhythm. The common clinical term 'alpha blocking' is probably incorrect, deriving from a time when the physiological basis of these rhythms was even less well understood. It is not an inhibition that flattens the alpha rhythm, rather the synchronized state of the EEG in the wakened but relaxed state results from inhibition by thalamocortical fibres of a higher frequency driving of cortical synapses by the mesencephalic reticular form-

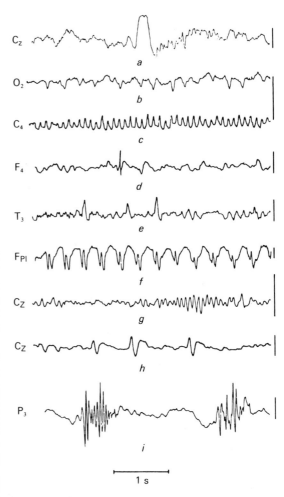

Fig. 16.1. Some examples of EEG waveforms (monopolar recording). (*a*) K-complex; (*b*) lambda wave; (*c*) mu rhythm; (*d*) spike; (*e*) sharp waves; (*f*) repetitive spike and wave activity; (*g*) sleep spindle, (*h*) vertex sharp waves, (*i*) polyspike discharges. Calibration marks all 100 μV, 1·0 sec.

147

ation. When the latter dominates during alerting, the alpha rhythm is desynchronized. Desynchronization of the motor strip mu rhythm occurs contralateral to a strong voluntary contraction of the muscles of a limb.

SLEEP STAGES

The transition from wakefulness to drowsiness is marked by increased amplitude of post-central alpha rhythm and its frequency may slow by 0·5–1·0 Hz. *Beta rhythm* (14 Hz or faster) may appear anteriorly especially when drowsiness is induced by a drug. (It is reasonably symmetrical unless thalamofrontal projections on one side are damaged.) With onset of true sleep a number of changes occur. For convenience these are described in accordance with the sleep stages (Chapter 15). The EEG stages merge into each other (*Fig.* 16.2).

SLEEP STAGE 1

The alpha rhythm disappears and low amplitude 2–7 Hz slow waves appear, randomly distributed and not rhythmic, but tending to group into irregularly spaced bursts. Quite modest but meaningful auditory stimuli will still arouse the subject causing reappearance of alpha activity (an apparent paradox if early sleep is not recognized). Electrical potentials generated by eyeball movements are recorded in anterior channels: these eyeball movements are slow and may last for several seconds. Muscle activity is otherwise diminished.

SLEEP STAGE 2

Alpha rhythm is now absent and 2–7 Hz waves more prominent, often bilaterally synchronous. Transient sharp waves, positive with respect to an 'indifferent' reference electrode, appear in occipital areas, usually not synchronously. Bilaterally synchronous negative sharp waves are recorded at the vertex of the skull. These are probably potentials evoked by an exteroceptive or interoceptive stimulus. *K complexes*, with a similar distribution, are certainly the result of sensory stimuli but not modality-specific (p. 151). Like the vertex

SLEEP

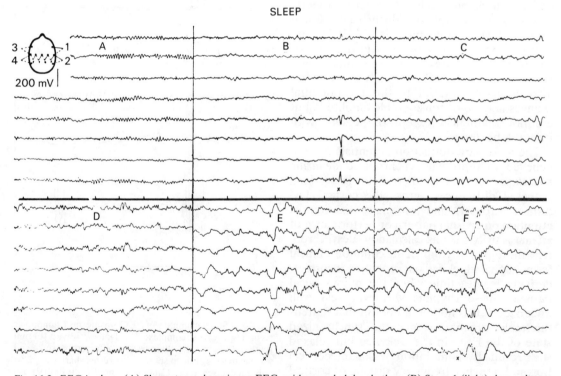

Fig. 16.2. *EEG in sleep.* (A) Sleep stage, drowsiness; EEG, widespread alpha rhythm. (B) Stage 1 (light); low voltage, mixed frequencies, vertex sharp waves (X). (C) Stage 1 (deeper); theta dominance. (D) Stage 2; delta activity: sleep spindles. (E) Stage 3; increasing irregular delta. (F) Stage 4; K-complexes in response to sound.

transient sharp waves, they are negative going but they are followed by a positive slow wave which is often followed by a sleep spindle. The *sleep spindle* is a short (few seconds) burst of 12–14 Hz waves of wide scalp distribution maximal over central regions and bilaterally synchronous and symmetrical. (The latter characteristics of an EEG phenomenon indicate that it is the result of *'projected' activity* from a common source near the midline and usually thalamic or lower in origin.) Sleep spindles are highly characteristic of forebrain sleep and the other transients just described show that the cortex is still rousable by afferent signals relayed through the thalamus.

SLEEP STAGE 3

Stage 3 is characterized by very slow (*delta*) waves of 2 Hz or slower frequency for 20–50 per cent of the time. They are of much higher amplitude than the 2–7 Hz waves of sleep stage 2. The evoked potentials and sleep spindles disappear as this stage deepens.

SLEEP STAGE 4

Delta activity dominates the record. It is polymorphic, not rhythmic, not bilaterally synchronous and, most importantly, not confined to one localized area of scalp (identified by phase reversals between adjacent recording channels with bipolar recording montages). K complexes are less easily identified and spindles and vertex sharp waves almost absent. Clearly the cortex is no longer responsive to thalamic projected activity.

During the sleep cycle, the subject then rouses through these stages, but from stage 2, commonly emerges into *REM stage sleep* instead of waking. As the name suggests, the characteristic feature is the rapid jerky eyeball movements, recorded on anterior channels of the EEG. Other muscular activity remains low but behavioural changes indicate that sleep is lighter and the cortical record loses the delta activity of deep 'slow wave' sleep. Low voltage waves of mixed frequency include an alpha-like rhythm but 1–2 Hz slower than the alpha rhythm of the waking state. The cortical EEG has the appearance of a state of arousal and sleep is certainly lighter but the threshold for

arousal by auditory stimuli is increased. This apparent paradox has caused REM sleep to be equated with the 'paradoxical' or hindbrain sleep of the cat (p. 143). From this stage the subject then wakens up or enters another cycle of deeper 'forebrain' sleep with thalamocortical fibres inhibiting the higher frequency driving of cortical neurones from the mesencephalic reticular formation.

EEG IN DELIRIUM, STUPOR AND COMA

The EEG changes may be surprisingly slight in the minor degrees of depressed consciousness which are associated with loss of awareness rather than loss of alertness (p. 140). Alpha rhythm is slowed but may remain within the normal range. It is gradually dominated by theta (4–7 Hz) and delta (0·5–3 Hz) activity. The theta activity is commonly post-central and the delta pre-central, both tending to become bilaterally synchronous, monomorphic and rhythmical as the level of consciousness decreases, quite different from the slow waves in the EEG of deep sleep.

Runs of delta activity may alternate with periods of faster rhythms, but as coma deepens and the patient becomes entirely unresponsive this 'background activity' disappears. The delta amplitude diminishes and appears as bursts followed by isoelectric periods (*burst-suppression activity*) and eventually as death approaches (medullary failure) the EEG becomes flat and featureless.

An almost identical series of changes occurs with deep barbiturate sedation, myxoedema coma, or severe hypothermia. It is reversible, with clinical recovery, if life is sustained by passive ventilation of the lungs while these conditions are corrected. With drug narcosis, the EEG provides the best measure of depth of narcosis. Blood levels of drugs show a poor correlation with both the clinical state and the EEG activity.

Certain EEG phenomena (eg *triphasic waves*) appear with some leuco-encephalopathies, metabolic or viral. Their physiological basis is not understood and they have little relevance to anaesthesia, but it is necessary to be aware of a condition described by electroencephalographers as 'alpha coma'. It is seen with brain stem lesions caused by head injury or pontine infarction. The EEG recording resembles a normal waking or sleeping pattern with absence of the typical delta activity which is usually associated with coma. Unlike true alpha rhythm the waves are not restricted to the post-central areas, do not attenuate with arousal stimulation, and may vary in frequency by several cycles/second. A type with anterior distribution has a graver prognosis than one with predominantly posterior alpha-frequency activity, especially if sleep patterns do not appear within a few days.

EEG in general anaesthesia

A number of papers have recorded the EEG changes corresponding to stages of anaesthesia induced by volatile anaesthetic agents. We have been satisfied with a six-point scale described in 1977 by Brierley and Prior (*Fig.* 16.3).

EEG stage 1 (continuous) EEG activity is continuous.

EEG stage 2 (mild suppression-burst) Periods of suppression, not quite isoelectric, last for less than 1.0 second and are followed by bursts (of delta activity) of 100–300 µV.

EEG stage 3 (moderate suppression-burst) Suppression epochs, total or almost so, last for 1–2 seconds and burst amplitude is 100–300 µV.

EEG stage 4 (severe suppression-burst) There is total suppression (iso-electric EEG) for more than 3 seconds between bursts of reduced amplitude (50–100 µV).

EEG stage 5 (low voltage activity) Total flattening for more than 3 seconds occurs between brief bursts of low voltage waves (50 µV).

EEG stage 6 (isoelectric) The recording is flat from all parts of the scalp with amplifier gains set not less than 300 µV/cm.

These phenomena indicate loss of reactivity of cortex, thalamus and reticular formation. Suppression-burst activity may appear locally over surgically isolated areas of cerebral cortex — it is a *deafferentation pattern*, found bilaterally with some encephalopathies or hypothermia as well as with hypnotic and anaesthetic drugs. With the latter it is reversible, but EEG stages 5 and 6 have a bad prognosis for survival except in controlled anaesthesia. The cortex is not inhibited as in sleep. It is disconnected from all corticopetal inputs.

Evoked potentials

The very small potentials of cortical neurones firing in response to a very brief sensory stimulus

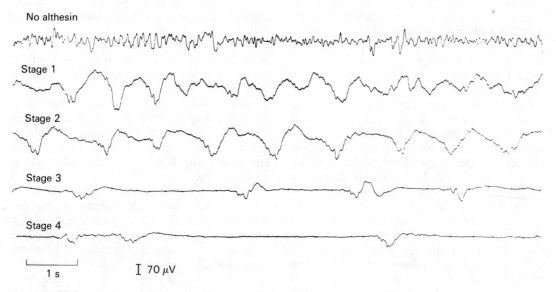

No althesin

Stage 1

Stage 2

Stage 3

Stage 4

1 s I 70 µV

Fig. 16.3. EEG stages in general anaesthesia: *see text* for description.

relayed through the thalamus are best seen by computer averaging techniques (isolating the evoked response which is time-locked to the stimulus from the spontaneous EEG which is relatively random when a large number of epochs are averaged). Some *primary evoked responses* may be of sufficient amplitude to be detected above the background activity, eg the *lambda waves* from photic stimulation (*Fig. 16.1*). Other primary cortical responses are too small to detect by contemporary methods, eg the response of Heschl's gyrus to a brief acoustic stimulus. Nevertheless, computer averaged vertex responses to a series of clicks applied to one ear show electrical potential shifts *before* the arrival of the thalamocortical signal. These are interpreted as volume conducted (not axonal conducted) *'far field' potential changes* generated at synapses at lower levels in the nervous system, summing algebraically potentials moving towards the cortex (vertex-positive) and others moving caudally (vertex-negative). By correlating the surface recording with others made from deep electrodes, and observing the latency shifts caused by local disease of the conducting pathways, it has been inferred that various wave peaks arise from electric events at identified anatomical sites, for example, in response to an acoustic signal, short latency potentials from auditory nerve, cochlear nuclei, olivary nuclei, inferior colliculi, lateral lemnisci, medial geniculate bodies, but doubtfully from Heschl's gyrus. It is for this reason that the waves recorded from the scalp are commonly termed *brain stem auditory evoked potentials*. The term 'cortical evoked potential' is, in fact, often a misnomer if by that is implied a thalamocortical discharge evoked from a lemniscal pathway.

LONG LATENCY RESPONSES

The response, whether seen or not at the primary receiving area, is followed by the *'secondary response'* of Forbes. It is oscillatory and affects the whole cortex bilaterally. In spontaneous or barbiturate-induced drowsiness the primary potentials increase in amplitude but the secondary late responses are decreased. These late potentials are probably cortical responses evoked by the extrathalamic route from the mesencephalic reticular formation (p. 49). The K-complexes and vertex-negative sharp waves seen in light sleep are similar *responses to startle*, not modality-specific (p. 139). The fact that the latter and the deliberately evoked responses are both decreased in amplitude in the alert state is further evidence for thalamocortical inhibition of spontaneous cortical activity (p. 123).

To increase the response from a primary afferent area fully awake it is necessary for the stimulus to be 'interesting' in a physiological sense. Local increase in amplitude is seen when attention is directed to a specific sensory modality (but soon habituates) and when appropriate patterned stimuli are used. This phenomenon is well seen with *visual evoked potentials* where sudden appearance or reversal of a pattern of luminance is more effective than an unstructured flash of light. The major positive component recorded over the posterior scalp at about 100 ms is mainly a foveal response corresponding to the lambda wave of classical electroencephalography which is associated with somatic eye movements. Secondary responses are also found but early 'far field' potentials are not clearly defined from retinal stimulation. Prolonged latency of the primary response is associated with conduction delays in the optic nerve, chiasma and tract.

SOMATOSENSORY EVOKED POTENTIALS

Electrical stimulation of a peripheral nerve, or natural stimulation of a skin area, evokes potential variation best seen over the contralateral Rolandic cortex where its arrival is signalled by a prominent negative wave with a latency of about 19 ms (depending on the site of stimulation). It is preceded by 'far field' potentials from the peripheral nerve, root plexus, dorsal column, medial lemniscus and thalamus. The evoked potential complex is also normally inhibited, possibly by the cerebellum, and the amplitude of the cortical response is strikingly increased in diseases associated with myoclonic jerking (Chapter 23) and in photosensitive epilepsy.

These phenomena have been described in some detail as they will certainly be used to explore the effects of anaesthetic drugs and other causes of coma or 'sleep'. This is not a method for the inexperienced: the 'far field' brain stem auditory evoked potentials may be recorded from the scalp when deep coma has caused the spontaneous EEG to become isoelectric. This is *not* an indication for persistence of a lemniscal thalamocortical response. Clinical conclusions on 'brain death' should only be made by a very experienced clinical neurophysiologist.

Slow potential shifts

Recording of slow potentials requires amplifiers with DC coupling or long time-constants. They are the result of either long acting neuromodulators or of the integrated action of the short axonal neurones in the cortex, responding to 'tonic' impulses from the deep midline structures. One of the best known of the slow potentials is the *contingent negative variation* (CNV) of Walter. It is a surface-negative slow potential which follows a warning stimulus until an expected stimulus occurs, ie it is associated with a learned response. This *'expectancy wave'* as it is sometimes called is typically frontal. Its origin is unknown but it is grossly similar to negative slow potentials evoked in the frontal cortex of experimental animals by stimulation of various sensory nerves.

All three cortical responses (spontaneous EEG, evoked potentials and slow potential shifts) are modulated by balanced activity of reciprocal effects from the *mesencephalic reticular formation* (MRF) and from a *mediothalamic-frontocortical system* (MTFCS) which projects from the medial thalamus via the inferior thalamic peduncle to the *frontal granular cortex* (p. 123).

ATTENTION AND VIGILANCE

The MTFCS produces positive cortical shifts of phasic type which are modality-specific, causing *selective attention* by inhibiting repetitive or irrelevant evoked potentials. The MRF produces negative cortical shifts of tonic type which are not modality-specific and it causes *change of vigilance* without selective attention. The balance of these actions determines the current conscious state of the subject by inhibitory ('gate') control of thalamocortical sensory relays at the thalamic reticular nucleus, a thin layer of cells surrounding the thalamus (p. 139). The 'gate' can be selectively controlled by the frontal cortex but this can be overridden (inhibited) by the MRF responding to a novel stimulus (general arousal). A pulsed output from this thalamic reticular

nucleus has been considered to generate the cortical EEG rhythm.

As a rule, the slow potential shifts affect both hemispheres to the same extent. The contingent variation obeys this rule in frontal and parietal areas, but over the sensorimotor cortex it is a few microvolts larger on the side contralateral to the subsequent (expected) movement. Its importance in psychophysiological research will be appreciated. There are other *movement related potentials* related to voluntary movement which do not require the contingent (expected) response to a previous warning signal.

SLOW CORTICAL POTENTIALS RELATED TO VOLUNTARY MOVEMENT

By averaging the cortical potentials preceding a voluntary movement (registered by electromyography) it is possible to detect consistent slow shifts of potential at remarkably long times before the motor response.

BEREITSCHAFTSPOTENTIAL (READINESS POTENTIAL)

This is a slowly increasing surface-negative potential recorded about 800 ms before the onset of a rapid finger movement from the anterior parietal and pre-central areas of both hemispheres, and not at all from the pre-frontal lobe. Unlike the contingent negative variation it is maximal in the parietal area. At the vertex (average amplitude $5 \cdot 3 \, \mu V$, scalp recorded) it is slightly asymmetric and it is enhanced by attention. Studies on Parkinson's disease suggest that it is an indicator of a diffuse regulatory function on area 6 caused by thalamocortical activity regulated by the basal ganglia (Chapter 22).

PRE-MOTOR POSITIVITY

Maximal in mid-parietal cortex ($1 \cdot 7 \, \mu V$), this positive wave occurs bilaterally 90–80 ms before the start of a rapid finger movement, possibly the mark of a 'command' signal for a ballistic type of movement.

MOTOR POTENTIAL

About 60–50 ms before the EMG record of the movement, a negative going potential ($1 \cdot 6 \, \mu V$)

may be recorded over the hand area of the contralateral hemisphere, not bilaterally. It presumably marks activation of the appropriate area of the motor cortex. With smooth goal-directed movement (as distinct from voluntary short movement) the pre-movement negativity continues into the movement phase until the goal is reached, without any pre-motor positivity. This slow potential (Zielbewegungspotentiale) is maximal contralateral to the moving hand in the pre-central cortex, but ipsilateral in parietal cortex.

POST-MOVEMENT POTENTIALS

A number of waves have been described (positive and negative) in the 50 ms following a movement, these are largest over the post-Rolandic area. As similar responses accompany passive movements it is believed that they are related to the termination of the movement and possibly proprioceptive ('reafferent potentials').

Although the interpretation of these slow waves must be tentative, it seems reasonable to conclude that preparation for a movement starts bilaterally and symmetrically and that the design and executive command of the movement are not elaborated in the motor cortex. Kornhuber advocates that motor commands of the cerebral cortex result from information processing in sensory, association and motivation areas, converted into spatio-temporal motor patterns by function generators in the basal ganglia and cerebellum. Clearly the frontal lobe can initiate and select from the available programmes in the conscious subject. In unilateral Parkinsonism all readiness potentials are reduced in amplitude and duration over the contralateral pre-central cortex except at the vertex (suggesting that there is a pallido-anterior thalamic gating control over the supplementary motor area).

Further reading

Dement W. and Kleitman N. Cyclic variations in EEG during sleep and their relation to eye movements, body motility and dreaming. *EEG Clin. Neurophysiol.* 1957; **9**: 673–90.

Halliday A.M. *Evoked Potentials in Clinical Testing*. Edinburgh: Churchill Livingstone, 1982.

PART 4 Interaction with the Environment

Chapter 17
Reflex activity

Fundamentally the term 'reflex' implies an invariant response to a standard stimulus. This is substantially true where the reflex arc consists of afferent and efferent neurones with a single synapse between them (monosynaptic reflex). The excitability of the reflex may be modified in various ways, but not its distribution. The term is still convenient when the response to a stimulus is substantially stereotyped though varying in detail as in the spinal polysynaptic reflex associated with withdrawal from noxious stimuli. It becomes more difficult to justify the term, apart from the involuntary aspect, in the righting reflexes utilizing the basal ganglia and other 'long loop' reflexes, where no two successive responses may be identical although the applied stimuli and initial postural set may seem to be standardized. An element of 'goal-directed' activity becomes apparent. When it comes to still higher stimulus–response relationships using the cerebral cortex, such as the 'conditional reflexes' of Pavlov, there are many who would deny the validity of the term 'reflex' to describe the complicated behaviour patterns which may be triggered by an appropriate stimulus, and which are so difficult to distinguish from the goal-seeking activity of 'voluntary movement' as to give rise to endless philosophical discussion.

It is worth examining the nature of these differences. With the introduction of interneurones between afferent and efferent neurones, an element of plasticity is introduced. An input may be directed into one or many efferent pathways. Alternatively, an effector unit may be activated from different areas of a receptive field. A pool of neurones may be involved *in toto* or only partially, leaving a *subliminal fringe*. As will be shown, the latter cells may undergo subthreshold excitability changes. If these cells in a motoneurone pool are accessible to afferent stimuli from another receptive field, the reflex appropriate to the latter will be either facilitated or inhibited according to the subthreshold excitability changes produced by the first reflex. Clearly, the response of a polysynaptic reflex will depend not only on the intensity, duration and localization of stimuli, but also on the immediately preceding excitation state of neighbouring neuronal pools. The interneurones which provide this plasticity of response are, in the main, short and non-myelinated. The increasing preponderance of grey matter towards the encephalic pole of the neuraxis is clearly highly correlated with the flexibility of the input–output relations appropriate to higher levels of the nervous system.

On the other hand, where any input can, in principle, be directed to any output there is a danger of mass reflex responses where a more discrete reaction would be more appropriate. The nervous system avoids this by means of *inhibitory control* at various levels, and especially at cortical. Examples will be shown of inhibition at input and output stages, but obviously the interneurones are well suited for this gating function.

From the functional point of view, reflexes may be classified as (*a*) postural, (*b*) protective, (*c*) appetitive, (*d*) autonomic, with different degrees of complexity within each category. The principal postural reflexes are (i) the stretch reflex, (ii) cervical reflexes, (iii) vestibular reflexes, (iv) righting reflexes. There are many protective reflexes and typical examples are (i) the muscle lengthening reflexes, (ii) flexion-withdrawal reflexes, (iii) viscera-protection reflexes, (iv) avoidance reactions. The appetitive reflexes for seeking and utilization of food and sexual satisfaction combine somatic and visceral responses and it is difficult to isolate the spinal from the conditional reflex components. Autonomic reflexes, with smooth muscle and glandular effector organs, are autoregulatory to maintain a homoeostatic balance. Basically so are the somatic reflexes, but obviously a perfectly functioning system would lead to virtual immobility, resisting the effort of other motor parts of the nervous system to impose different postures and movements. These are rendered possible by supraspinal projections which modify the balance of reflexes. This introduces flexibility into the system. At the same time it introduces the possibility of achieving motor responses indirectly by energizing or inhibiting part of the reflex system which will then permit (? induce) movement to restore a new balance. The possible importance of this concept will be discussed in the chapter on voluntary movement (Chapter 22).

Postural reflexes

STRETCH REFLEXES

The reflex responses of skeletal muscle to stretch are the best understood because they are most easily investigated. The studies of

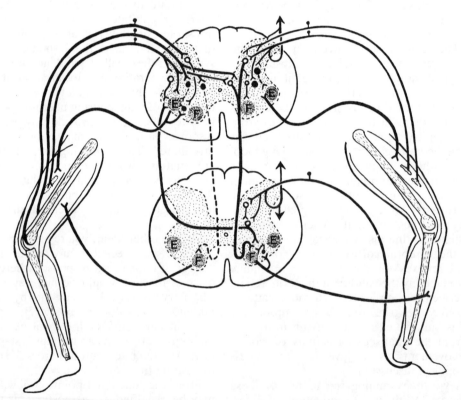

Fig. 17.1. *Segmental control of muscle tone.* The diagram indicates the facilitatory (right limb) and inhibitory reflexes (left limb) on quadriceps tone. On the right, annulospiral endings in quadriceps send group Ia afferent fibres to the cord which end monosynaptically and disynaptically on efferent motoneurones (only alpha shown) to the same muscle and collaterals to inhibitory interneurones suppressing the ipsilateral antagonists (hamstrings). The contralateral flexor muscles are facilitated. Excitatory fibres are also shown from the capsule of the right knee joint.

The left quadriceps illustrates segmental polysynaptic reflexes: inhibitory reflexes from the secondary endings of spindles (Ib afferents) and tendon organs (II afferents), and facilitation of the flexor muscles at different segmental levels, evoked by excessive tension in quadriceps. The sacral spinal segment (*lower*) also shows proprioceptive group III afferents to the flexor muscles (plantar reflex for withdrawal). The activity of the extensor (E) and flexor (F) motoneurones is limited by negative feedback through Renshaw interneurones.

recent years have revealed that there is not a 'simple' spinal reflex, but rather a family of reflexes. Although it is convenient to deal first with the shortening reaction, in life this is always accompanied or modified by one or more of the lengthening reactions described in the section on protective reflexes. Probably every skeletal muscle shortens reflexly in response to stretch. This is most apparent in the antigravity muscles such as the extensor muscles of the lower limbs and the flexors of the upper, and least apparent in the extraocular muscles, where many physiologists have denied the existence of stretch reflexes. In many muscles not directly concerned with maintaining posture against gravity, the stretch reflexes are only apparent when their excitability is increased, as when the pyramidal tract is damaged. The main stretch reflexes are negative feedback responses of two types; in one (group Ia afferent) extension of the receptor opposes extension, in the other (group Ib afferent) tension of the receptor opposes tension. Higher threshold (groups II and III afferents) receptors permit extension. The systems are highly asymmetrical and the balance between them is different for extensor and flexor muscles (*Fig.* 17.1, *Table* 17.1).

The shortening response to induced stretch of muscle is a device to maintain muscle length (and hence body position) when it is passively displaced. Muscle shortening of greater degree, with a 'jerk' of the related limb, only occurs if the lengthening stimulus is applied abruptly. Apart from the clinical testing situation, this occurs on landing after free fall and it is implicated in stepping reactions. The reflex elicited by the tendon jerk is monosynaptic. It is simple for the beginner to understand and it has been the subject of detailed functional studies. For these reasons there is a widespread belief that the *monosynaptic stretch reflex* is the most important mechanism for maintaining equilibrium length and the tone of muscle, despite the common observation that tendon jerks are poorly correlated with muscle tone. In light anaesthesia the stretch reflex tends to disappear when the monosynaptic tendon jerk is still present or even enhanced. Conversely, 'areflexic' patients may have perfect muscle tone. Certainly the resistance to passive stretch, the basis of *muscle tone*, is due to reflex shortening of muscle, but the reflex arc involved is *polysynaptic*. Whereas the monosynaptic reflex is a very local response to a local stimulus, simple

Table 17.1. Motoneurone responses to stretching an extensor (E) or flexor (F) lower limb muscle

Threshold	Low	→		High		
Receptors	Spindle primary	Golgi tendon	Spindle secondary	Pressure– pain		
Afferent c.v.	Fast	→		Slow		
Fibre type	Ia	Ib	II	III		
Muscle stretched					Motoneurone response	
Extensor {	+	−	−	−	E	ipsi
	−	+	+	+	F	ipsi
	−	+	○	○	E	contra
	+	−	○	○	F	contra
Flexor {	−	○	−	−	E	ipsi
	+	−	+	+	F	ipsi
	+	−	○	○	E	contra
	−	+	○	○	F	contra

The motoneurone is facilitated (+), inhibited (−) or unaffected (○). Note that ipsilateral and contralateral reciprocal effects are similar for extensors and flexors (though differing quantitatively) but the secondary endings of spindles and the nociceptors in both muscle groups evoke ipsilateral flexor (withdrawal) synergy.
Based on Granit, 1970, from cat muscle.

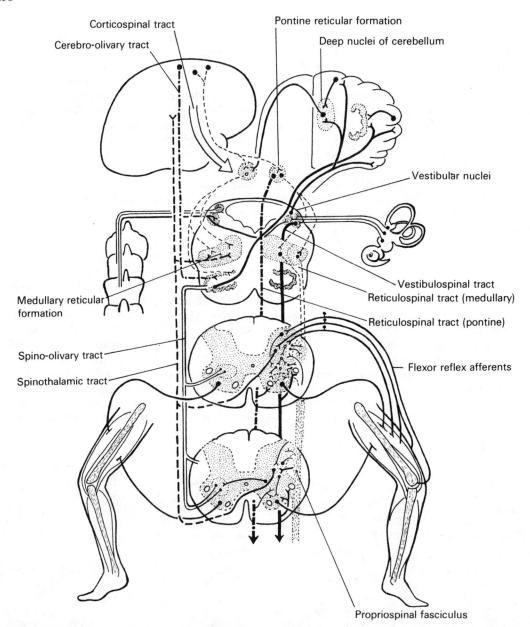

Corticospinal tract

Cerebro-olivary tract

Pontine reticular formation

Deep nuclei of cerebellum

Vestibular nuclei

Vestibulospinal tract
Reticulospinal tract (medullary)

Reticulospinal tract (pontine)

Flexor reflex afferents

Medullary reticular formation

Spino-olivary tract

Spinothalamic tract

Propriospinal fasciculus

Fig. 17.2. *Supraspinal and segmental modulation of reflex postural tone.* The interneurone pool of the spinal grey matter, with facilitatory and inhibitory neurones, modulates the alpha motoneurones of the anterior horn directly and by biasing muscle spindles through gamma motoneurones. The interneuronal pool receives groups II, III and IV afferent fibres (flexor reflex afferents) from the muscles, skin and high-threshold joint receptors of the limbs. Supraspinal controls are on the right side of the diagram. The vestibulospinal tract is facilitatory to extensor muscles and is activated by vestibular and neck receptors. Medullary reticular neurones are inhibitory (medial) and facilitatory (lateral) to the gamma motoneurones (through the propriospinal fasciculus at lower levels). Their neurones are controlled bilaterally by fibres from the pontine reticular formation which also projects a medial reticulospinal pathway (mixed facilitatory and inhibitory) (*see Fig* 4.1).

The pontine (and mesencephalic) reticular formation receives extrapyramidal corticospinal fibres (areas 6 and 4), bilaterally carried in the corticospinal tract, they are mainly inhibitory to postural reflexes. The pyramidal tract fibres concerned with voluntary movement inhibit protective reflexes and may switch dominance from flexion to extension synergies. An important cerebellopontine projection controls alpha–gamma linkage, another switch.

observation shows that if one muscle is stretched there is a motor response in other muscles, particularly in those which normally cooperate synergically with the stretched muscle. In both forms of myotatic reflex the antagonistic muscles are inhibited (*reciprocal inhibition*). As this probably requires an inhibitory internuncial neurone (*Fig.* 17.2), it would appear that the excitatory monosynaptic pathway is a special case for rapid and localized response to stretch. Most reflex pathways are polysynaptic, and there is increasing evidence that some of the intercalated neurones may pass through the brain stem and possibly the cerebellum and cerebral cortex. To distinguish the two main types of stretch reflex they are sometimes referred to as the 'phasic' and 'tonic' reflexes respectively.

THE PHASIC STRETCH REFLEX

The tendon jerk or 'pluck reflex' is a brief short latency contraction of an abruptly stretched muscle most easily elicited from the antigravity muscles but not confined to them. The natural stimulus is a sudden stretch of the previously unloaded muscle. A tap over its tendon does this efficiently for test purposes, applying an almost synchronous stretch to receptors in the muscle and tendon. The stretch-sensitive organ is the *primary ending in the muscle spindle* which is placed in parallel with the power-producing extrafusal muscle fibres so that it measures the amount of their passive stretch but stops producing signals when the extrafusal fibres contract. The transduction mechanism is described on p. 87.

The nerve fibre passing centrally in a peripheral nerve from muscle spindle to spinal cord is a large diameter, rapidly conducting Ia fibre. It has a cell body in the dorsal root ganglion (or its cranial nerve homologue) and passes into the spinal cord by a dorsal nerve root. Note that there is no synapse in the root ganglion. The central extension of the axon enters the cord grey matter in the dorsal horn.

Some fibres do not end there but pass forward to their first synapse with an anterior horn cell of the efferent limb of the reflex arc (*see Fig.* 9.1). A synchronous electric stimulus to the afferent nerve has much the same effect as a tap on the tendon. The resulting monosynaptic reflex is termed the Hoffman reflex (shortened to the *H reflex*). There are no interneurones: the reflex arc is monosynaptic.

The afferent fibre terminates in the anterior horn on the soma and dendrites of one or a limited number of motoneurones which emerge from the cord in the anterior nerve root as fast conducting group I fibres innervating motor units close to the muscle spindle supplying the afferent limb of the reflex arc. There is evidence that some afferent fibres (or their collaterals) terminate on gamma motoneurones and so influence the muscle by altering the bias of intrafusal muscle fibres of the spindles (p. 92).

As the phasic reflex is a local response to a local stimulus it follows that different degrees of stretch of a whole muscle will evoke proportional muscular contraction. The tendon jerk is not 'all or none'.

THE TONIC STRETCH REFLEX

Readers are warned that some writers, especially Continental, restrict the terms 'stretch reflex' and 'myotatic response' to this type. The appropriate stimulus is a slower stretch of the muscle than that which evokes the phasic reflex jerk. It is more suited to maintaining postural equilibrium when the muscles are being stretched by gravitational and similar forces.

Like the phasic reflexes, the stretch-sensitive organ is the *primary annulospiral ending* of the muscle spindle. Afferent nerve fibres are of the same class as for the phasic reflex (Ia) but after entering the dorsal grey horn they synapse with one or more interneurones (*Fig.* 17.2). The interneurones are distributed to motoneurones in an extensive column on both sides of the

Fig. 17.2. (*contd*)

Peripheral influences on the medullary centres are from the flexor reflex afferents, relayed to the contralateral spinothalamic tracts from which collateral fibres pass to the medullary reticular formation. The internuncial pool of the cord projects by the spino-olivary tract to the inferior olive for relay to the 'spinal' cerebellum (*see Fig.* 23.2). The ascending tracts are shown on the left side of the diagram.

cord, innervating synergic muscles *bilaterally*. Some of the interneurones are inhibitory and these terminate on the motoneurones of ipsilateral muscles antagonistic to the stretched one. On the other hand, the interneurones distributed to contralateral motor centres are connected in the opposite sense. That is to say, on the side of the stretched muscle there is an excitatory drive to its own motoneurones (and those of its synergists) with reciprocal inhibition of its antagonists. On the contralateral side the opposite situation applies — the partner of the stretched muscle (and its synergists) is inhibited and the partner of the antagonist is facilitated, though not necessarily enough to evoke contraction of the muscle (*Figs* 17.1, 17.2).

With these polysynaptic connections, the latency of the reflex response to stretch is slightly longer than with the monosynaptic reflex, but the drive to the motoneurones is less synchronous and hence more prolonged and possibly continued by reverberative feedback. An *after-discharge* is common. The numerous synapses, facilitatory and inhibitory, offer opportunities for modulation of the response according to the stimulation status elsewhere in the nervous system and hence for integration.

The motoneurones innervate skeletal muscle in the same way as the tendon jerk. Indeed it is a tenet of the Sherringtonian analysis of reflex activity that all motor influences to the muscle, including the other types of reflex responses to be described later, use the same '*final common path*': the lower motor neurone being the ultimate integrator. Modern studies on different types of motoneurones and muscle fibres (p. 242) suggest that this may not be so, phasic and tonic reflexes utilizing fast and slow-twitch muscles respectively. This matter is still debatable.

MODIFICATION OF THE STRETCH REFLEXES

The excitability of the stretch reflex arcs is modified by the balance of facilitatory and inhibitory impulses acting at the soma-dendritic region of their motoneurones (p. 240) and also by adjustment of the bias stretch of the muscle spindles caused by the gamma

motor system (p. 92). Since the combined effects may cause a very powerful shortening reaction of the stretched muscle, the integrity of its muscle fibres may be endangered in states of hyper-reflexia. Damage is prevented by inhibitory reflexes based on *tension and pain receptors* in the tendon and muscle which limit the contraction or even permit lengthening (p. 89). This is sometimes described as *autogenic inhibition*. As these are protective reflexes their discussion is postponed until after the other postural reflexes are described.

EXTENSOR THRUST AND POSITIVE SUPPORTING REACTION

These are probably different though functionally related reflex responses. The extensor thrust is seen in the spinal dog when the sole of the foot is stimulated by pressure, and not by a noxious stimulus. It is a phase of the gallop reaction (p. 210) and is probably involved in the standing posture in the normal human adult.

Receptors responsible for the *extensor thrust* are believed to be stretch receptors of the intrinsic muscles of the foot. The reaction, shortening of the muscles causing plantiflexion of toes and tarsus and of the antigravity muscles of both lower limbs (all physiological extensors though the toe movements are described as 'flexion' for historical reasons), stabilizes the lower limbs and fixes the plantar arches for the standing posture. The central connections are unknown but are probably polysynaptic at segmental level. It is the basis of a number of reflexes familiar to the neurologist as the reflexes of Rossolimo, Mendel and others.

A light touch of the sole of the foot evokes similar downward movement of the toes and tarsal arches, with first an ipsilateral and then a bilateral extensor muscle contraction throughout the lower limbs. This is the *positive supporting reaction*. The radiation of this reflex indicates that its central connections are polysynaptic. The receptors and afferent nerve fibres involved are uncertain.

The cutaneous plantar 'flexor' response, equated with the positive supporting reaction of the animal decerebrated at a low level, may be so marked that if the foot is touched lightly on the sole it follows the finger like a magnet. The *magnet reaction* is probably the lowest threshold plantar reflex, being reinforced by the proprioceptive reflex just described once the extremity encounters active resistance. It has not been well studied in man, in contrast with the reflex to noxious cutaneous stimuli described later. Like the stretch reflexes, both of these plantar postural reflexes are easily masked and replaced by the response (withdrawal) to painful stimuli. The dominance of the postural reactions is considered to depend on the integrity of fibres running in the pyramidal tract (p. 238). Clinical evidence suggests that corticospinal 'extrapyramidal' fibres inhibit extensor (postural) tone while the pyramidal fibres proper inhibit flexor tone (protective reflexes). The downgoing toe response elicited by stroking the medial side of the sole of the foot with a sharp object is not part of the weight bearing response. Although the toes turn down, proximal lower limb flexors contract rather than extensors. It is a protective reflex and will be described in the appropriate section.

Neck reflexes

It is a general principle that the postural reflexes work to bring the body posture into conformity with the orientation of the head. Distribution of limb muscle tone appropriate to the upright posture is inappropriate if the head is flexed, extended or rotated at the neck. Adjustments to compensate for neck flexion and extension are particularly important in quadrupeds, but are detectable even in the human. Flexion of the neck increases extensor tone in the lower limbs and flexor tone in the upper; neck extension does the reverse. Neck rotation is more important in man. Rotation turning the jaw to the right shoulder produces extension of the right upper and lower limbs, flexion of the left limbs and rotation of the rest of the vertebral column. These postures are best seen when the reflexes are exaggerated as in the decerebrate state, otherwise the responses are obscured by other reflexes such as the propping and contact reactions and by the vestibular reflexes.

It is generally accepted that the main (? sole) receptors initiating the neck reflexes are in the intervertebral joints but surprisingly little is known about them (*Fig.* 17.2). They are probably Ruffini spray endings, but a possible contribution from receptors in ligaments cannot be excluded. They project to the lateral vestibular nucleus. The wide distribution of muscular responses indicates that the central connections are polysynaptic via the vestibulospinal tract and medial longitudinal bundle (*Figs.* 17.2, 23.1).

Static vestibular reflexes

In this section only the static vestibular reflexes affecting body posture will be discussed. Those concerned with righting responses and with eye movements are described in later sections, but it should be noted that both groups of reflexes are designed to orientate the head and the eyes with respect to the vertical as indicated by the direction of gravity and to compensate for rapid movements of the head in space. Obviously they interact with the neck reflexes (*Fig.* 17.2). The labyrinthine positional reflexes adjust the forces in the antigravity muscles to keep the skull correctly orientated with respect to gravity.

The classic studies of Magnus suggested that the otolith organs of the labyrinth evoke simultaneous effects on all four limbs but a more convincing model described by Roberts associates activity in the otolith receptors on one side with activation of the antigravity muscles of the limb diagonally opposite to the quadrant of the head which is tilted down, with reciprocal effects from the vertical semicircular canal, the latter dominating over the otolith influence.

To summarize, the static upright posture is maintained by stretch reflexes (monosynaptic and polysynaptic) which are modified by neck and vestibular reflexes to keep the centre of gravity of the body over the feet and the head (and eyes) horizontal in space.

It is now necessary to consider other reflexes designed to protect the body from damage and to restore posture when these static reflexes prove insufficient or inappropriate.

Protective reflexes

Like the postural reflexes, the reflex movements for protection of parts of the body have both proprioceptive and cutaneous receptors. All are polysynaptic, with multisegmental and bilateral responses, and many have 'long-loop' connections.

LENGTHENING REACTION

As described above, the appropriate stimulus for the postural stretch reflex is a change in length of the primary afferent receptor of the muscle spindle. The reflex shortening of extrafusal muscle fibres rapidly raises tension transmitted through the muscle tendons. At some point the applied stretch and its reactive resistance must endanger the integrity of the muscle fibres. To avoid the overloading effect there are tension sensitive organs which reflexly inhibit the stretched muscle, allowing it to lengthen passively — a form of autoregulation. The most important receptors for this reflex are the *Golgi tendon organs* which are in series with the extrafusal muscle fibres (in contradistinction to the 'in parallel' arrangement of the length receptors of the spindles). The tendon organ transmits through Ib afferent fibres, only slightly slower than the primary spindle afferents. Like the latter, the Ib fibres have reciprocal actions on antagonist muscles and on contralateral homologous muscles (*Figs* 17.1, 17.2).

In addition to its primary sensory ending, the spindle also has *secondary sensory endings*. (These were formerly referred to as 'annulospiral' and 'flower-spray ending' respectively but these descriptive terms are more appropriate to the cat than to man.) They are considered to be tension receptors and to reflexly inhibit the extrafusal muscle fibres by slowly conducting group II afferent fibres. The functional significance is uncertain. As they are in parallel, they may limit the firing rate of limited bundles of muscle fibres but they are unlikely to cause a lengthening reaction like the series-linked tendon organs. The latter are certainly responsible for the marked lengthening and fall of tension of the 'clasp-knife' response when a spastic muscle is stretched passively. Stimulation of *intramuscular pain nerve endings* connected with small diameter group III slowly conducting sensory nerve fibres, elicits withdrawal reflex responses. Unlike the group I fibre reflexes, the group II

and III responses have not been shown to act contralaterally (*Fig.* 17.2).

Withdrawal reflexes

Excitation of pain receptors in the skin elicits polysynaptic multisegmental and bilateral responses which tend to withdraw the stimulated area from the stimulus. In the limbs this commonly evokes contraction of flexor muscles but sometimes of extensors. The responses are not stereotyped but depend on the site and intensity of the stimulus which is of a noxious type and so presumably stimulates pain receptors. The contralateral response is dominantly extensor ('crossed extensor reflex') to maintain posture when the stimulated limb is withdrawn.

The area of skin surface innervated by a single afferent fibre is termed its *receptive field* which overlaps with the receptive field of other afferent fibres. An area of skin is functionally connected, through polysynaptic spinal cord relays, with a muscle which lies under it. The muscle is excited by stimuli within its own skin area and inhibited from adjacent areas of skin. The reflex is said to have *local sign*. Muscles antagonistic to the muscle stimulated are reciprocally inhibited. The net effect is locally to withdraw the skin from the stimulus.

PLANTAR REFLEXES

The response is that which would be appropriate for the standing position. To lift the sole of the foot from a 'dangerous' stimulus, the foot is arched by contraction of the small plantar muscles which, additionally, flex and adduct the toes. Plantiflexion is physiologically an extensor response, the digital flexor muscles being misnamed for historical reasons. With stronger, and especially moving stimuli (spatial and temporal summation), flexion at ankle, knee and hip withdraws the whole limb from the stimulus and the contralateral limb is extended.

This well known plantar reflex is only one of a wide range of lower limb protective reflexes appropriate for removing the skin from the noxious stimulus — it is irrelevant whether the muscles are flexors or extensors. Stimulation over extensor muscles (eg glutei, quadriceps, anterior tibial muscles) causes them to contract, though more distant joints may be flexed. Painful stimulation of the heel pad evokes plantiflexion of the foot (an extensor reaction) to lift the heel off the ground.

There must be circumstances where the only effective response is to move the lower limb as far from the ground as possible, by flexion at all joints, including the metatarsophalangeal joint of the hallux. The upgoing, so-called 'extensor', hallux response is a minimal *flexion withdrawal reflex*. It is a normal response which can be demonstrated by electromyographic recording, and its reflexogenous zone includes the whole lower limb, anterior abdominal wall and bladder mucosa. But, as already indicated, there are other protective reflexes with more local sign and these are of lower threshold. They are often at least partially antagonistic to the Babinski response just described. The hallux response is an obvious example. However, the balance is shifted in favour of the upgoing-toe response if the ipsilateral pyramidal tract, or some of its fibres (p. 238), is not functioning. When this happens, a noxious stimulus moving distally along the outer border of the foot and then across the metatarsal pads to the base of the big toe, evokes the so-called 'extensor' response. It is not a 'pathological reflex', but a normal one disclosed by alteration of dominance. As the pyramidal tract lesion increases, more and more of that response's reflexogenous zone becomes apparent and the response can be obtained by stimulating the medial side of the planta, then the dorsum of the foot and, progressively, up the anterior surface of the limb to the abdominal wall and (with the most severe lesion) bladder mucosa. At that stage the response occurs to quite small stimuli within that wide area. Even a bladder contraction may be enough to evoke 'spontaneous' *flexor spasm* of the lower limb.

When receptive fields for two reflexes overlap, it is common for one of them to be 'concealed' by the dominant one, but for reversal or variability to occur with modification of body posture or on simultaneous stimulation in other receptive fields. Concealed reflexes are also disclosed by *reflex rebound*. This term is applied to the contradictory movement which sometimes follows immediately after a reflex excitation or inhibition of muscle. Thus an 'extensor' hallux response may follow immediately after a 'flexor' response in normal subjects. It is for this reason that the clinical neurologist concentrates on the *first* hallux movement as this indicates which of the conflicting reflexes is dominant.

ABDOMINAL AND ERECTOR SPINAE SKIN REFLEXES

Similar reflex responses to skin stimulation are found in the trunk muscles. Like those of the lower limbs just described, they are multisegmental responses with some local sign in the segment stimulated and with the purpose of inducing a movement away from the stimulus. In addition to a contraction of muscles adjacent to the stimulated skin, the erector spinae muscles relax. A large number of allied abdominal and erector spinae reflexes are harmoniously knit together in a single mechanism for the protection of the trunk and the underlying abdominal viscera. As with the lower limb reflexes, the response to a given stimulus may be altered by a change of posture or by an appropriate voluntary contraction. Reciprocal inhibition is an important element and is not confined to one side of the body. Reflexes evoked by simultaneous stimulation at two opposite points of the trunk inhibit one another.

Unlike the lower limb protective reflexes, the effective stimulus is not always noxious. There is evidence (based on latency measurements) that touch receptors connected to fast conducting afferent nerve fibres initiate the reflex which is then continued by slower fibres, presumably from pain nerve endings (*Fig. 17.2*).

They are spinal polysynaptic reflexes. It is possible that there are long-loop connections, but the prolonged asynchronous muscle discharges can be adequately accounted for by the contribution of slow nerve fibres to a polysynaptic central spinal mechanism. Interruption of the pyramidal tract in the spinal cord causes diminution or loss of the reflex ipsilaterally and it may be augmented in extrapyramidal disorders, but these modifications are probably due to changes in reflex excitability rather than to interruption of a cerebral reflex arc. Even when no abdominal skin reflex can be elicited by scratching the abdominal skin, the response may still be elicited by electrical stimulation of an intercostal nerve.

This cerebral influence on reflex excitability causes marked plasticity of the abdominal skin reflexes. They can be modified by training, expectancy of pain and other emotional stimuli and they tend to habituate when tested repeatedly. Indeed they may show many of the characteristics of a conditional reflex. They are particularly potentiated by pain in abdominal viscera, and irritation of peritoneal nerve endings causes tonic contraction which is familiar to the abdominal surgeon. Sensitization widens the receptive field and also causes the reflex contraction to irradiate to the flexor muscles of the limbs, by supraspinal influences brought to bear on the interneurones.

PERINEAL PROTECTIVE REFLEXES

Similar protective reflexes occur if the skin of the upper medial aspect of the thigh is stroked, pinched or pricked. The dartos muscle contracts, drawing up the ipsilateral side of the scrotum, and the ipsilateral testicle is elevated towards the inguinal canal by contraction of the cremaster muscle. The reflex 'centre' is in the upper lumbar segments of the cord and, like the abdominal reflexes, the reflexes are often abolished by lesions of the corticospinal tract.

Cerebral modulation of protective reflexes has not been reported for the anal and penile reflexes. Stimulation of the perineum or of the anus with a needle causes contraction of the external anal sphincter. The reflex is probably polysynaptic with central integration in the S5 segment of the spinal cord. This reflex is therefore usually maintained except with cauda equina lesions.

BULBOCAVERNOSUS REFLEX

The bulbocavernosus muscle contracts palpably if the glans penis is squeezed. The spinal segments concerned are S2, 3, 4. It is also frequently abolished in lesions of the cauda equina. It is not strictly a protective reflex but is related to a sexual reflex; the muscular contraction compresses venous networks in the cavernous bodies of the penis to promote erection.

PROTECTIVE REFLEXES OF FACE AND EYES

The head, and especially the face, shares in the protective reflexes of the trunk, the head being jerked away from a painful or threatening stimulus, especially when the eyes are threatened, in which case the eyes are also closed. It is difficult to decide whether these are conditional reflexes or learned responses. They disappear with light sedation or mental disorder, leaving only the responses to actual contact stimulus and to flashes of light or sudden noise. They also show habituation (p. 165) with repeated stimulation, but this is typical of nociceptive reflexes and does not indicate a 'voluntary' element.

CORNEAL REFLEX

A light touch to the cornea of one eye evokes a long asynchronous reflex discharge of the orbicularis oculi bilaterally, causing the eyes to blink. The latency is 25–40 ms, indicating a polysynaptic pathway since the afferent (trigeminal nerve, first division) and efferent (facial nerve) pathways are short. If the stimulus is continuing and painful the eye closure becomes tonic. The reflexogenous zone extends to the area of facial skin supplied by the supraorbital nerve.

BLINK REFLEXES TO LIGHT AND SOUND

Like the corneal reflex, the blink response of orbicularis oculi occurs bilaterally and with long latency to stimulation with a flash of light (receptor is the retina, afferent nerve the optic, reflex centre in the mid-brain) or a sudden noise (receptor is the cochlea, afferent nerve the acoustic and reflex centre in the pons).

BLINK REFLEX TO GLABELLA TAP

The blink response to tapping the skull near the eyes (notably at the glabella) evokes similar long latency (27–40 ms) bilateral responses of orbicularis oculi, but these are preceded by a short latency response with the characteristics of a stretch reflex (fixed latency, 15 ± 4 ms, and relatively constant amplitude). Electrical stimulation of one supraorbital nerve shows that this myotatic component of the blink response is ipsilateral and has a lower threshold than the second 'nociceptive' response. The afferent fibres of the first component (presumably originating in the muscle spindles of the eyelids) pass centrally in the facial nerve and those of the second component in the trigeminal nerve. Thus the two components of the glabella tap response may be affected differentially by disease of the Vth and VIIth cranial nerves.

Habituation of the second component causes the glabella tap response to disappear if the glabella is tapped repeatedly in the normal subject. In Parkinsonism and in many disorders associated with cerebral atrophy both components are increased and the second component fails to habituate ('persistent glabella reflex'). Apparently *habituation* requires corticofugal nerve fibres and the basal ganglia are involved. A cholinergic system has been suggested. Habituation of behavioural responses to recurrent stimuli which have lost their startle significance involves the reticular formation.

TEAR REFLEX

Intimately linked with the corneal blink reflex is a conjunctival reflex (afferent trigeminal nerve, first division) with an efferent limb in the facial nerve to the lacrimal gland via the pterygopalatine ganglion. Stimulation of the conjunctiva causes production of tears.

The pupillary reflexes have already been discussed (p. 94) as they are feedback control of afferent input rather than true protective reflexes.

Protective reflexes of nose, mouth and throat

SNEEZING REFLEX

Tactile stimulation of the nasal mucous membrane reflexly initiates deep inspiration followed by forced expiration through a closed glottis, closure of the eyes, lacrimation and head movement (first extension as the chest expands then flexion along with expiration). The afferent limb of the reflex arc is the second division of the trigeminal nerve, the reflex centre (polysynaptic) is in the medulla and the efferent pathways are the facial nerves (bilaterally), the spinal nerves to the internal costal muscles and probably to the diaphragm.

Other stimuli (which may summate with the nasal one) are bright light (optic nerves) and stimulation of skin of face or nose. The effect of the reflex is to expel foreign matter from the upper respiratory tract and nose.

COUGH REFLEX

The upper respiratory tract is protected by a similar reflex induced by irritants affecting the epiglottis, larynx and trachea. The afferent limb is the vagus nerve to the medulla, and efferent fibres pass by vagal, phrenic and thoracic intercostal nerves to laryngeal, diaphragmatic and intercostal muscles. The reflex has three phases: (i) deep inspiration, using all the accessory respiratory muscles; (ii) closure of the glottis; (iii) rapid expiration with passive opening of the still contracted glottis, the burst of air under high pressure expelling foreign matter from the upper respiratory tract.

GAG REFLEX

Irritation of the mucosa of the posterior pharyngeal wall and posterior third of the tongue induces contraction of the pharyngeal constrictor muscles and tension of the soft palate. The afferent nerves are the trigeminal (maxillary division) and glossopharyngeal (IX) and the efferent are the pharyngeal rami of the vagus (X). The reflex excitability is very variable and readily modified by central influences such as apprehension or hysteria (the latter traditionally abolishes it).

THE DIVING RESPONSE

This name has been given to an important interaction of reflexes which have survival value for diving mammals but which may endanger life if evoked in man. Sudden entry of cold water, irritant chemicals, or foreign objects such as an endotracheal tube or endoscope into the nose or larynx, and cold stimulation of the muzzle area stimulate a variety of receptors of the trigeminal (V) and glossopharyngeal (IX) nerves which relay in the medulla oblongata to the medulla respiratory automatism mechanism (Chapter 20) causing sudden inhibition of respiration. The afferent signals also evoke a strong vagal (X) discharge resulting in laryngeal spasm, bradycardia and constriction in all vascular beds except those of the cerebral and coronary circulations. This upper airways reflex, for protection against entry of water etc. into the lungs, interacts with the reflexes from the carotid bodies. Hypoxia, hypercapnia and acidaemia stimulate chemoreceptors of the glossopharyngeal (IX), with efferent vagal (X) and sympathetic responses (ie cholinergic and adrenergic responses together). This normally increases the ventilatory excursion (p. 193), but interaction between the nasal/laryngeal reflexes and the carotid body reflexes prevents the respiratory drive and potentiates the bradycardia and vasoconstriction. Apnoea persists and cardiac arrest is common. Blood pressure depends on variable balance between lowered cardiac output and peripheral vasoconstriction. The reflex interaction is increased and the anti-apnoeic action of the carotid bodies is reduced if the reflexes are induced immediately after a period of hyperventilation.

Excessive diving response is a probable cause of many deaths from drowning, inhalational anaesthesia, aerosols and intubation without adequate preparation, and possibly for some cot deaths in infancy. The laryngeal reflexes are particularly potent in the newborn. Passive inflation of the lungs may reflexly counteract the diving response.

The protective reflexes of the upper respiratory tract, nose and mouth are of particular importance to the anaesthetist. It may be advantageous to reduce their excitability by local anaesthesia of receptive mucosae to allow toleration of artificial airways. Conversely, a patient cannot be considered fully recovered from general anaesthesia, or other forms of coma, until these essential reflexes have returned.

Grasp, feeding and coital reflexes

The reflexes considered up to this point have had the function of maintaining body posture in a stable upright position or protecting the whole or part of the body from damage by noxious stimuli applied to skin or mucous membranes. There is a further large series of reflexes for the preservation of the individual and the race by holding food (or sexual partner) and initiating feeding or sexual behavioural patterns. Like the reflexes already discussed, some of these are simple and localized; others are so complex as to make their reflex status debatable. The simpler ones tend to disappear after infancy but reappear with certain brain disorders (notably ablation of area 6a), indicating that they have been suppressed by higher nervous activity in the normal individual after infancy.

GRASP REFLEX

Whether evolved to allow tree-living animals to hang from the branches or so that their infants can cling to the mother's hair, a grasp reflex is dominant in the newborn. On closer study there are a number of reflexes described under this rubric. A non-moving strong pressure to the palmar surface of the infant's hand or fingers evokes tonic grasping. It disappears after six months of life. The appropriate stimulus appears to be a combination of stretch of muscles and contact with skin.

A similar *tonic grasp response* is evoked by a firmly applied object moving distally across the palm to the base of the index finger. Here the main (? only) stimulus is tactile at the onset, but the initial 'closing reaction' of the fingers is reinforced by traction on the long flexor muscles of the fingers. It is rarely seen unless the contralateral frontal lobe is damaged.

INSTINCTIVE GRASP REACTION

This is a term used by Denny-Brown to describe a somewhat different grasp reflex, sometimes named 'forced groping'. The appropriate stimulus is again contact with skin, but the reflexogenous zone is wider, including parts of the lateral and dorsal aspects of the hand and wrist. The response is a movement of extension followed by flexion with pronation or supination, and protraction or retraction of the forearm to bring the touched object into contact with skin nearer the palm of the hand. In other words, a randomly detected object is then orientated with the part of the hand which elicits the closing reaction and exploratory finger sensation (p. 94). This is a basis for exploring space. It is probably under parietal lobe control.

INSTINCTIVE TACTILE AVOIDING REACTION

Contactual stimuli (not necessarily noxious) may evoke complex withdrawal movements of the whole hand. The receptive zone is the terminal phalanges. These reflexes are more apparent if the contralateral parietal lobe is damaged. They are avoiding reactions and are probably under frontal lobe control.

GRASP REFLEX OF THE FOOT

Normal infants show a tonic grasp reflex of the toes in response to light pressure or a stroking movement applied to the distal half of the sole and plantar surface of the toes. It occurs with contralateral frontal lobe lesions and in many children with Down's syndrome (mongolism).

There are a number of interpretations of these contactual reflexes of the hands and feet. Some authors consider them to be defence reactions functionally related with the body-righting reactions, others as the basic reflex mechanisms for exploration of external space. The latter concept is clearly important in speculations about the development of cortical control of movement.

Hand–mouth reflexes

For further evaluation of external space, an identified object has to be brought within the receptive field of sensory organs specially adapted for detecting environmental changes at some (limited) distance from the body surface. The same response is clearly appropriate for bringing possible food to the mouth. The baby shows a strong tendency to bring its hand, or any object held in the hand, to its mouth.

THE PALMO-MENTAL REFLEX

This is a persisting element of such a reflex. During tactile stimulation of the palmar surface of the hand there is ipsilateral contraction of the depressor muscle of the lower lip or of the mentalis muscle. They are supplied by the mandibular division of the facial nerve. This vestigial reflex tends to vanish but reappears in association with subcortical lesions.

SUCKING AND ROOTING REFLEXES

Other oral reflexes (described as 'primitive reflexes') associated with feeding in the newborn and which normally disappear until 'released' by disintegration of higher nervous functions, are those appropriate to rooting and sucking. Rooting means that the lips move towards a stimulus applied to nearby parts of the face, the head turning towards it and the lips pouting — a response pattern to bring the infant's mouth to the nipple when its face touches the breast. Stimulation on and near the lips then evokes a sucking response: the tongue is moved downwards and backwards and the lower jaw depressed, at the same time as the lips are tightly closed. The afferent fibres from the reflexogenous zone (lips, tip of tongue, cheek, chin) run in the trigeminal and glosso-pharyngeal nerves and the efferent fibres in the trigeminal, facial and hypoglossal nerves. The reflex centre is in the medulla and adjacent pons.

MASTICATION AND BITING

The masticatory and tongue muscles and salivary glands are reflexly excited (motor division of V, VII and XII) by stimuli within the mouth (V) via the medulla. Chewing may also be voluntary (from the cortical masticatory area) (p. 204) or involuntary from the lateral part of the substantia nigra, a movement pattern commonly seen in patients over-dosed with levodopa or phenothiazine drugs.

SWALLOWING

There are a number of reflexes involved in deglutition. They are extremely vulnerable to anaesthesia or other causes of loss of consciousness. They are best understood by following the passage of a bolus of food from the mouth. First the oral cavity is closed (orbicularis oris muscle, facial nerve) and the jaws closed (masticatory muscles, trigeminal nerve). Then the base of the tongue is pressed against the hard palate, pushing the bolus towards the pharynx. Once behind the anterior arch of the palate the bolus is moved downwards by the three pharyngeal constrictor muscles while escape to the nasal cavity is prevented by upward and posterior movement of the soft palate (tightened by tensor palati) combined with contraction of the superior constrictor of the pharynx.

To prevent the bolus passing into the respiratory passages the laryngeal orifice is closed by fixing the lower jaw while the larynx is lifted forwards under the arched root of the tongue by elevation of the hyoid bone. The backward movement of the tongue depresses the epiglottis over the laryngeal orifice and the glottis is reflexly closed. At the same time respiration is arrested. The bolus is thus directed downwards and prevented from passing into the larynx or nasal cavity. The middle and inferior constrictors of the pharynx then pass the bolus into the oesophagus where peristalsis carries it to the stomach. Throughout the transport from mouth to stomach, the passage is lubricated by mucous secretion.

Initiation of swallowing is under voluntary control but once the bolus passes through the palatine arch it becomes entirely reflex. The afferent nerves are the glossopharyngeal (IX) and vagus (X) and the efferent nerves are the trigeminal (V motor), facial (VII), glossopharyngeal (IX), accessory (XI) and hypoglossal (XII) with the vagus (X) taking over when the bolus reaches the oesophagus. This multiple reflex is organized in the medulla. When coordination of the various components is impaired by bulbar diseases or anaesthesia the most important disturbance is that oral contents may pass into the respiratory tract during deglutition.

Coital reflexes

The feeding and swallowing reflexes are fundamental for preservation of the individual. For preservation of the race, the coital reflexes are of almost equal biological importance. Indeed some of the orofacial and upper limb gripping responses have sexual as well as feeding functions. Like feeding responses, reproductive behaviour is more dependent on higher nervous activity (p. 127) (modified by endocrinal status) than on spinal reflexes in its initiation. For completion of coitus reflex activity is complementary, but not essential. Nevertheless the paraplegic male patient is capable of maintained penile erection and ejaculation on manipulation of the genitalia.

It is doubtful whether human subjects display the treading and pelvic elevation behaviour which precedes copulation of quadrupeds. The pelvic thrusting movements of both partners during intercourse are almost entirely voluntary but at orgasm may be reflex as in the spinal animals studied by Sherrington. Autonomic reflexes are, however, important for the tumescence and mucus secretion of the genitalia of both sexes, and for ejaculation in the male, though these components of the sexual response may also be evoked from mid-brain, hypothalamic and rhinencephalic levels of the brain.

Chain and alternating reflexes

The two fundamental principles of organization of spinal reflex activity, (i) reciprocal innervation, (ii) the 'final common path', carry the implication that muscles (or their motor units) may be driven reflexly by stimuli which combine or conflict in their demands. 'Allied' reflexes evoking the same movement pattern may show simultaneous or successive combination. Thus a firm, slightly noxious, stimulus moving distally across the sole of the foot evokes extensor thrust, plantar grasp and local withdrawal of plantar arch, all causing downgoing toe responses. Stretch and vestibular reflexes combine to promote the standing posture. 'Antagonistic reflexes' on the other hand cause rivalry for control of the final common path and the outcome depends upon which of the two is dominant, a situation which clearly varies at different stages of development, presumably due to inhibitory control by later maturing nerve circuits. In general, nociceptive reflexes dominate except in those situations where summation of allied reflexes prevents this. Antagonistic reflexes may also show simultaneous or successive combination.

Polysynaptic reflexes commonly exhibit

after-discharge with persistence of excitatory or inhibitory synaptic potential after the motor response has stopped and this facilitates or inhibits response to an immediately following stimulus which would otherwise be subliminal. Thus the scratch reflex tends to repeat itself, especially if a parasite travels across the receptive surface. In chewing, the jaw reflex restimulates itself. These are examples of *chain reflexes* and many elaborate behavioural responses may be essentially similar for the train of allied reflexes may change slightly with each repetition. In fact, the examples given are *alternating reflexes* since the direction of movement holding for a phase in one sense is followed by a phase of opposite direction and this in turn by reversion to the earlier phase, and so on, though the stimulus remains unaltered.

The coital reflexes just described are alternating reflexes in this sense and so also are the stepping reflexes seen in young infants.

STEPPING REFLEX

We have already described the positive supporting reaction by which the stiffened leg supports the body's weight when the foot is in contact with a suitable support (p. 160). If now the support is slowly moved backwards, the supporting reaction suddenly melts, the formerly extended leg is flexed, the foot is picked up and swung forward to be replaced on the ground ahead of the original point of contact. The supporting reaction then reappears. The change from extensor to flexor response is believed to depend on stimuli from the hip joint and its related ligaments and muscles. This is the stepping response. A similar lateral stepping sequence (the *sway reaction*) occurs if the body is displaced latterly beyond certain limits. With big displacements the reaction is a *sideways hop*. Propping, stepping and hopping reactions counteract the effect of externally applied forces including the forward and downward fall of the body in normal locomotion. They are not 'reflex walking' but are incorporated into walking automatisms (p. 207). Twisting of the body axis (neck as well as lumbar spine) also stimulates the hip and neck receptors which initiate reflex stepping. In short, the stepping responses restore body posture when the normal postural reflexes are inadequate to maintain the centre of gravity over the feet.

In the successive phases of the alternating reflex of stepping, reciprocal innervation is present. Alternation of reflexes results from a combination of spinal cord and supraspinal effects. When antagonistic reflexes requiring the same final common path are stimulated simultaneously, the dominant reflex (usually nociceptive) excludes the other, but when they use the lower motor neurone in succession, the expression of the first reflex facilitates the second ('*successive induction*'). If both stimuli overlap but one response has after-discharge, the facilitated response of the latter appears as '*rebound*'. If both stimuli persist the response becomes rhythmical (eg scratching, stepping, chewing and coitus). In experimental animals the *rhythm of alternation* persists after deafferentation of the entire limb. Clearly the 'turning point' (from extension to flexion and back again) must be centrally operated though phasing can be influenced by proprioceptive or cutaneous stimulation (pp. 197, 209). Indeed, the rhythm of the phase is synchronous throughout the musculature involved. The two lower limbs are opposed in phase (but in quadrupeds strong stimulation causes galloping, with both hind limbs in phase). The turning point is determined by the balance of excitatory and inhibitory influences brought to bear on the motoneurones of the limbs and does not require rhythmic stimulation. The supraspinal source of these influences is not known for certain but is likely to be some part of the extrapyramidal motor system of the basal ganglia and reticular formation. The latter is at present considered to be essential for the righting reflexes though Magnus, who made the fundamental studies, favoured the red nuclei.

Righting reflexes

Stepping and hopping reactions may be considered as special examples of a righting reflex but there are many others, such as (i) labyrinthine righting reflexes, (ii) body righting reflexes acting upon the head, (iii) neck righting reflexes, (iv) body righting reflexes acting upon the body, (v) optical righting reflexes. Information derived from vestibular organs, eyes, neck and body surface reflexly evoke movements required to bring first head and eyes, and then the rest of the body, into the normal position with respect to gravity. At the same time, the position of all four limbs must be adjusted to promote the balanced posture. Some of these reflex adjustments are familiar to the clinician as 'associated movements', for example the swinging of the arms during walking. The complicated afferent inputs and motor outputs require integration and coordination of a chain of reflexes, and this probably takes place in the circuits of the basal ganglia acting through the reticulospinal system, though a considerable amount of limb–limb coordination (ipsilateral and contralateral) is effected by long spinal reflexes using the *propriospinal system* of connections between the lumbosacral and cervicothoracic segments of the cord which run in the white matter immediately enclosing the central grey matter of the cord (*Fig.* 17.2). Lloyd has suggested that spinal motoneurones receiving their basic activity from interneurones of the anterior horn are under the control of the short propriospinal pathways. When there is an afferent input to the posterior horns, their basic activity is received from the dorsal interneurones of the cord and they then come under the control of long bulbospinal and reticulospinal neurones and these prepare the motoneurones for pyramidal tract influence.

Cervico-ocular reflexes

Proprioceptive signals from receptors in the ligaments and joints of the first three cervical vertebrae (*Fig.* 17.2) ascend and cross in the medulla oblongata to the contralateral vestibular nucleus and the medial longitudinal bundle and act in combination with signals from the labyrinth to maintain ocular stability during simultaneous head and neck movements and to adjust the postural muscles to maintain the upright posture during axial rotation. From the vestibular nucleus inhibitory stimuli are sent to the ipsilateral VIth nerve nucleus and facilitatory stimuli to the contralateral (ie back to the side originating the cervical signals). Turning the head to the left stretches ligaments in the right side of the neck, exciting the left vestibular nucleus and, through it, the right abducens nucleus, with inhibition of the left nucleus. The direction of conjugate gaze is to the right, with reference to the head, but towards the original point in external space.

In man, full gaze stabilization requires integration of neck, vestibular and visual information. The visual reflexes override the vestibular nucleus control. Thus head rotation produces *compensatory eye movement* (gaze fixed to same point in space) in the dark, but in the light it does not do so if the subject can fixate on a target moving in phase with the head. The integration of visual and vestibular signals is carried out in the *floccular lobe of the cerebellum* (Chapter 23). If the signals conflict there is a sensation of movement and reflex stimulation of the vomiting centre (motion sickness). It is reduced by either eliminating the visual input or depressing the vestibular signals by anticholinergic drugs or general sedation.

Further reading

Angell-James J.E. and Daly M. de B. Nasal reflexes. *Proc. R. Soc. Med.* 1969; **62**: 1287.

Creed R.S., Denny-Brown D., Eccles J.C. et al. *Reflex Activity of the Spinal Cord*. Oxford: Oxford University Press, 1972.

De Gail P., Lance J.W. and Neilson P.D. Differential effects on tonic and phasic reflex mechanisms produced by vibration in man. *J. Neurol. Neurosurg. Psychiatry* 1966; **29**: 1–11.

Granit R. *The Basis of Motor Control*. Academic Press: London and New York, 1970.

Hunt C.C. and Perl E.R. Spinal reflex mechanisms concerned with skeletal muscle. *Physiol. Rev.* 1960; **40**: 538–79.

Paulson G. and Gottlieb G. Developmental reflexes: the reappearance of foetal and neonatal reflexes in aged patients. *Brain* 1968; **91**: 37–52.

Roberts T.D.M. *Neurophysiology of Postural Mechanisms*, 2nd ed. London: Butterworths, 1978.

Chapter 18
Vestibular function

THE LABYRINTH

The labyrinthine endorgans, closely related to the cochlear organ in the inner ear, transduce mechanical force to nerve action potentials by special adaptation of *hair cells*, a device adopted early in evolution to detect shearing forces by converting the bending of a cilium into polarization changes of the cell from which the cilium (hair) arises. The hair cell is depolarized by displacement of the cilium in one direction, hyperpolarized by opposite displacement. Movement of the cilium modulates leakage of electric current from the hair cell in a local circuit. This induces a *generator potential* (also termed 'microphonic' potential as it exactly follows the displacement of the cilium). The hair cells are in synaptic contact with the afferent terminals of the *vestibular nerve*. The cell bodies of the latter have spontaneous activity and the generator potential of the hair cell regulates this — increasing the firing rate with one direction of displacement, lowering it with the other, and this without any refractory period. The inputs to the vestibular nuclei of each side of the brain stem are exactly balanced. This basic system for detecting displacement is adapted in two ways in the labyrinth.

UTRICLE AND SACCULE

The *utricle and saccule* have *maculae* consisting of groups of hair cells with a relatively heavy load, the *otolith*, placed on the free end of the cilia. It is calcareous material in a gelatinous matrix, all in a watery medium. The mass of the otolith is accelerated by the gravitational pull of the earth and therefore signals the direction of the vertical through the centre of the earth. When the head is tilted the displacement of the otolith bends the hair cells. The effective stimulus is its *acceleration*. By mathematical integration the vestibular nucleus converts this into *head velocity*, and by further integration into a signal of *head displacement*. Thus the utricle and saccule primarily signal *linear* acceleration of the head and this information is used to activate motor responses which dynamically oppose the force acting on the head. The derived signal, position, is used to adjust the position of the eyes, a 'static' otolith reflex.

Compensatory torsional movements of the eyes (counter-rolling) are minimal in the human unless *g*-forces are increased (as in diving aircraft). Version movements are best seen when the brain stem is disconnected from higher centres. The so-called '*doll's head movements*' are prominent if the vestibular and oculomotor nuclei and the connecting *medial longitudinal bundles* are intact. The utricle responds to movement of the head in different planes. When the head is flexed the eyes are tonically deviated upwards. When the head is hyperextended, the eyes are deviated downwards. When the head is inclined to either shoulder the two visual axes are rotated in the opposite direction. Rotational changes about a vertical axis do not produce otolith reflexes since the relation to gravity is not altered, and this excludes the neck receptors from the afferent side of the ocular reflex as major contributors. (Nevertheless, positional nystagmus has been reported after upper cervical rhizotomy.)

Positional nystagmus occurs when, owing to imbalance of the otolith and/or neck induced ocular reflexes, the drive to the VIth nerve nucleus is excessive. The abducted eye then receives inhibitory signals from the *reticular formation*, briefly bringing the eye back to the central position. The other eye is entrained to move in parallel by the connections of the medial longitudinal bundle (p. 178). *Imbalance* of the central connections of the otolith reflex also causes positional nystagmus. As a rule the slow component of positional nystagmus is opposite to the direction the head is displaced, but there are some ill-understood clinical circumstances in which the direction may change.

The macula of the utricle is curved so that its hair cells detect head tilts in all directions. The macula of the saccule is in a sagittal plane, detecting dorsoventral movements. It is also possible that different types of hair cells transduce ocular and postural reflexes.

THE SEMICIRCULAR CANALS

The *semicircular canals* of the labyrinth have similar hair cell receptors specialized in a different way. Unlike the maculae of the utricle and saccule, their *cristae* hair cells have their cilia embedded in the *cupula*, a gelatinous substance of the same specific gravity as that of the surrounding fluids. Therefore the cupula, unlike the otolith, does not exert a force on the cilia in the direction of gravity. The semicircular canals have no significant static function. Movements of the surrounding fluid stimulate the hair cells by displacing the cupula.

Fluid movement is induced, with a time lag, by moving the head or by heating or cooling the labyrinth ('*caloric stimulation*') to cause convection currents. Thus each crista responds to *relative* movement of the *endolymph* within the canal which leads to the chamber (ampulla) containing the crista and cupula. All the hair cells within each crista are orientated in one direction so each canal system detects endolymph movement in one direction of space.

Each labyrinth has three such canal systems which are arranged orthogonally and so are able to detect movement in any direction of space because of the inertia of the endolymph which 'lags' behind the wall of the labyrinth, causing the cupula to move like a pendulum until the fluid movement matches that of the head (a matching which has to be restored when the head stops moving). Like the otolith macule, the cupula/crista responds to *head acceleration*, but viscous friction converts this into a *velocity signal* to the hair cells and their polarization changes modulate the resting firing rate of *vestibular nerve* afferents, but in this case the message used by the vestibular nucleus remains related to velocity. It is not translated to position information and the cupula returns to its null position when the flow of endolymph in a canal has a steady velocity. For these reasons the semicircular canals detect *onset and cessation of movement of the head* in any plane of space but do not monitor constant velocity or static posture of the head.

The motor responses to this information are phasic (kinetic) and have a marked tendency to adapt. They include eye movement and skeletomotor responses similar to the otolith reflexes just described but with different temporal characteristics. Both act in concert, the otolithic organ is active during *linear* acceleration and the semicircular canals during *angular* acceleration. For the present purposes it will be adequate to consider them together as 'the vestibular organ'. Anaesthetists specializing in otolaryngology should consult appropriate specialized literature.

The endolymph of the vestibular organ is continuous with that of the cochlea (Chapter 11), with a membranous labyrinth lying in a series of hollow channels in the petrous temporal bone (the bony labyrinth) from which it is separated by a space containing perilymphatic fluid and vascular connective tissue. The perilymphatic fluid provides a channel for the exchange of chemicals and to balance the pressure between the endolymphatic and subarachnoid spaces. Endolymph is secreted by cells in the membranous labyrinth and cochlea and re-absorbed in an endolymphatic sac. Disorders resulting in excess fluid (hydrops) interfere with labyrinthine and cochlear function (Ménière's syndrome). Endolymphatic fluid resembles intracellular fluid (high potassium, low sodium, high protein) and perilymphatic fluid resembles extracellular fluid (low potassium, high sodium, low protein).

The hair cells of the labyrinth receive a small number of terminals of *efferent vestibular neurones*. One is reminded of the gamma motor innervation of the other system of static and dynamic position receptors, the muscle spindles. By analogy, it seems probable that these efferent neurones modulate the excitability of the receptor cells, but their mode and circumstances of functioning are not understood.

VESTIBULAR NERVE

The efferent neurones, with the afferent neurones receiving synaptic (? neurotransmitter) signals from the hair cells, pass through a lamina cribrosa into the internal auditory canal along with the fibres of the cochlear nerve to the cistern of the cerebellopontine angle. The afferent neurone resembles those of spinal nerves in having its ganglion cell (perikaryon) outside the brain stem and then continuing centrally, ie it is a bipolar ganglion cell. It is situated in *Scarpa's ganglion* within the internal auditory canal. The primary afferent vestibular neurone maintains a constant baseline firing rate of action potentials which is increased or decreased according to whether its controlling hair cell is depolarized or hyperpolarized by deflection of cilia. The imposed firing rate tends to adapt towards the resting rate. This *adaptation* is additional to the viscous inertial properties of the acceleration transducers described above. It is particularly marked in a group of neurones with irregular firing rates, suggesting that there is a differentiation for static and dynamic functions.

After crossing the cerebellopontine cistern, the primary afferent neurones enter the brain stem at the inferior cerebellar peduncle and divide into ascending and descending branches to a group of four *vestibular nuclei* in the floor of the IVth ventricle lateral to the pontine reticular formation. Some primary afferent neurones pass directly up the inferior cerebellar peduncle to the 'vestibulocerebellum' (p. 223). They are accompanied by second order neurones from the vestibular nuclei. The cerebellar deep nuclei send fibres back to the vestibular nuclei — in fact a greater input to those nuclei than the fibres originating in the labyrinth (p. 225).

There is considerable topographic and functional specialization within the nuclei (*Fig.* 18.1). The superior and interstitial vestibular nuclei are mainly concerned with vestibulo-ocular reflexes, the lateral nucleus (Deiter's) with vestibulospinal reflexes, particularly to the upper limbs, and the medial nucleus with coordination of eye, head and neck movements. The descending vestibular nucleus integrates postural information from the utricle and saccule with proprioceptive signals from the spinal cord, all under cerebellar control. Both sides are linked by commissural fibres and with the reticular formation, forming a pontine area for modifying postural reflexes.

The outputs of the vestibular nuclei are by (i) *vestibulospinal tract* to extensor motoneurones of the spinal cord; (ii) *medial longitudinal bundles* to the extraocular muscles (p. 117) and via the *interstitial nucleus* of Cajal and the cerebellum; (iii) *vestibulocerebellar fibres* to the flocculonodular lobe of the cerebellum (p. 223); (iv) connections to the *pontine reticular formation*; (v) *vestibulocortical* fibres to the cerebral cortex relayed by the thalamus. Probably some thalamic afferents join kinaesthetic fibres and pass to the striatum for righting reflexes (Chapters 9 and 17). Disorders of the vestibular input to this system cause dystonic torticollis. Clinical experience (vertigo, basilar migraine and pontine vascular disorders) suggests a linkage between the vestibular and vagal nuclei so that vertigo commonly leads to vomiting. Conversely, drugs suppressing the vestibular centres are used as anti-emetics (eg metoclopramide, cyclizine, prochlorperazine etc.). In a considerable number of subjects, these drugs induce a dystonic state, presumably through the vestibulo-thalamo-striatal system described above.

The efferent second order neurones to motor control systems are of two types, tonic and phasic (kinetic), with mutual reciprocal inhibition through interneurones. The nuclei of the two sides are connected by commissural neurones in a manner similar to that described for the spinal cord grey matter (p. 160). They function as a balanced system. Both sides are disturbed by unilateral loss of labyrinthine input but this can be compensated. The nystagmus, past pointing and loss of equilibrium caused by labyrinthectomy is compen-

174

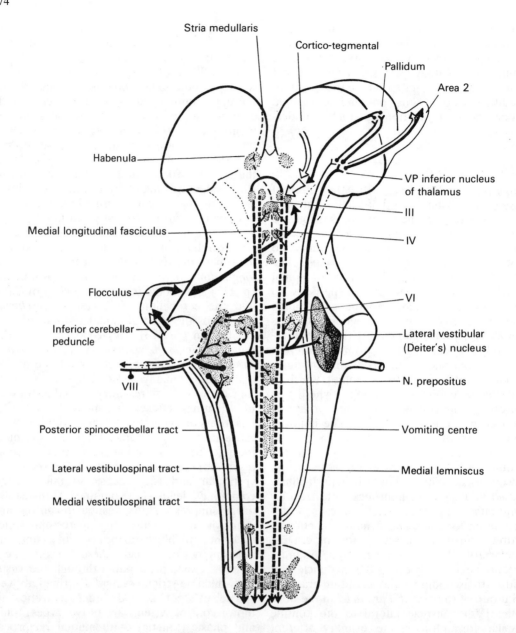

Fig. 18.1. *The central vestibular apparatus*. The right vestibular nerve afferent neurones are shown entering the group of vestibular nuclei at the pontomedullary junction. A major bundle of second order neurones enters the inferior cerebellar peduncle (*see Fig.*23.1) and is relayed through the vermis to the contralateral vestibular nuclei and to the contralateral thalamus (VP inferior) which they enter along with the proprioceptive fibres of the medial lemniscus and are relayed further to the lower end of the interparietal sulcus (area 2) for central appreciation of space orientation and movement. Other fibres relay to the pallidum (*see Fig.* 9.1) and are distributed to the tegmental nuclei for movement of the head and eyes. The cortex also projects to the tegmentum (open arrows) from the motor area 4 and the cortical centres for gaze (*see Fig.* 19.2). Also shown is the stria medullaris from septum to habenula where it relays in the fasciculus retroflexus to the interpeduncular nucleus (*see Fig.* 14.1), probably for head movement.

Important second order vestibular neurones join the medial longitudinal bundle of both sides to enter the apparatus in the middle of the diagram, the circuits controlling eye movements. They are omitted from this diagram and more fully pictured in *Fig.* 19.1: the second order neurones pass directly or after reticular relay into the VI nuclei bilaterally, sated within a few days. This has been attributed to tonic input from the cerebellum and reticular formation which gives a 'fine tuning' to the vestibular mechanism.

The vestibulocortical projection constitutes a pathway for providing subjective awareness of vestibular information and for modifying voluntary movements of the eyes as well as reflexly.

PERCEPTION OF MOTION AND OF THE VERTICAL

When moving fast around a wide curve (in a train or aeroplane) external objects are seen as if inclined. This indicates subjective appreciation of the interaction between gravity and centrifugal force. There is a sensation of turning. On a swing arranged to remain parallel with the ground, or in an elevator, one is aware of net increases or decreases of gravity (strictly the accelerative component of the change). The afferent signals clearly arise in the labyrinths and derivations from the vestibular nuclei interpreted at a point accessible to introspection.

The primary vestibular projection (closely associated with kinaesthetic fibres, Chapter 9) is through the *thalamus* to the contralateral suprasylvian gyrus just anterior to the auditory area, and the upper lip of the extraparietal sulcus. This is at the area representing facial sensation in the *second somatosensory area* and the interparietal sulcus (area 2) (p. 85). The vestibular field has a distinct cytoarchitectural structure. Collaterals of the thalamocortical projection go to the pre-central and post-central gyri.

Studies on the subjective interpretation of tilt and movement are increasingly important in space flight (with zero *g*) or in high speed aircraft (with greatly increased *g* while looping). It is remarkably sensitive. The 'after sensation' when angular rotation is stopped lasts for about half a minute, ie as long as the labyrinthine signal, because of the inertia of the endolymph/cupola and the adapting vestibular neurones. In some forms of migraine and epilepsy a discharge from this area of the cerebral cortex is experienced as *vertigo* (sensation of spinning). *Sensation of linear movement* within the head, sinking sensation, light-headedness and dizziness are sensations of altered orientation in space, an integration of visual, proprioceptive and vestibular signals. They are non-specific sensations with respect to localization of a disorder of function and they are common after hyperventilation, sedative drugs or general anaesthesia.

Conscious perception of orientation in space is a late development of a system evolved to control head and eye positions in order to provide a stable retinal image when the body is moving relative to the external environment. The primary function of the vestibular system is to derive velocity and position signals from the labyrinths and reflexly to control the position of the head (to stabilize it in space regardless of the orientation of the trunk and limbs) and to move the eyes in compensation for uncorrected head movements in order to limit apparent movement of the seen part of space. The vestibular nuclei are important sites for integration of signals from proprioceptive receptors in the neck with visual signals directly or indirectly from the retinae, a prototype for the cerebellum. The complex integrating circuit, requiring mainly polysynaptic pathways, sends efferents by the vestibulospinal and reticulospinal tracts to modulate the spinal postural reflexes and to the brain stem system for moving the eyes. It will be convenient to describe oculomotor control first

---

Fig. 18.1. (contd)
excitatory to the ipsilateral VI nerve and inhibitory to the contralateral (reciprocal innervation). Crossing fibres also inhibit the contralateral vestibular nuclei. The two vestibular complexes therefore act as a push–pull balanced pair.

Descending branches pass to the nucleus prepositus and ascending ones to the interstitial nucleus of Cajal bilaterally, the lower and upper ends of the oculomotor complex, sending collaterals to the III, IV and VI nuclei. The ascending bundles (— — —) and descending fibres from Cajal's nucleus (---) and a medial vestibulospinal descending bundle constitute the medial longitudinal fasciculus. There is also a lateral vestibulospinal tract from the lateral vestibular nucleus to the spinal cord (shown on right of medulla). Caudal to the prepositus nucleus in the midline, the vestibular nucleus projects to the 'vomiting centre' of the dorsal motor nucleus of X and apparently to other bulbar autonomic centres.

because, though complicated and not completely understood, it illustrates some general principles required for proper appreciation of other aspects of motor control.

Further reading

Balch R.W. and Honrubia V. *Clinical Neurophysiology of the Vestibular System*. Philadelphia: FA Davis, 1979.
Rudge P. *Clinical Neuro-otology*. Edinburgh: Churchill Livingstone, 1983.
Wilson V.J. and Melville Jones G. *Mammalian Vestibular Physiology*. New York. Plenum, 1979.

Chapter 19

Movements of the eyes and fixation of gaze

Each eyeball is moved by six muscles which, acting reciprocally, are able to rotate the globe in the orbit to direct the line of gaze horizontally to right or left and vertically (up and down). In addition to these *version movements*, the muscles causing vertical movement are inserted obliquely and this adds movements of rotation. *Rotation* of the eyes is necessary to stabilize the retinal image with respect to the horizon or direction of gravity. The motor control is required to coordinate the 12 muscles of the two eyes in such a way as to limit movement of a visual stimulus across the retina ('*image slip*'). In primitive chordates without binocular vision this is sufficient. The primary controls are therefore for linkage of the three *oculomotor nuclei* (III, IV, VI) with reciprocal inhibition between, for example, abduction and adduction, and for compensatory version and rotation movements to limit image (or retinal) slip. This is possible because the ocular muscles have tonic activity in the resting position which can be regulated up or down. This activity gradually ceases during surgical anaesthesia. The eyes then assume a divergent position.

With the development of binocular vision it was necessary for the reciprocal control to be bilateral and the required compensatory movements became complex. This is achieved by an important tract, the *medial longitudinal fasciculus* or bundle, one for each side (linking III, IV and VI nuclei) and connected bilaterally at upper and lower ends by the *interstitial nuclei of Cajal* and the *interpositus nuclei* respectively (*Figs.* 19.1, 19.2). Each of these nuclei is connected with its opposite by commissures running between the vestibular nuclei. Thus any input drive into the system evokes bilateral eye movements. These are not necessarily symmetrical. Ipsilateral drive to the abducens nucleus (VI) appears to be dominant in man.

The polysynaptic connections make the system vulnerable to disruption by anaesthesia, resulting in skew deviations and uncoordinated eye movements, but normally the eyes move as a pair because of the interneuronal systems of the cross-connected vestibular nuclei and related parts of the pontine reticular formation, regulated by the cerebellum. Some authorities identify a *pontine gaze centre* in the paramedian reticular formation of the pons caudal to the VI nucleus which integrates vestibular input with descending corticobulbar fibres from the contralateral hemisphere. Into this system are projected secondary afferent neurones from the neck proprioceptors and from the otolith and canal receptors of the labyrinths as described in Chapter 18, *both* types converging and relaying in the vestibular nuclei.

Signals of retinal slip are generated by directional sensitive cells of the retina (p. 97). In lower animals these signals pass in the optic nerve fibres but instead of going to the lateral geniculate nucleus for visual perception, they traverse the upper brain stem to the ipsilateral superior colliculus. Some fibres are believed to pass directly to the vestibular nuclei and cerebellum, but the superior colliculi are mainly responsible for visuo-oculomotor reflexes.

The *superior colliculus*, on the roof (tectum) of the mid-brain, receives primary optic afferents from the retina and also from certain cells in the visual cortex, from the acoustic nuclei and inferior colliculus, and from the spinal cord (*Fig.* 19.3). Most of the primary visual afferents cross in the chiasma. Each superior colliculus receives bilateral fibres, but

178

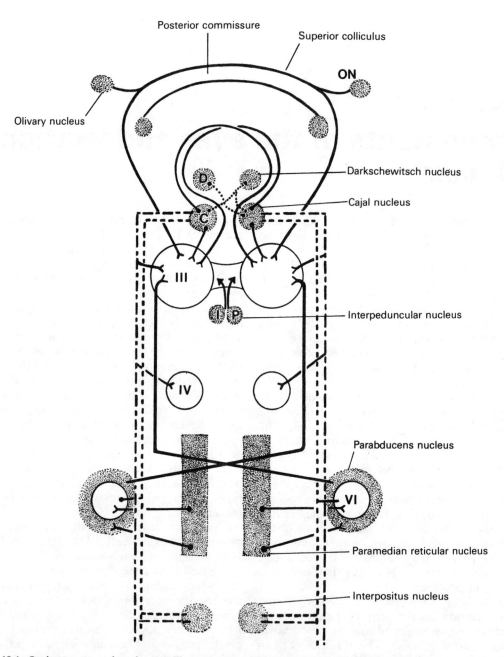

Fig. 19.1. *Oculomotor control mechanism.* The oculomotor (III), trochlear (IV) and abducens (VI) nuclei are linked by fibres descending (—·—·) and ascending (---) in the medial longitudinal fasciculus. The ocular fibres terminate at the interstitial nucleus of Cajal (C) and descending fibres (vestibulospinal and tectospinal) project to the spinal cord (*see Fig.* 18.1). The ocular control fibres end caudally at the interpositus nuclei (which may be linked). The VI nuclei are connected with the contralateral III for conjugate gaze. This group of lower centres is driven by the two pontine areas, the parabducens nucleus adjacent to VI which provides tonic innervation driven by the vestibular nerve and the pontine paramedian reticular nucleus which also evokes saccades. This is the main site of corticobulbar input, especially from the frontal eye fields of area 8.

The mesencephalic control linking eye movements with head movements (and other afferent inputs through the superior colliculus which is above the posterior commissure) is shown *top*. The occipitoparietal projection for pursuit gaze and optokinetic responses enters the system from each side at the olivary nuclei (ON) of the mesencephalon, ipsilaterally and through the posterior commissure. The commissure also links both of the interstitial nuclei (C). The closely related nuclei of Darkschewitsch (D) and the midline interpeduncular nucleus relay optic and olfactory stimuli for combined movements of the head and eyes. The interpeduncular nucleus relays impulses from the habenular nucleus which reach it by the fasciculus retroflexus (*see Fig.* 19.2).

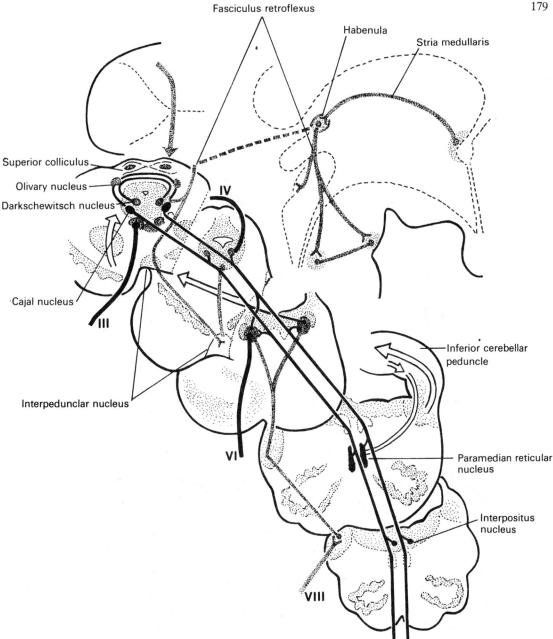

Fasciculus retroflexus

Habenula

Stria medullaris

Superior colliculus

Olivary nucleus

Darkschewitsch nucleus

Cajal nucleus

III

IV

Interpedunclar nucleus

VI

VIII

Inferior cerebellar peduncle

Paramedian reticular nucleus

Interpositus nucleus

Fig. 19.2. The oculomotor mechanism of *Fig.* 19.1 in anatomical site. The parallel lines indicate the medial longitudinal fasciculi. The IIIrd, IVth and VIth nerves are identified (note that the IVth nerve decussates on the dorsum of the mid-brain). Other nuclei shown are (*from above downwards*) superior colliculi, olivary nuclei, nuclei of Darkschewitsch and interpeduncular nucleus in the mesencephalon. Indicated in black are the important regulatory nuclei related to the ocular components of the medial longitudinal bundle — the interstitial nucleus of Cajal at the upper end, interpositus nuclei in the medulla and the paramedian reticular nuclei in the pons (the main target for corticofugal impulses).

Some regulatory inputs linking gaze with position of head and neck are indicated in grey. Inferiorly the vestibular second order neurones pass bilaterally to VI nuclei. Olfactory linked stimuli from the septal area (*upper right of diagram*) pass in the stria medullaris to the habenula and are relayed to the tectum and tegmentum. The important fasciculus retroflexus is also shown on the brain stem sections. It passes anteriorly between central grey and red nucleus to the interpeduncular nucleus which relays dorsally to the oculomotor nuclei. The open arrows represent vestibulo-cerebellar connections with efferent neurones decussating in the mid-brain to enter the upper oculomotor control area. Efferent fibres in the inferior cerebellar peduncle pass to the paramedian reticular formation (*see Fig.* 23.1).

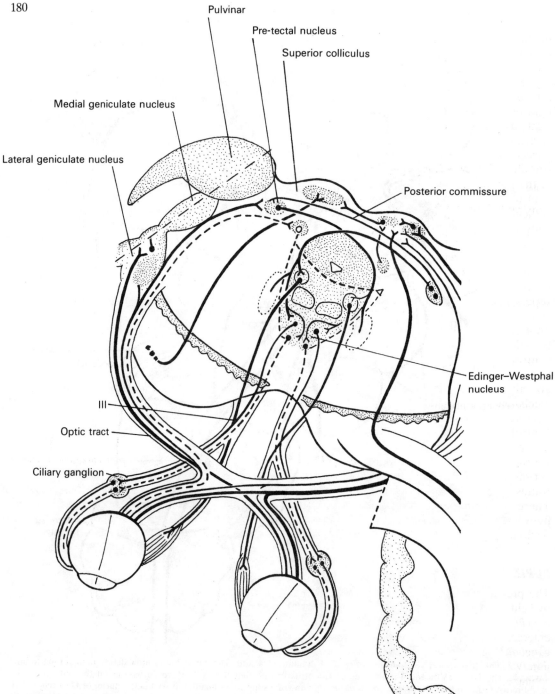

Pulvinar

Pre-tectal nucleus

Superior colliculus

Medial geniculate nucleus

Lateral geniculate nucleus

Posterior commissure

Edinger–Westphal nucleus

III

Optic tract

Ciliary ganglion

Fig. 19.3. *The pupil reflexes. Left*: the reflex arc for the light reflex. Optic nerve fibres from both eyes pass directly to the tectum of the mesencephalon and are relayed bilaterally in the nuclear zone of the superior colliculus to the pre-tectal area on both sides of the central grey matter and then to the Edinger–Westphal nuclei of the IIIrd nerve complex from which pupillomotor fibres pass in the oculomotor nerve for a short distance and then pass to the ciliary ganglion. The reflex pathway from the right retina is shown (----) with ipsilateral and consensual efferent paths. The solid lines indicate the optic and mid-brain pathways involved in visual accommodation. This is a synkinetic movement rather than a reflex and is more fully depicted in *Fig.* 19.4.

mainly from the contralateral side of both retinae — ie concerned with the ipsilateral homonymous visual fields. There is a strict topographic representation in lower animals, not confirmed in primates. Although a flash of light evokes responses (possibly the source of light awareness in patients with complete cortical blindness) most of the units are 'direction-specific' and respond to a light stimulus moving in the visual field, particularly at the periphery.

From the surface layer of the superior colliculus, the afferent fibres enter an underlying nuclear zone where visual and acoustic signals are integrated for reflex control of eye movements to direct the eyes towards a moving visual or acoustic target. Second order neurones pass to a deeper cellular layer of the superior colliculus, continuous with a specialized part of the reticular formation, the *pre-tectal area*, which in turn projects bilaterally to the spinal cord (*tectospinal tract*) for reflex control of head and neck movements, to turn towards a visual or acoustic target. The eyes are also moved by an input to the central mechanism described above, via the *interstitial nucleus of Cajal* at the upper pole of the ocular control circuits, and the vestibular nuclei at the lower pole. There is a parallel indirect route via the tectopontine fibres, pontine nuclei and vermis of the cerebellum. Note that all of these routes entrain the whole oculomotor synergy. There is no evidence for direct connections between the superior colliculus and individual oculomotor nuclei.

PUPIL REFLEXES

The pre-tectal area also relays impulses evoked by light to the *Edinger–Westphal nuclei* bilaterally (*Fig.* 19.3). The pupilloconstrictor nerve emerges with the IIIrd nerve fibres to the *ciliary ganglion* where the postganglionic neurones innervate the smooth muscle of the pupillary sphincter. As the connections are bilateral, light shone on one retina evokes both *direct and consensual light reflexes*. The direct response is commonly greater than the consensual.

Two important evolutionary developments have provided command systems for the oculomotor mechanism which are so powerful that they can over-rule the vestibulo-ocular

and visuo-ocular reflexes just described. These are the linked development of foveal vision and an analytic visual cortex. As with other examples of encephalization of sensori-motor linkage to be described later, the cortex not only adds a new dimension of control, it inhibits the lower level reflexes. In man the vestibulo-ocular and visuo-ocular reflexes are best seen in the unconscious or decorticate patient. They function to maintain the constancy of *the whole visual field* during movement in space. The emergence of foveal vision requires an added precision of compensatory movement — to direct gaze towards a peripherally detected *target*, even if it is not moving, and the cortex has provided a mechanism to *explore* visual space with eyes and hands. These are more than 'search and report' functions; they are controls of directed gaze, reflex and voluntary.

Control of gaze movements

These movements bypass the collicular–pre-tectal–oculomotor reflex by 'long-loop' reflexes through the cerebral cortex and the cerebellum to the same basic oculomotor mechanisms distributed to both eyes. For this purpose it is reasonable to regard the interconnected mid-brain interstitial nuclei of Cajal and the *interpositus nucleus* (near XII) as 'centres' for conjugate gaze in the vertical axis, and the vestibular-reticular apparatus (p. 175) as a 'centre' for conjugate horizontal gaze since the cortical and cerebellar influences are injected into the basic system via Cajal's nucleus and the pontine reticular and vestibular nuclei on each side.

NYSTAGMUS

Gaze may be driven reflexly from the retina, labyrinth, neck proprioceptors and cerebral cortex. Strong, imbalanced driving from any of these sources may give rise to nystagmus, especially where the input into the oculomotor mechanism is by the vestibular nuclei. They drive the eyes slowly to one side. With continuing drive the conjugate deviation of gaze is not maintained. The eyes return abruptly to the mid position then resume the slow version which is the active response. The alternation of slow and fast movements is termed *nystagmus*. The movements are conjugate unless the linking medial longitudinal bundle is damaged when monocular nystagmus occurs, with internuclear ophthalmoplegia (disconnection of the contralateral medial rectus from the dominant ipsilateral lateral rectus muscle).

The quick phase of jerk nystagmus is not understood. (Pendular nystagmus is an oscillatory scanning movement associated with defective foveal vision.) An *eye centering movement* observed in animal experiments has been attributed to the reticular formation, activated by tonic neck reflexes. Collaterals from the secondary vestibular neurones to the oculomotor nuclei are directed to inhibitory neurones in the *paramedian reticular formation* caudal to the VI nuclei and produce bursts of firing during the quick phase. This would briefly interrupt the tonic drive from the vestibular nuclei, but the driving source of the quick re-setting movement is unknown. Various authors describe *burst–tonic neurones* related to the quick phase in VI nucleus, apparently activated from the vestibular nuclei.

We have avoided describing the movements as 'saccades' since they may differ materially from the saccades of voluntary movement. The fast component of nystagmus is abolished by anaesthetics and tranquillizers but the slow tonic deviation is relatively preserved.

PREVENTION OF RETINAL SLIP

From the foveal area of the retina, optic nerve afferents are relayed in the lateral geniculate nucleus by the geniculocalcarine tract to area 17 of the cortex on one or other side (perhaps both, *see* Chapter 10). Intra- and subcortical connections via *the prestriate areas* 18 and 19 to the *angular and supramarginal gyri* of the parietal lobe, activate command neurones which project near the inferior medial aspect of the geniculocalcarine tract to the *contralateral tectum* of the mid-brain and so into the 'gaze centres' (*Fig.* 19.4). This constitutes an *optokinetic system* for direction of gaze towards the visual field containing an object of interest. It is not for gaze fixation (it is found in animals without a fovea) but supplements the vestibulo-

ocular reflex from the semicircular canals to prevent retinal slip with head movements at frequencies too low for the vestibulo-ocular reflex to function (less than 0·01 Hz). It appears that the visual association cortex computes an error signal from the apparent movement of the visual image and feeds back motor control signals proportional to the error. This supplements the vestibulo-ocular reflex as a 'back up' which persists when the canal cupula returns to its resting position and the canal signal falls back to zero. By different detectors, both signals interpret head velocity.

In most circumstances the reflex outputs (measured by intensity and duration of optokinetic or vestibular nystagmus) have equal time constants. It is probable that optokinetic and canal signals converge on the same second order vestibular neurones (presumably not the medial longitudinal bundle as the vestibulo-ocular and optokinetic nystagmus are not abolished by bundle lesions). Neurologists value the *optokinetic response*, tested by moving a striped pattern across the visual field, as a test of posterior hemisphere function (*Fig.* 19.5). Note that it is not necessarily abolished along with hemianopia. Conversely, no response occurs unless *attention* is directed at the moving pattern.

When the discrepancy between vestibular signals or apparent movement of visual space indicates that the head is turning to the right, the eyes are driven conjugately towards the left — ie to watch a visual area disappearing towards the left. This relatively slow movement is the active response. If the error signal persists, the gaze rapidly but briefly returns to the mid resting position and then resumes its slow movement. This alternating movement of gaze is *nystagmus*. Unfortunately, although the reflexes drive the slow component, the direction of the more spectacular fast, resetting, component has been used to define the direction of nystagmus. One reason for this is that the response is increased if voluntary gaze is directed away from the direction of apparent movement. Thus, a reflex driving the eyes to the left is more evident when gaze is directed to the right, the direction of the fast phase. In consequence, mild pathological nystagmus is first evident on looking to the side of the fast phase. The example just described would be defined by a clinical observer as 'right-beating

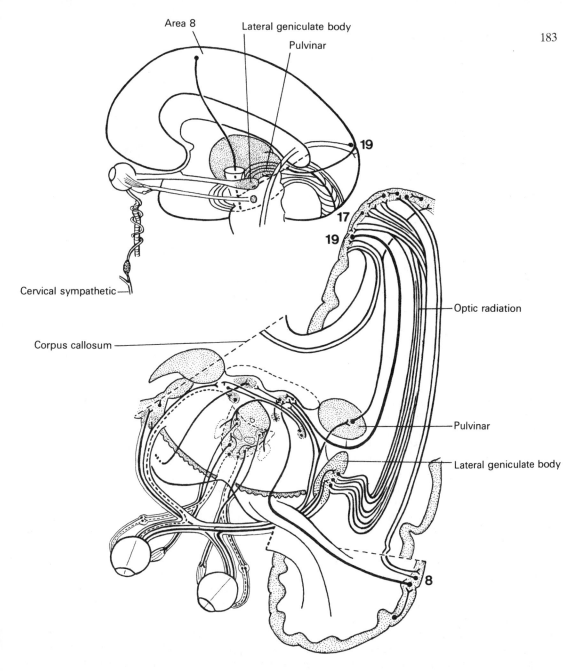

Area 8

Lateral geniculate body

Pulvinar

19

17

19

Cervical sympathetic

Corpus callosum

Optic radiation

Pulvinar

Lateral geniculate body

8

Fig. 19.4. The mid-brain mechanism for light reflex (----, *Fig.* 19.3) is shown *lower left*. Accommodation of the lens and associated pupil modulation is tightly coupled with convergence of the eyes to minimize image blurring. This is detected by the visual cortex which then 'commands' the convergence mechanism, through corticobulbar fibres. Optic nerve fibres are shown passing bilaterally to the superior colliculi and also to the lateral geniculate body and pulvinar where they are relayed in the optic radiations to the striate area of each hemisphere. (As the horizontal brain section may be unfamiliar, the right hemisphere has been detached by section of the corpus callosum at the dashed line indicated.) Note the transoccipital linkage across the splenium of the corpus callosum, joining peristriate areas (19), not primary receiving areas. Peristriate cortex is also connected longitudinally to the pre-central area 8. From areas 19 and 8, corticobulbar motor neurones (▬) descend to the superior colliculus and also to the contralateral pontine gaze centre. These areas entrain the gaze mechanism. The connections shown from superior colliculi to III complex bilaterally evoke convergence (▬ to medial recti) and the autonomic (ciliary ganglion) response of the ciliary muscle (——) and pupillary constriction (----). The sympathetic pupillodilator control from the cervical sympathetic chain is indicated (*upper part of diagram*).

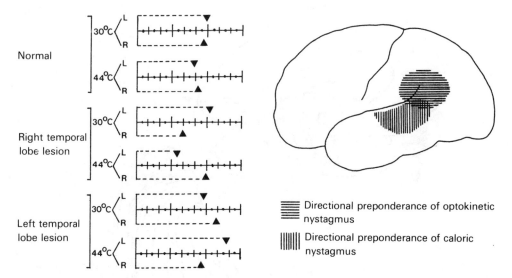

Fig. 19.5. Directional preponderance of caloric nystagmus (to the side of the cerebral lesion) occurs with lesions in the posterior halves of the temporal lobes. Directional preponderance of optokinetic nystagmus occurs with lesions in the region of the supramarginal and angular gyri. Caloric nystagmus is evoked by Hallpike's method. The nystagmus durations are denoted by the interrupted lines. Each continuous line represents a 3-minute interval.

nystagmus on right lateral gaze'. In fact, the abnormality is the slow gaze shift towards the left, driven by the right 'supranuclear opto-kinetic centre' and the vestibulo-ocular reflex from the cupula of the dominant of one pair of semicircular canals (depending on head position). Stimulation of one horizontal canal, for instance, drives the eyes slowly to the opposite side and the quick phase is directed towards the side stimulated. Opposing muscles are reciprocally inhibited.

With two intact labyrinths the input to the vestibular nuclei summates algebraically (excitation + inhibition). Damage of one side (receptor or nuclei) unbalances the system so that nystagmus is induced by slower head movements. If the cupula is stimulated by inducing thermal convection currents in the endolymph with the canal vertical there will be *directional preponderance* in favour of the intact canal and 'canal paresis' of the diseased one. With a hot stimulus, the intact canal produces slow eye movements to the other side which have greater peak velocity, amplitude, frequency and duration of response than the movements evoked from the damaged canal. A cold stimulus drives nystagmus in the opposite direction — to the stimulated side. (Since most people find it easier to observe the quick

phase, a mnemonic for the quick movements is the word 'cows' — cold, opposite; warm, same.) A cortical centre modulating vestibular nystagmus is in the posterior temporal lobe. It overlaps with but is distinct from the area regulating optokinetic nystagmus (*Fig.* 19.5).

If the *direction* of nystagmus is opposite to that expected, or if it is monocular, or reversing, the disorder is central, either in the vestibular nuclei or in the cerebellum which should inhibit the response. The anaesthetist rarely requires to localize a vestibulo-ocular disorder. His main interest is in the fact that the reflex is at pontine level. Bilateral loss of caloric responses indicates severe depression of pontine function — either from deep sedation or from 'brain stem death'. The same significance applies to otolith vestibulo-ocular reflexes. The 'dolls head' response (p. 171) is released by disconnection from higher levels, and abolished by pontine sedation or death.

In the conscious subject, the degree of attention is important. Optokinetic nystagmus may be absent if the subject does not direct attention to the striped drum or tape moving across his visual field. Conversely, vestibular nystagmus is inhibited if the eyes are open and fixating. Inhibition is due to a higher level gaze reflex.

THE FIXATION REFLEX

This is not the same as the optokinetic reflex, which is a compensation for head movement to minimize retinal slip. With the development of foveal vision and alerted attention, a necessary refinement is to shift the gaze (against the compensatory direction if required) so that an *interesting* object in the peripheral visual field with defined contours and usually moving with respect to the background is brought into the foveal field, for better discrimination. The foveal gaze must then be fixed on that target until its arousal value is lost. Little is known about this reflex in man. Like the optokinetic response, it utilizes the visual pathway to the striate cortex (area 17). It is generally stated that the efferent path is the corticocollicular path described above for the optokinetic response but it should be stressed that few authors differentiate between the latter and the foveal fixation response. The only clinico-pathological report we can trace is a case of Gordon Holmes: 'Disease involved the dorsal portion of the thalamus, including the pulvinar.' Though he regarded this as an interruption of corticotectal fibres, it could have been in the afferent limb of the reflex (*see Fig.* 19.4).

The fixation response is remarkably powerful, overriding the neck and vestibular reflexes. The ocular axes are not completely locked to the target. A *microtremor* at 30–50 Hz and irregular flicks keep the edge of the visual image moving across the cones of the fovea. This opposes adaptation of the receptor mechanism. Disease of the fovea permits greater ocular tremor, to the extent of visible oscillation of the eyes (*pendular nystagmus*). Visual contrast is impaired by movements which are excessive or of too low frequency but also by very fast movements of the eyes. Even the fast movement of normal saccades is associated with depression of visual acuity.

VERGENCE AND FOCUSING

Closely associated with fixation is the neurological control for true *binocular vision*, bringing a selected target to homologous points of both foveas by converging the eyes until the visual axes meet at the point of interest (*Fig.* 19.6). Like the optokinetic and fixation responses, vergence only occurs in the alerted subject. Perhaps 'response' is a better term than 'reflex'. Vergence is a learned response. It appears at about the third month of life and is readily modified by placing prisms in front of the eyes. A lesion between the oculomotor nuclei in the upper mid-brain will cause convergence paralysis, but no single brain stem site of stimulation evokes convergence. There is no evidence for an unpaired nucleus of Perlia. Asymmetric convergence movements with an accommodation response have been reported from unilateral stimulation of points in the primate pre-occipital cortex and it is suggested that bilateral activation 'at the highest level of nervous activity' using the splenium of the corpus callosum, utilizes command neurones projecting independently to both sides of the pre-tectum and tectum for integration at brain stem level (*see Fig.* 19.4).

A foveal specialization of the retinal slip control would be sufficient. All objects lying on a three-dimensional curved circle (the *horopter*) through the fixation point and the lenses of both eyes will be seen as single, being projected to homologous areas of each retina (*Fig.* 19.6). Binocular fusion does not occur for objects inside or outside of the horopter circle. It is, therefore, functionally important to select targets on the horopter for presentation to the retina but to retain the other signals for depth perception (*stereoscopy*).

ACCOMMODATION

The fixation point, and hence the horopter circle, is adjustable by altering the curvature of the lenses of the two eyes identically. Focusing is produced by the *accommodation response*. The curvature of the crystalline lens of the eye, and hence its refractive power, depends on the tension exerted on its capsule by the circular fibres of the ciliary muscle inside the eyeball, counteracting the passive elastic tension of the choroid and sclera. In near accommodation (focus on a near point) the ciliary muscle contracts and, because of its connection with zonule fibres, counteracts the elastic force of the choroid, decreases the tension on the capsule, and permits the lens to become more convex (until age or disease hardens the lens). The ciliary muscle is part of a muscle forming

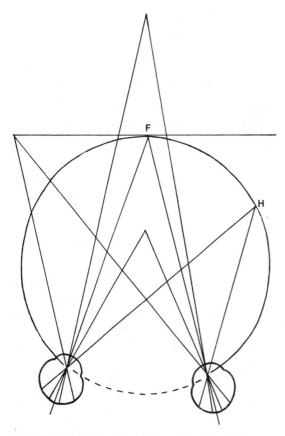

Fig. 19.6. Depth disparity in binocular vision. Both eyes view an object at F (fixation point). The visual axes are projected backwards. The image falls on corresponding retinal areas, and this is true for any object in a three-dimensional curved surface (horopter) through the fixation point and the foci of refraction of each eye (e.g. H). The images of all objects on either side of the horopter are disparate. The diplopia is greater for near than for distant objects. Diplopia is uncrossed for objects outside the horopter and crossed for objects within it.

the ciliary nerve branches of the IIIrd cranial nerve, a part of the parasympathetic nervous system (Chapter 26). These are relayed in the ciliary ganglion from the Edinger–Westphal nucleus in the mid-brain (*see Fig. 19.3*). (There may be separate fibres for accommodation and for the light reflex. More than 90 per cent of ciliary ganglion neurones are for accommodation.) As it is an autonomic nerve, the innervation of the pupil is unusual since accommodation is linked to a somatic response, near vision, and indeed it is under some voluntary control through this linkage.

The accommodation response is an *associated movement* tightly linked with convergence of the eyes. In constant ambient light the pupils do not constrict or the lenses focus unless the eyes converge. Accommodation is part of a *near fixation synergy*. (Unfortunately for patients with myotonic pupils, the smooth muscle contracts and relaxes more slowly than the adductors of the eyeballs.) The eyes are converged and the ciliary muscle contracted to minimize retinal blur as perceived by the visual cortex (*see Fig. 19.4*). It has been described as an 'even-error servo system' and the correction oscillates detectably at about 2 Hz. It is only in this sense that the accommodation response is reflex. The pupil response is certainly a synkinesis. The supranuclear control of fusion and accommodation is unknown but, as they are sometimes associated with defective fixation reflex, it is probable that they involve similar pathways from the occipital visuomotor area.

Exploratory eye movements

Searching movements of the eyes are carried out by two types of movement. Like all movements, the ocular muscles function synergically with modification of postural control reflexes. These are described as saccadic and pursuit movements (*Fig. 19.7*).

SACCADIC EYE MOVEMENTS

Saccadic eye movements are rapid 'flicks' of the eyes for scanning visual space and for rapidly directing the foveas to an interesting target. They are conjugate *search movements*, often described as ballistic. This adjective is not

the sphincter of the pupil. When it contracts, the pupil constricts. For optical reasons, this also improves the depth of focus of the lens during near vision, reducing the requirements for exact focusing.

The ciliary muscle is a smooth muscle with *muscarinic acetylcholine receptors*. It is contracted by cholinomimetic drugs such as the anticholinesterases (Chapter 2) which cause spasm of accommodation, and transmission is blocked by atropine-like drugs. The latter dilate the pupil and cause blurred vision by preventing the accommodation response. The muscle is innervated by a plexus of nerves from

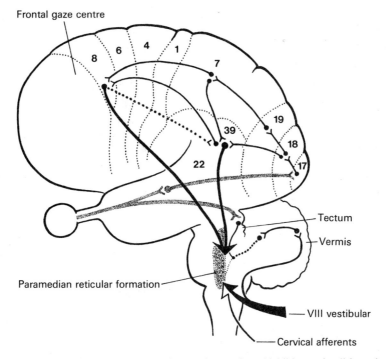

Fig. 19.7. *Control of gaze.* Paramedian reticular formation receives tonic and inhibitory stimuli from the vestibular nuclei and neck proprioceptors and also from area 39 which integrates visual and vestibular signals received from areas 17 and 22. The optic radiation (----) to area 17 is also relayed through visual association areas 18 and 19 to parietal area 7 which has 'command' neurones to a frontal gaze centre in area 8. This area is shown as having reciprocal inhibitory connections with area 39 but its main outflow is by corticobulbar fibres to the tegmentum, at the upper end of the oculomotor control system. Ocular movements evoked from area 39 are tonic 'pursuit' movements, those from area 8 are ballistic 'saccades'. Both efferent tracts evoke bilateral ('gaze') movements, the appropriate innervation of extraocular muscles being organized by the oculomotor apparatus illustrated in *Fig.* 19.1. They are coordinated by the superior colliculus which receives first order optic neurones (*grey*) (*see Fig.* 19.2) and by the cerebellar vermis (*see Fig.* 23.1). The cerebellar control is inhibitory. Vertical gaze requires the joint action of both cerebral hemispheres.

Not included in the diagram is a pathway from the septal area via the habenula and interpeduncular nucleus to the tegmentum (*see Fig.* 14.1). It directs head and eye movements towards olfactory targets. Head and eye movements and the cranial nerve motor nuclei are closely linked through internuclear fibres of the medial longitudinal bundle.

exact as it is possible to arrest a saccade before completion. During these fast (600–700 degrees/second) movements of the eye, vision is suppressed by an unknown mechanism. Experiments on the monkey suggest that saccades are evoked by command neurones in area 7 of the *parietal lobe, acting through the frontal eye fields* to a saccade generator area in the *paramedian reticular formation of the pons.* In that area there are neurones which excite or inhibit bursts of firing of the oculomotor neurones. They are sometimes designated *burst neurones* and *pause neurones* and are at present believed to be exclusive to saccades, not to pursuit movements of the eyes or to steady fixation which is probably controlled by

tonic neurones of the pontine reticular formation. Studies on Parinaud's syndrome (various palsies of vertical gaze) in man indicate a similar vertical saccade generator in the reticular formation of the *upper medial mid-brain,* dorsal to the red nucleus. The vertical saccade centres of each side are linked by the *posterior commissure.* It is very vulnerable to pressure by pineal tumours, III ventricle tumours and hydrocephalus.

The burst of very high frequency impulses (up to 1000/s) from the burst neurones drives both eyes rapidly until the burst is cut off by a complementary discharge of pause neurones in the midline of the pons and in the contralateral medullary reticular formation. The timing of the burst is extremely accurate, bringing the central gaze on to the target, and indeed it may be modified in mid flight.

Speculatively, the burst duration must be pre-programmed at a supranuclear level as it is difficult to conceive of a negative feedback control acting with sufficient speed. Unlike limb movement where inhibitory feedback from position receptors is an adequate solution, eye movement control is unusual in that the movement to the target is carried out precisely, whatever the starting position of the eyes in the orbits. Stretch and tension receptors which are present in the extraocular muscles are considered to play a minor role. Feedback through the visual pathway would be a possible mechanism if it could be compared with an efference copy signal proportional to the eye position (*see* Corollary discharge, Chapter 24).

A unilateral lesion of the pontine reticular formation causes a dissociated ipsilateral palsy of conjugate gaze with loss of saccades to the contralateral half field, but *oculocephalic response* is preserved (probably through the vestibular nuclei), permitting both eyes to be driven beyond the midline to the side of the lesion in response to turning the head. In reading or scanning a face, scene or picture, the eyes make saccadic movements to direct gaze to 'interesting parts' of the visual field.

PURSUIT EYE MOVEMENTS

When an interesting target has been located, the foveas are kept on target by a smooth pursuit movement system which inhibits further saccades. (Continuous slow drift and quick flick micromovements are either noise in the system or fine corrective movements to compensate for receptor adaptation, Chapter 10.) If the object moves, the eyes pursue the target, presumably by the optokinetic and fixation responses of the occipital eye fields and coupled there with the convergence–accommodation focusing responses. How this posterior motor command system is brought under voluntary control is not known. A clinical aphorism is that *the occipital eye fields generate smooth pursuit and the frontal eye fields generate saccades*. Normal goal-directed vision uses both together and doubtless the

basal ganglia and cerebellum are involved in their coordination. It is possible, for instance, that the saccade 'burst' neurones are inhibited by the 'pause' neurones of the reticular formation until the latter are inhibited by the superior colliculus or the cerebellum, as with other ballistic types of movement (Chapter 23). Perhaps surprisingly, the pursuit movements are more vulnerable than the saccades to barbiturates.

GOAL DIRECTED AND VOLUNTARY CONTROL OF GAZE

The involuntary systems described to this point have indicated a hierarchy of reflexes stabilizing the retinal images by (i) compensation for head movement, (ii) following a peripheral target, (iii) locking on to a selected target, (iv) discriminating it by reducing image blur. With the encephalization of vision these basic homoeostatic reflexes are put at the disposal of the goal-seeking brain to explore visual space actively. This requires a capacity to unlock the eyes from the powerful postural and fixation reflexes and to put them at the disposal of association areas of the cortex acting through the later developed corticobulbar system. It is suggested by Mountcastle that the fixation and tracking neurones of parietal area 7 receive processed signals (? error correction) from the visual association cortex and project them through the frontal eye fields (*Fig.* 19.7) to the saccade generator for control of *directed gaze* (as distinct from searching) as part of the system for directed attention when motivated, or conditioned, by the limbic system (Chapter 14).

The occipital eye movement field of areas 18 and 19 is connected by a subcortical fibre tract, the superior longitudinal bundle, to an ipsilateral *frontal eye field* in the second frontal convolution (area 8). Both ends of this major projection are connected with the contralateral areas by an extensive fibre system in the *corpus callosum* (*Fig.* 19.4) (there is doubt about interconnection of the frontal eye fields). These interhemisphere links are necessary for vertical gaze and for convergence. The frontal eye fields send fibres back to the occipital and pre-occipital eye fields of both sides to *inhibit* the optokinetic and fixation responses (*Fig.*

19.7), releasing the brain stem oculomotor mechanism from postural fixation at the onset of a goal-directed movement. Because of the cross-modality linkages of the cortex, the visuo-motor system is then put at the disposal of the integrative cortex, frontal and other, to search for a *desired* target even though the head and/or external space are moving.

The efferent projection from the frontal eye fields to the oculomotor mechanism is closely linked with command signals to move the head and, to some extent, the body. Electrical stimulation or epileptic excitation commonly evokes head turning along with conjugate deviation of the eyes. From areas 8, 1, 4 and 6 of the frontal cortex efferent corticobulbar fibres pass through the genu of the internal capsule to the mid-brain, where they join pyramidal tract fibres and cross to the contralateral oculomotor area adjacent to the VI nucleus (for horizontal gaze) and the reticular formation of the mid-brain tegmentum for vertical gaze. Although the two hemispheres normally work together, each hemisphere is mainly responsible for exploratory gaze to the contralateral side, which it 'sees'. Thus irritative pre-central lesions cause *conjugate deviation* of the eyes and head to the side opposite the lesion, paralytic lesions cause deviation towards the side of the lesion, but never vertical deviation. There is, however, sufficient bilateral representation to permit recovery of voluntary gaze to the opposite side even after hemispherectomy.

It is the bilaterality of impulses (from frontal, parietal or occipital cortex or from the labyrinths) which evokes vertical eye movements, travelling in the pre-tectum or posterior commissure for upward gaze and the fasciculi retroflexi for downward gaze and the ventral periaqueductal grey matter of the mid-brain, medio-dorsal to the red nucleus.

Further reading

Bach-y-Rita P., Collins C. and Hyde J.E. (ed.) *The Control of Eye Movements*. New York: Academic Press, 1971.

Bender M.B. Brain control of conjugate horizontal and vertical eye movements. A survey of the structural and functional correlates. *Brain* 1980; **103**: 23–69.

Blackwood W., Dix M.R. and Rudge P. The cerebral pathways of optokinetic nystagmus: a neuro-anatomical study. *Brain* 1975; **98**: 297–308.

Chapter 20

Motor automatisms of respiration and feeding

An important reason for the extended account of the relation between vision and eye movement control is to prepare the reader for some general concepts of sensori-motor control. Particular attention is drawn to the corticofugal pathways outside the pyramidal tract. It is difficult to find a suitable heading for this section which will not perpetuate the widespread belief that the cerebral cortex, and specifically a specialized 'motor area', originates command instructions for movement, overriding a primitive 'extrapyramidal' system and entraining a cerebellar system for co-ordination of muscle synergies.

In the following chapters it will be shown that the basal ganglia and cerebellum are involved between the formulation of an intention to move and the activation of the neurones of the pyramidal tract and that the latter are in the main outflow pathways from both of these 'inferior' structures. They are certainly involved in the control of eye movements and are only omitted from the last chapter for convenience of presentation. Rhythmical movements that are capable of reflex and voluntary modification illustrate the links between peripheral and cerebral motor controls. The concept has been introduced in the preceding chapter on eye movements and will now be followed by an introduction to the mid-brain regulation of axial movement, respiration and feeding and then gait as a transition to goal-directed movement of the limbs.

The mid-brain and its extension into the diencephalon has a central core of grey matter extending from the periventricular area of the IIIrd ventricle to the periaqueductal area of the mid-brain. Dorsal to the aqueduct it is specialized in the *tectum* (colliculi) for integration of eye, head, and trunk movements involving vision and hearing (Chapters 10 and 11). Ventral to the aqueduct are the upper nuclei of the medial longitudinal bundle (the nucleus of Darkschewitsch and the interstitial nucleus of Cajal, *see Fig.* 19.1). More ventrally and laterally, the central grey differentiates into the more discrete nuclei of the mid-brain reticular formation in the *tegmentum*. Efferent connections from the hypothalamus (*see Fig.* 25.2) to this region are relayed through the facial nuclei bilaterally to the muscles of facial expression and to the pneumotactic centre for respiration (*see Figs* 20.1–2).

The tegmental nuclei, which include the red nucleus and substantia nigra, control the medial pontomedullary reticular formation distributed to the axial muscles and responsible for motor automatisms including respiration (*see* later) and locomotion (Chapter 21), linking these areas with the primary motor activating system, the periventricular grey matter. All of the motor automatisms (including the autonomic system, Chapter 26) are bilateral, being cross-linked at numerous levels, and cannot be activated unilaterally. Many of them are initiated by a movement of the head and trunk, with displacement of the centre of gravity of the body and entrainment of a series of head-on-body and body-on-body righting reflexes (Chapter 17). The role of head movement is crucial, probably consistent with the later evolution of the vestibular system and cerebellum.

The *control of head movement*, despite its importance, is not fully understood, but it seems likely that it involves tegmental nuclei specialized for displacement in different planes of space. From studies in lower animals it is likely that the *ventral tegmentum* extends the neck dorsally (part of the orientation arrest response), the *dorsal tegmentum* flexes the neck (feeding and forward movement response), the *nuclei of Darkschewitsch and Cajal* rotate the neck (and also direct gaze in response to the tectum) and the *substantia nigra* pars reticulata flexes the neck and trunk laterally for turning the body to one side. They are reciprocally connected for alternating automatisms (released in disease as tremors).

All of these tegmental nuclei receive indirect signals from distance receptors via the colliculi, habenula and corticotegmental fibres but they are integrated by the *subthalamic nuclei* which include the nucleus of the field of Forel, the subthalamic nucleus of Luys and probably the inferomedial part of the pallidum.

Superimposed on this system for head–trunk control and especially for the lateralized movement of turning to one side is the striatum. A *paleostriatum* relaying downwards to the subthalamic group of nuclei receives afferents from the intralaminar and centromedian nuclei of the thalamus relaying nociceptive, proprioceptive and vestibular signals (*see* Fig. 9.2), some relayed secondarily from the cerebellum (*see* Fig. 23.1). This is the reflex arc for the *righting reflexes* (Chapter 17). It is inhibited and brought under cerebral control by the *neostriatum* (Chapter 22).

Pontomedullary control of motor automatisms

Movements of the jaw, face, pharynx, larynx and respiration are of particular interest to the anaesthetist. They are also important for a proper understanding of motor control of the limbs since they represent a class of movement intermediate between the innate postural and protective reflexes and the 'encephalized' movements typical of the limbs. *Figs* 20.1 and 20.2 (*see below*) are general diagrams to show the structural components of the brain stem reticular formation relevant to supraspinal control of rhythmical involuntary motor activity. The areas of reticular formation relevant to cerebellar regulation are omitted (*see* Chapter 23). The same basic mechanisms control respiration and gait. The systems are difficult to dissect because they are distributed and the chains of control are not entirely from above downwards so that experimental dissection or

disease by cross-section at an anatomical level gives a confusing picture.

These 'automatisms', as they are sometimes called to distinguish them from reflex involuntary movements, show the following general properties: (i) cortical control is bilateral and mainly inhibitory; (ii) linked reflexes with a tendency to cyclical repetition are involved and largely bilateral (entirely bilateral in respiration); (iii) parallel descending neurones converge on brain stem and spinal neurones (interneurones and motor neurones) which integrate the supraspinal drives by summating their excitatory and inhibitory synaptic potentials (Chapter 3). The sum may be insufficient to produce adequate depolarization of the 'final common path' until segmental inputs are added. In this way a common central drive is finely regulated at segmental level instead of producing an all-or-none response.

The latter principle applies to single motor units as well as to whole muscles. For instance, the timing in relation to the respiratory cycle, and the duration of burst discharge of respiratory neurones, is strongly influenced by afferent feedback. Individual units may respond entirely differently to a common central drive, such as changes in Pco_2 or Po_2 and lung inflation.

The general principles of alpha–gamma linkage and the role of muscle spindles in voluntary movement, described in Chapter 22, apply to all movement systems both 'voluntary' and 'automatic'.

Respiration

Fundamentally the essential vital process of respiration is a cyclical muscular activity of spinal motoneurones driven by reticulospinal fibres from a central pattern generator controlled by sensory feedback loops and reflexes to optimize the oxygen and acid-base levels of arterial blood and to adapt the breathing to a number of non-homoeostatic behaviours. Respiration is arrested during chewing, swallowing and vomiting (p. 204). Breathing is also arrested in full inspiration during defaecation and urination, and temporarily arrested during alteration of trunk posture and strong muscular effort. Inspiration is increased in rate and volume as a gasp, and expiration is slowed in a controlled manner during phonation and in sniffing for olfactory orientation and exploration (p. 203). Respiration is arrested by stimulation of parts of the pre-motor area (6b) associated with chewing, swallowing and vocalization and of the orbitofrontal cortex (area 13) involved in the arrest reaction of the orientation response (Chapter 14). Thus, although the fundamental rhythm of respiration has a bulbospinal control, it is strongly modulated by motor commands originating in the cerebral cortex and basal ganglia and these are predominantly inhibitory (*Fig. 20.3*).

Voluntary respiration is possible. When the bulbospinal centres with their reticulospinal projection to the motoneurones of the respiratory muscles are damaged by disease (eg bulbar poliomyelitis) or surgery (eg high cervical section of the anterolateral column of the spinal cord for relief of pain), it is possible for respiration to continue under voluntary control. This is believed to use the corticospinal (pyramidal) tract. Voluntary control is effective while the subject is awake but sleep abolishes this voluntary control and the subject is then liable to stop breathing unless ventilated passively.

Ventilatory excursion is reduced even in normal sleep. During the rapid eye movement phase of sleep (Chapter 16) the hypoventilation may be sufficient to cause episodes of hypoxaemia in patients with chronic bronchitis and cor pulmonale, and in patients breathing spontaneously following intermittent positive pressure respiration. Reactive stimulated respiration in the presence of muscle hypotonia (or airway obstruction) causes *snoring*.

It is evident that corticospinal fibres, the mesencephalic reticular formation and collaterals from ponto-medullary reflexes may modify the rhythmic motor output of the medullary central pattern generator for respiration, temporarily abrogating its homoeostatic function. Other, more important, sensory feedback loops and reflexes are homoeostatic, adjusting the pattern of respiration according to prevailing requirements.

NORMAL RESPIRATION

In normal breathing, inspiration is active. The diaphragm is drawn down and the ribs flared by the external intercostal muscles to increase the thoracic volume. The negative pressure created draws air into the lungs through the upper respiratory tract. In expiration the relaxing muscles allow the ribs to fall back and the diaphragm rises. Air passes out through the glottis. The driving force is mainly the elastic recoil of the lungs and rib cage, but a certain amount of expiratory force is applied by contraction of abdominal muscles. If there is increased resistance to outflow of air, a positive expiratory effort is applied by the abdominal and internal intercostal muscles. The cross-section of the rib cage becomes more circular (instead of elliptical). Activity of expiratory muscles is also required during exercise of medium intensity. The expiratory force is applied earlier in the cycle as exercise increases and becomes dominant during coughing, sneezing, phonating and vomiting. The inspiratory and expiratory muscles are reciprocally innervated at spinal and possibly medullary levels but the expiratory motoneurones are inhibited by the tonic CO_2 drive during quick respiration.

The recruitment of inspiratory and expiratory muscles is governed by reflexes sensing intrapulmonary pressure and passive stretching of the intercostal muscles which are superimposed on a breathing frequency determined by chemoreceptor driving of a central generator. The optimal breathing frequency is that which requires the minimum average muscular force. *The amount of innervation* of the inspiratory muscles (recruitment and firing frequency of neurones and order of recruitment of muscles, from upper intercostal spaces downwards with increasing tidal volume), is pre-programmed within the nervous system to reach a predetermined endstate of *tidal volume*. If the diaphragm and intercostal muscles are insufficient to achieve the required volume, the nervous system recruits the 'accessory muscles of respiration', such as the sternomastoid and scalene muscles.

Excluding the cortical respiratory controls described above, which override spontaneous respiration, we have to examine the neurological mechanisms of quiet breathing and its reflex modification for changed circumstances within the physiological range. The primary drive for quiet breathing is chemical, inspiration being activated by raised arterial P_{CO_2}, lowered P_{O_2}, or lowered pH. The medullary centre responds mainly to P_{CO_2}, the carotid bodies to decreasing P_{O_2}. In non-REM sleep (*see* Chapter 15) the rhythm is maintained but slowed and with reduced tidal volume (allowing mild hypercapnia and hypoxia). In REM sleep breathing is irregular with more shallow than deep breaths. The reduced response to hypercapnia is more marked in males.

CHEMORECEPTORS FOR RESPIRATORY DRIVE

INTRAMEDULLARY

Chemosensitive structures in the ventral medulla include receptors that respond to changes in blood gases, driving neurones in the *lateral medullary reticular formation*. The efferent cells are clustered dorsal to the nucleus ambiguus and are referred to by some authors as the *nucleus retroambigualis*. Some receptors adjacent to the pia mater and ependyma respond to changes in the hydrogen ion concentration of the cerebrospinal fluid (Chapter 28). The extracellular pH in the brain is currently believed to be the main chemical signal determining ventilation, by modulating transmission of cholinergic neurones on which there is convergence of neurones from peripheral chemoreceptors and unspecified peripheral receptors. The exact site of the main receptors (if indeed they are localized) has not been determined. Some authors favour the *area postrema* (p. 35). (For diagrammatic purposes this area is marked in *Fig.* 20.1 as the CO_2 (or pH) sensitive site, and the locus coeruleus as oxygen-sensitive, but the chemosensitive zone probably extends between these points on the median eminence of the floor of the IVth ventricle.) They can also be fired by certain drugs — veratrium alkaloids, nicotine and acetylcholine — and suppressed by procaine. Calcium channels may be involved. The response to CO_2 tension is slowly modified during *acclimatization* to altitude or to submarine depths (acute effects are due to altered partial pressures of alveolar gases).

Animal experiments, and the relatively insignificant loss of respiratory drive from lesions affecting the other ventilatory drives in man, indicate that this system provides the major stimulus to the pontomedullary respiratory neurones, but the dendrites of the latter integrate the hypercapnic/hypoxic drive with others derived from peripheral chemoreceptor and proprioceptive reflexes. Some of the latter also operate at segmental level.

CAROTID BODIES (GLOMUS)

A carotid body lies behind the bifurcation of each common carotid artery. It contains receptors susceptible to variations in the gaseous content of arterial blood and also pressure-sensitive receptors (Chapter 8). Both types, but particularly the chemoreceptors, send signals by the glossopharyngeal (IX) and vagus (X) nerves via relays in neck ganglia to the medulla where they end in the respiratory and vasomotor 'centres'. Stimulation of the chemoreceptors by hypoxia, hypercapnia and acidaemia results in a reflex increase in respiration but also causes bradycardia and peripheral vasoconstriction. Doxapram is a stimulator of peripheral chemoreceptors. It has a modest pressor effect due to catecholamine release and the increase in both systolic and diastolic blood pressure is accompanied by an increase in heart rate. An important interaction of carotid body receptors with the protective reflexes of the nose and larynx is described on p. 165. The inspiratory stimulation by anoxia is relatively insignificant except at peak of CO_2 driving. The carotid body may also have O_2-sensitive 'off-switch' neurones which limit inspiration when blood oxygen content is adequate. This can be of practical significance in treating ventilatory failure with high CO_2 levels (chronic bronchitis) when high O_2 in inspired gas may decrease the tidal volume. (It seems surprising that this example of the 'off-switch' mechanism has been so little studied in an easily accessible organ.)

AORTIC BODIES

Mesodermal structures similar to the carotid bodies are situated between the aortic arch and the ligamentum arteriosum and probably function like them. Aortic bodies lying on each side of the abdominal aorta are different. They are

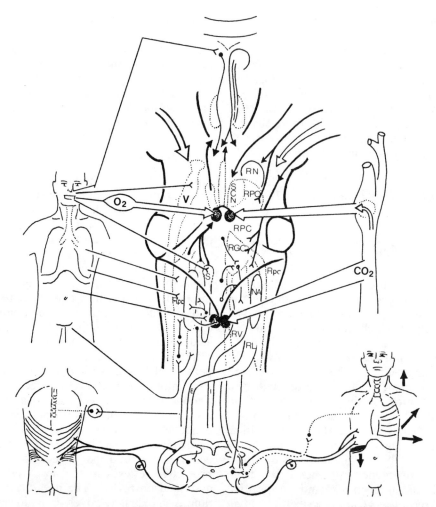

Fig. 20.1. *Central control of respiration*. The brain stem, with some cranial nerve nuclei (*left*) and the main nuclei of the reticular formation (*right*). The afferent signals affecting respiration are listed from above downwards but the important regulators are P_{CO_2} (or pH) and P_{O_2} detected at the lower and upper end of the median eminence of the IVth ventricle and chemoreceptors (including O_2) in the carotid bodies (*right*). The lower black area is the area postrema and the shaded area above is the locus coeruleus.

Afferent signals are shown from olfactory receptors, via the habenula, the face (V), lung (to the lateral medullary reticular area Rpc), taste receptors and abdominal viscera to upper and lower solitary nucleus (S) and pain fibres. They project to the area inhibiting inspiration and to the nucleus ambiguus (NA), for autonomic responses. The cerebral peduncle (*right of diagram*) indicates higher inputs from the cortex and diencephalon to the mesencephalic reticular formation. The central inspiratory area is in the gigantocellular area of the pontine reticular formation (RGC) and projects through ventral and lateral medullary reticular centres to the contralateral (partly ipsilateral) reticulospinal tracts to terminate at the spinal motoneurones for inspiratory and expiratory muscles.

The lower sketches illustrate inspiration (*right*) and expiration (*left*), with indication of the associated autonomic controls of the bronchioles. The diagram on the right illustrates sympathetic bronchodilatation and on the left, parasympathetic bronchoconstriction from the dorsal nucleus of X (between S and NA).

Key: RN, red nucleus; SCN, superior central nucleus; RPO, oral pontine reticular nucleus; RPC, central pontine reticular nucleus; RGC, gigantocellular reticular nucleus; Rpc parvicellular reticular nucleus; NA, nucleus ambiguus; S, solitary nucleus; RV, ventral reticular nucleus; RL, lateral reticular nucleus; E, expiratory pathways; I, inspiratory pathways.

paraganglia containing chromaffin cells of neuro-ectodermal origin, producing catecholamines. Their function is not clear and they are unlikely to be concerned with respiration.

PULMONARY CHEMORECEPTORS

Chemoreceptors in the alveolar walls do not induce normal quiet respiration. Rather than blood gases or pH, their effective stimuli are phenyl diguanide and serotonin. These substances reflexly induce expiratory apnoea followed by hyperpnoea, suggesting that the receptors have a protective rather than a respiratory function. Termed J-receptors, they evoke lung deflation in pathological conditions and may inhibit monosynaptic spinal stretch reflexes of the limbs.

RECEPTORS IN MUSCLE

If evolution has selected a central integrated drive for respiration based on homoeostasis of blood gases and acidity, it might be expected that some local control would also be evolved (in analogy with the control of body temperature). Indeed there is good evidence that both active and passive exercise of skeletal muscles stimulate the rate and amplitude of respiration. The respiratory response to CO_2 is potentiated. Surprisingly, the exact mechanism remains unknown. The possibility of a chemical stimulus is debated, with chemoreceptors sensing metabolites of active muscle rather than local changes in blood gases. No adequate stimulus or receptor has been identified. A receptor system in veins has been postulated. Chemosensitive nerve endings for pain seem no differerent in muscle from those of other tissues. Some experimental evidence favours a reflex from muscle proprioceptors. This should be distinguished from the undoubted role of proprioceptors of the thoracic cage in providing segmental control of the ventilatory cycle. This is not a primary driving depolarization and will be described after the mechanisms responsible for quiet rhythmical breathing.

MEDULLARY RETICULAR MECHANISM FOR RESPIRATION

The neural basis for the rhythmic component of quiet breathing is by no means certain. In the 1960s it was generally believed that two 'centres' in the medullary lateral reticular formation sent impulses to the inspiratory muscles and the expiratory muscles respectively, each reciprocally inhibiting the other and so giving rise to rhythmical alternation of inspiration and expiration. At the present time the concept of inspiratory and expiratory neurones is still accepted but no longer grouped discretely and with doubts about the mutually inhibitory system at medullary level. Reciprocal inhibition at spinal level is, however, clearly demonstrable. It is not known whether there is an autorhythmic 'pacemaker' cell or a complex of neurones. In *Fig. 20.2* the symbol for the central inspiratory apparatus should not be interpreted as representing a single cell. Most of the neurones that fire periodically in some phase of the respiratory excursion are in the *lateral reticular formation of the medulla*, around the nucleus ambiguus (motor nucleus of X), the expiratory motoneurones a little caudal to the inspiratory motoneurones. Each side of the medulla projects to both sides of the spinal cord in the anterior portion of the lateral column and lateral portion of the ventral column, but mainly contralaterally. Crossing is at spinal level as well as just below the obex. This *reticulospinal path* is mixed with vestibulospinal and spinothalamic fibres. (It is liable to section if spinothalamotomy is carried out at C_1–C_3 levels. Respiration may be maintained by crossing fibres from the contralateral tract and by corticospinal fibres but, as pointed out above, ventilation is impaired, particularly during sleep.)

The lateral medullary reticulospinal projection is responsible for periodic respiration, but when descending and bulbar reflex controls are interrupted by a lesion of the dorso-medial medulla at or above the obex the movements are not rhythmical nor do they have the sinusoidal characteristics expected of an interacting mutually inhibitory driving system. The tidal volume varies in amplitude and rate and the pattern — described as *ataxic breathing* — is dominated by gasps. The response to P_{CO_2} and pH is reduced and easily suppressed by sedative drugs. A similar de-centralization may occur in deep sleep, one cause of sleep apnoea.

196

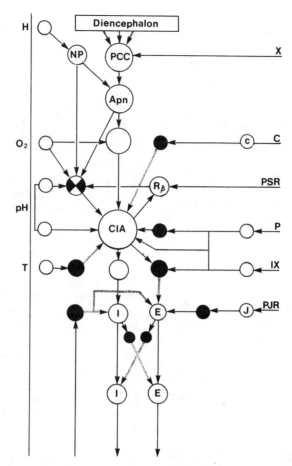

Fig. 20.2. *Schematic diagram of respiratory control.* Inspiratory (I) and expiratory (E) motoneurones are reciprocally connected by inhibitory interneurones (●) only in the spinal cord and are driven by the central inspiratory apparatus (CIA), the expiratory being inhibited by 'early burst' interneurones in the nucleus retroambigualis. The respiratory pattern generator in the pontomedullary area, part of or adjacent to the nucleus of the solitary tract, consists of a group of neurones (CIA) driven by pH receptors in the median eminence of the IVth ventricle but modulated by 'off-switch' neurones (⊗) which integrate inputs from the pH-sensitive cells and R_β neurones relaying signals from pulmonary stretch receptors (PSR). Chemoreceptors in the same area, near the locus coeruleus are O_2-sensitive and contribute to the dendritic input to the 'off-switch'. Oxygen receptors and others in the carotid bodies (C) inhibit the CIA. The drive to inspire is facilitated by the apneusis area (Apn) under control of the pneumotactic control centre (PCC) of the mesencephalon and the 'off-switch' neurones are facilitated by the nucleus parabrachialis (NP). The mesencephalic centres are further modified by various diencephalic areas such as the basal ganglia and the hypothalamus (H), including the thermoregulatory area.

The central regulator is inhibited during tasting (T), swallowing and coughing (IX) or an inspiratory gasp is followed by prolonged active expiration. Pain (P) may evoke a similar reflex especially if it is visceral. Chemoreceptors in the pulmonary alveoli responsive to toxic material stimulate pulmonary J receptors (PJR) which inhibit expiration. The vagus nerve (X), shown as projecting to the PCC, probably modifies the system at all levels.

An inhibitory neurone (*lower left of diagram*) suppresses both inspiration and expiration during severe contraction of skeletal muscles. It is shown as receiving ascending signals but the source is unknown and could be a corollary discharge from the pyramidal tract. Between CIA and the medullary neurones the pathways cross to the other side of the spinal cord and the fibres then descend in reticulospinal pathways closely related to the ascending spinothalamic tracts.

Realization that most of the expiratory phase is a passive elastic response of the thorax (and that expiratory bulbospinal neurones can be silent in experimental animals under certain circumstances in which normal breathing is maintained) is forcing a reassessment of the reciprocal driving system described above. Expiratory neurones are normally biased near their firing thresholds by continuous synaptic bombardment but they are periodically inhibited during inspiration. The expiratory reticulospinal neurones certainly receive inhibitory signals from the inspiratory neurones (probably via inhibitory interneurones), but there is no satisfactory evidence that the inspiratory neurones (which are normally biased by a continuous inhibition) are further inhibited by the expiratory neurones. They are indeed turned off during the expiratory phase, but this is effected by a group of 'off-switch' neurones (*Fig.* 20.2). These medullary neurones are apparently activated progressively by the inspiratory neurones which are then suppressed when the total activity of 'off-switch' neurones (an integration of firing rates and recruitment) reaches a theshold roughly proportional to the chemical drive on the inspiratory neurones — ie higher P_{CO_2} evokes more inspiratory activity and raises the switch-off threshold. Inspiration is terminated abruptly and passive expiration then occurs.

Thus the main variable in the cycle is the inspiratory phase, not what would be predicted from pure reciprocal inhibition. The 'off-switch' neurones are presumably excited by a corollary discharge from the inspiratory neurones. They may also receive inhibitory fibres from pulmonary stretch receptors but it is the fact that the neurones switching off inspiration are also dependent on the chemical drive that makes it possible for tidal volume to increase in response to increased drive for ventilation despite the Hering–Breuer and other reflexes described below.

Presumably once the inspiratory neurones are switched off, the effect of the controlling neurones decays in a non-linear manner until insufficient to suppress the appearance of the next inspiration, but the pause can be prolonged by the pulmonary stretch reflexes or shortened by receptors for gasp and cough which act as gating mechanisms. The latter reflexes, and also voluntary exhaling and phonation, use *expiratory reticulospinal neurones*. They undoubtedly exist, even though the reciprocal control model is abandoned for normal breathing. Strong stimulation of pulmonary chemoreceptors induces expiratory spasm (*expiratory apnoea*). (A word of caution is required. It will be shown below that respiratory motoneurones appear to receive both facilitatory and inhibitory synaptic signals from the medullary respiratory driving system. A truly effective 'off-switch' device in the medulla would make the inhibitory bulbospinal projection unnecessary.) This reassessment of the respiratory rhythm generator raises interesting speculation about the control of expiratory muscles and their normal role.

PONTINE RETICULAR FORMATION

The inspiratory–expiratory antithesis suggests an either–or situation, which is not correct. Respiratory neurones vary in the duration of burst discharge, number of spikes per burst, timing in relation to the respiratory cycle and order of recruitment. Some units (known as *phase-spanning units*) start to fire near the end of one phase and continue into the other. Most of these units are found in the *pontine reticular formation* rather than in the medulla. Their activity smooths out the change from inspiration to expiration and vice versa.

A small number of neurones fire in all phases of respiration, without burst activity. These phase-spanning and *'tonic' neurones* are responsible for smoothing a respiratory excursion which would otherwise tend to have a 'saw-tooth' configuration. Although some are present in the medulla, tonic and phase-spanning units are most characteristic of a higher level of downward projecting reticular formation neurones in the medial and lateral parts of the pons, the lower part favouring transition from expiration to inspiration, and the upper (near the locus coeruleus) favouring transition from inspiration to expiration. Some upper potentine neurones strongly facilitate inspiration, ie they potentiate the medullary response to a standard chemical drive.

Vagal reflexes regulate breathing at this level as well as in the medulla, via the nucleus solitarius and nucleus ambiguus (sensory and motor nuclei of the vagus). The exact site of the 'central pattern generator' is uncertain. A single group of neurones, probably in the reticular formation near the CO_2-sensitive zone of the *area postrema*, governs medullary 'centres' for inspiration and expiration. Without a vagal input, the tonic facilitatory effect of the pontine reticular nucleus holds the medullary ventilatory drive in the inspiratory phase. This inspiratory spasm or cramp ('apneusis') has been described as 'the decerebrate rigidity of the respiratory musculature'. If it is interrupted sufficiently to maintain life, the respiratory pattern is termed 'apneustic breathing'. Inspiratory spasm may last for 1–2 minutes and is followed by a single expiration or several phasic breaths. The powerful expiratory efforts which intervene between periods of prolonged inspiratory apneusis are attributed to disinhibition of lower medullary expiratory neurones which are also tonically driven by CO_2. Another inspiratory spasm follows, successive apneustic periods becoming progressively shorter. Small phasic breaths may be superimposed on the inspiratory spasm ('cluster breathing'). In human disease or head injury, apneustic breathing is rare. It indicates decerebration at the upper pontine level. Even with lower pontine lesions the inspiratory phase predominates.

The anterior pontine reticular formation has a neuronal system which inhibits the 'apneustic centre', ie its activity prevents tonic inspiratory activity of the medullary neurones. It has been described as a *'pneumotactic' control centre*, possibly by having a high proportion of phase-spanning neurones. It is responsible for permitting rhythmical breathing in most decerebrate patients. Apneustic breathing only occurs if it is destroyed or isolated from the pons. Some authors consider that in addition to inhibiting the 'apneustic centre' of the pons, it activates the expiratory reticulospinal neurones of the medulla which are not spontaneously active. (While deprecating the use of 'centres', this term is convenient to avoid circumlocution where the usage is, we hope, clear.)

Table 20.1. The respiratory pattern results from the released function of levels below the lesion

	Function	*Mechanism*	*Effect of lesion*
Neocortex	Voluntary expiration (vocalization etc.)	Selective inhibition of inspiration and active expiration	Dysphasia
Pallidum	Gating of axial musculature	Switch of 'set'	Respiratory dyskinesia
Limbic	Ventilation for anticipated activity	Respiration for action	Inappropriate ventilation
Hypothalamus			
Anterior	Metabolic regulation	Rate control	Bradypnoea
Posterior	Thermoregulation		Tachypnoea
Mesencephalon	O_2 inhibition	Feedback control (minute volume)	Periodic breathing
Isthmus	CO_2 drive, with volume-sensitive switch	Amplitude control (tidal volume)	Hyperventilation
Pons	Smoothing	Phase spanning	Ataxic breathing: hiccup
Open medulla	Peak limiting reflexes	Off switch	Inspiratory apnoea
Closed medulla	Inspiration/expiration 'flip-flop'	Cycle	Cluster breathing; gasping Sleep apnoea
Cervical spinal cord	Load correction of volume Distribution to muscles	Reciprocal innervation of muscles	Ventilatory paresis Complete apnoea

The threshold or set-point of the phase-spanning system is controlled by a reticular 'off-switch' just ventral to the aqueduct of the mid-brain and floor of the rostral part of the IVth ventricle. Lesions here cause central neurogenic hyperventilation with low threshold to $P\text{CO}_2$ and pH associated with loss of the response to O_2, suggesting a target area for the carotid body input.

The control of respiration rate is uncertain, but probably diencephalic. Respiratory movements are not controlled by the cerebellum. Its homologue at this primitive level of motor control is the pneumotactic centre with input from the vagus in place of the vestibular nerve. The ventilatory cycle tends to 'hunt' (Cheyne–Stokes respiration), with bilateral diencephalic lesions, indicating some higher control, presumably inhibitory (*Table* 20.1).

It is probably through the two pontine systems that emotional (hypothalamic) and sniffing (cortical, p. 203) control are exerted on rhythmical breathing. These influences are minor compared with those of the reflex inputs from stretch receptors in lungs and thorax. Most other respiratory-related movements, such as chewing, swallowing and speaking, are supported by complete arrest of inspiratory activity until the hypercapnic/hypoxic drive dominates over the higher level inhibition.

FETAL BREATHING

In the fetus, quiet breathing movements occur of a type considered 'paradoxical' in the adult. The diaphragm moves downwards and the abdomen enlarges but the chest wall is drawn in unless the intercostal muscles are recruited by hypercapnia. This pattern persists in premature infants or those with respiratory distress syndrome due to deficiency of pulmonary surfactant. Further hypercapnic drive recruits the laryngeal abductor muscles (causing the fetus to inhale meconium). The rhythm of quiet breathing is irregular: with the increased drive it becomes regular and deeper. In the adult, respiration is mainly abdominal in the male with more intercostal muscle activity in the female. Hypercapnia recruits upper thoracic muscles and then the 'accessory muscles of respiration' of the thoracic inlet and snout.

The episodic breathing pattern of the fetus is associated with EEG and eye movement features characteristic of REM sleep (Chapter 16). They are not completely linked and probably indicate independent activation of the mesencephalon. A linkage between depth of sleep and regularity of breathing persists in the adult but the linkage is looser except in some clinical disorders. The transition from fetal to neonatal pattern of breathing may be associated with disinhibition of the carotid body response to hypoxia. In the fetus, hypoxia arrests breathing unless the brain stem is transected at the isthmus when it then causes increased depth and, particularly, rate of respiration. It could be an important protective device in utero to prevent inhalation of amniotic fluid in response to placental hypoxaemia. How this protection is switched off after birth (so that hypoxaemia becomes a secondary inspiratory stimulus) is not known, but inflation of the pulmonary alveoli by the first gasp may be important. The midwife can then relax, having administered a sharp cutaneous stimulus if the snout reflex is not sufficient.

Anaesthetists should consider that the hypoxic response may not be well established in the newborn. Fetal movements are arrested by smaller doses of pentobarbitone than in adults, at a level which may be insufficient to anaesthetize the mother, and this effect is on the suprapontine control. During the birth, fetal breathing is arrested. This has been attributed to prostaglandins of the E series (and may be potentiated by use of prostaglandins in labour). The effect is more caudal than that of pentobarbitone, probably at the medulla. Inhibitors of prostaglandins synthesis, such as salicylates, indomethacin and meclofenamate, stimulate the volume of the respiratory cycle even in the adult, so it is unlikely that the suppressive effect on fetal breathing is related to patency of the ductus arteriosus. The central action of prostaglandins on neonatal breathing (and other fetal effects) makes prostaglandin administration potentially hazardous to the baby at full term labour or in presence of hyaline membrane disease of the lungs since it seems to raise the threshold of the respiratory rhythm generator. The threshold for breathing and its volume are not naloxone sensitive but opioid peptides and somatostatin (acting near the nucleus of the solitary tract) reduce the frequency of the periodic breathing and 5-HT may stimulate episodic breathing in the fetus (as well as provoking non-REM sleep).

Isocapnic hypoxia in the late gestation fetus also suppresses other pontomedullary automatisms such as heart beat regulation and fetal movements — providing valuable clinical signs for the obstetrician.

PATHOLOGICAL RESPIRATORY RHYTHM

The brain stem reticular formation provides a very adequate suprasegmental control for the respiratory rhythm based on relatively small variations in the chemistry of the perfusing blood. If the diencephalic control of medullary centres is depressed due to decreased blood flow, chronic alveolar underventilation or to hypnotic drugs, the respiratory rhythm becomes periodic (*Cheyne–Stokes respiration*). Ventilation waxes and wanes from apnoea to hyperventilation and back to apnoea. Higher lesions interfere with the control of air flow through the larynx and oral cavity (basal ganglia) or its patterned control (cerebrum) by modulating the suprapontine control (*Fig. 20.3*). Thus general anaesthesia affects speech and vocalization before ventilation.

Intracranial lesions causing Cheyne–Stokes respiration are always bilateral and deep in the hemispheres or diencephalon. In this type of breathing the hyperventilatory phase is due to an excessive response of the medullary reticular formation to the chemical drive, followed by post-hyperventilation apnoea. It is associated with hyperactive ventilatory response to CO_2 stimulation and the de-repressed centre is driven to excessive response even with moderately lowered CO_2 and normal O_2 pressures in the blood.

Periodic breathing without hyperventilation is found in patients with posterior fossa com-

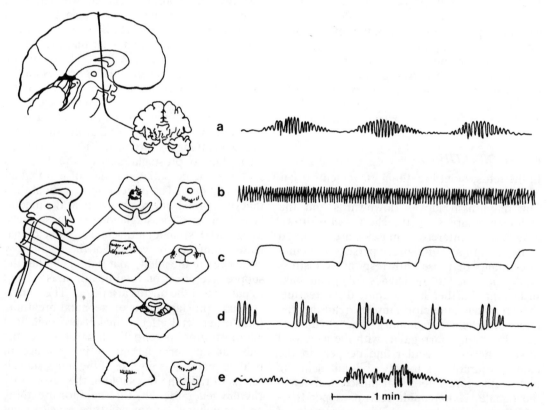

Fig. 20.3. Pneumographs of abnormal respiratory patterns associated with pathological lesions (shaded areas) at various levels of the brain (inspiration up). *a*, Cheyne–Stokes respiration; *b*, central neurogenic hyperventilation; *c*, apneusis; *d*, cluster breathing; *e*, ataxic breathing.

pressive lesions. The respiratory rate is increased and the rhythm less regular, often exhibiting *cluster breathing* with irregular pauses. Other types of pathological respiratory rhythm are mentioned above. *Biot's breathing* is a type of ataxic breathing in which episodes of apnoea are followed by a series of inhalations of irregular amplitude. It occurs when the upper pontine (pneumotactic) centre is disconnected from the lower pontine/medullary centres but some vagal reflexes remain intact. It has been described in cases of meningitis. If the afferent vagal control is also removed by a bilateral lesion of the dorsolateral pontine tegmentum, apneustic breathing (p. 198) occurs. The most common lesion in man is pontine infarction, but it is rare.

Respiratory failure occurs with acute bilateral lesions of the medulla or its respiratory neurones (eg bulbar poliomyelitis). Conversely, the sensitivity of the medullary respiratory centre to P_{CO_2} and P_{O_2} is increased by pyrexia (and by aspirin in large dosage). Rarely, destructive lesions of the mid-brain and pons cause *hyperventilation*, with low inspiratory threshold to CO_2. A respiratory alkalosis results unless oxygen is supplied but this procedure does not influence the pattern of deep, regular, rapid inspirations. Head injury causes a constellation of respiratory patterns, none being consistent or typical.

REFLEX MODIFICATION OF RESPIRATORY VOLUME

Clearly, the major factor controlling the range, rate and regularity of the respiration is the chemosensitive brain stem system which can be temporarily overridden by the pyramidal tract commands to the respiratory muscle motoneurones. This generalization is true if airflow takes place through a low resistance airway. When this does not apply, load compensatory inflation and deflation reflexes modify the response to the chemical drive.

INFLATION REFLEX

Inflation of the pulmonary alveoli activates *pressure receptors* on vagal afferents which pass centrally in the *vagus nerve* to the medulla and up the tractus solitarius to the caudal portion of the ipsilateral nucleus solitarius (a few fibres cross to the contralateral nucleus). They are relayed (by R_β neurones) through the nucleus ambiguus (motor nucleus of vagus) to 'off-switch' neurones in the pontine reticular formation 'pneumotactic' centre. In man the inflation reflex is not initiated until the alveoli are almost fully expanded. This stimulus reflexly inhibits the inspiratory muscles and prolongs expiration, with activation of expiratory muscles (*Hering–Breuer reflex*). This reflex facilitates *active expiration* as distinct from the passive elastic recoil which is normally adequate. Note the vagus-stimulating effect of positive pressure ventilation. 'Fighting the machine' is not altogether a willed movement. During anaesthesia, positive pressure ventilation may cause passive inflation followed by active (reflex) expiration, especially if the rib-cage reflexes are stimulated.

DEFLATION REFLEX

Full deflation of the lungs stimulates a reciprocal *vagal reflex* through the lower pons with *activation of inspiratory muscles* and inhibition of expiratory muscles. It is inactive in normal circumstances but may stimulate a dangerously uncontrolled inspiration in divers without breathing apparatus. The vagal reflexes compensate for load variations in the airways but are not primary determinants of the phases of respiration as was formerly thought.

A general principle is that *the pons* acting through the medulla *regulates the amplitude of inhalation*, the expiratory rate being determined by passive neuronal and musculoskeletal relaxation. The vagal reflexes from *pulmonary receptors control the frequency of respiration* by limiting inspiratory and expiratory peaks and regulating the balance between inspiratory and expiratory activity. Other modifications of the central respiratory rhythm are imposed by stretch reflexes of the rib cage which are more localized in their action. In man these are probably more significant than the Hering–Breuer reflex.

LOAD COMPENSATING REFLEXES FROM THE CHEST WALL

The work produced by the inspiratory and expiratory muscles is greater than would be predicted from the displaced volume of air. The extra work is to overcome the impedance and elastance of the airways (breathing through the nose involves twice the load imposed by mouth breathing), apparently to stabilize lung volume within a 'normal' range. When inspiring against a positive intra-alveolar pressure, the expiratory muscles do not completely relax; when expiring against negative pressures, the inspiratory muscles do not completely relax, indicating that the 'switch' can in some way sense the lung volume regardless of the direction of flow.

An important contribution is reflex activation of the expiratory muscles when the chest expands, by length and tension receptors of the spindles of the intercostal muscles and diaphragm, and probably by reflexes mediated by position receptors of the rib joints. They are both monosynaptic and polysynaptic reflexes, some segmental, others acting more diffusely by propriospinal anterolateral column paths linking intercostal and phrenic motoneurones to proprioceptors from all parts of the thoracic cage.

The reflexes are not simple stretch reflexes to resist muscle lengthening, though this may play a part in terminating inspiration. Tracheal obstruction at the onset of inspiration causes increased discharge from the spindles of inspiratory muscles, though they are contracting. This could only occur if these spindles are being forced to shorten by fusimotor nerve fibres (Chapter 9). (The misalignment between intrafusal fibre length and that demanded of the extrafusal fibres by the medullary chemosensitive drive is detected by the spindle and reflexly excites additional alpha motoneurone activity to cancel the misalignment, according to the servo theory of motor control. The theory is under attack so far as voluntary movement of limb muscles is concerned, p. 240, but the experiments by Sears and others on respiratory muscles appear to be compatible with it.)

The soma of the lower motoneurone to an intercostal muscle or the diaphragm integrates the reflex input of the chest proprioceptors with that of sensory fibres from the abdominal muscles, neck (head movement), from splanchnic afferents from abdominal viscera, and from the skin of the chest. It thereby facilitates or inhibits the central respiratory drive descending from the medulla. Recent research attributes a greater role to spinal control than was previously suspected.

Slow potential changes of the presynaptic potentials of intercostal and phrenic motoneurones occur in phase with respiration. This implies that the brain stem respiratory centres exert an alternating excitatory and inhibitory influence on them. The central drive (including the vagal reflexes) activates both fusimotor and alpha motoneurones with typical cerebellar controlled alpha–gamma linkage. In the cat diaphragm it is found that most spindles act as passive stretch receptors while some are fusimotor driven and others intermediate. The role of the gamma loop in regulating respiratory muscles is still debatable. The precise control of airflow despite varying loads may be required for phonation and sniffing, rather than for breathing.

GASP, COUGH AND INHIBITING REFLEXES

The main stimulus to the first inspiratory movement of the newborn is probably the anoxia resulting from deprivation of the oxygen supply from the placenta, but an important stimulant to an inspiratory gasp is believed to be the effect of cold on the snout area when the fetal head is born. Abrupt cold stimuli of the face may evoke a *gasp* in the mature human, familiar to the layman treating syncope but sometimes forgotten by the anaesthetist. Sudden immersion of the body in cold water is an equally effective stimulus. Rapid maximal inspiration (gasp) is immediately followed by inhibition of respiration until the CO_2 drive resumes dominance. Sudden pain evokes a similar reflex, especially if it is facial or thoracic and thoraco-abdominal pain causes prolonged inhibition of inspiration. (Note that expiration is relatively unaffected so that the peak flow rate measurement may be little reduced.)

COUGHING AND SNEEZING

These are protective reflexes (p. 165) which also originate from the trigeminal afferents and also from stimuli within the respiratory tract from the nasopharynx to the branches of the main bronchi (the bifurcation zones are said to be particularly sensitive). Deep inspiration is followed by explosive expiration through the closed larynx (*cough*) or glottis (*sneeze*) to expel a potential foreign body. All expiratory muscles including the accessory muscles are recruited.

SUFFOCATION REFLEX

Irritant vapours (including some volatile anaesthetics) stimulate trigeminal receptors in the nose. Breathing is temporarily inhibited in the expiratory posture and mucous flow in the respiratory tract is stimulated. It is a component of the 'diving response' (p. 165).

ASSOCIATED MOVEMENTS

Not truly reflex, but as part of the movement synergies, breathing is arrested during drinking, swallowing and (less completely along with less complete glottal closure) in expressional sounds associated with emotion (groaning, sighing, sobbing). Conversely, swallowing may be impossible if the respiratory rhythm is imposed by a machine. (Associated with a peculiarity of pharyngolaryngeal anatomy, the suckling infant is able to suck and swallow without, apparently, arresting respiration.)

The respiratory arrest resulting from swallowing can occur in any phase of respiration. The exact mechanism of interaction of trigeminal, glossopharyngeal and vagal afferents with the central generator for rhythmic respiration is unknown. Laryngospasm and vomiting are less likely during rhythmical respiration than during uncoordinated respiration.

SNIFFING RESPONSE

A primitive mechanism for orientation of the leading ('head) segment in response to olfactory stimuli is the septum–stria medullaris–habenula–interpeduncular pathway connected with mid-brain centres for movement of the head. It survives as part of the arousal system (Chapter 15). A barely detectable olfactory stimulus may be increased by causing inspired air to eddy into the upper olfactory area of the nose, the nostrils being flared by the facial (VII) nerve. This is largely a voluntary behaviour. The respiratory rhythm is interrupted by a forced inspiration with closed lips, followed by delayed expiration. The upper motoneurones to facial and phrenic nerves appear to originate in cortical area 6b, bilaterally.

ENVIRONMENTAL EFFECTS ON RESPIRATION

The immediate response to an abrupt change in the environment is the arrest reaction with inhibition of respiration. With continuing stress, emotional or body cooling, the rate and tidal volume are increased by higher controls of the mid-brain from the septal nuclei and hypothalamus. These are driving pressures which may be influenced by the anaesthetist.

PHONATION AND VOCALIZATION

Defence and rage reactions from the amygdaloid and septal areas, via hypothalamus, and medial forebrain bundle to the periaqueductal grey matter of the mid-brain activate a vocalization area in front of the pontomedullary reticular formation (Chapter 14). Forceful expiration through the mouth causes a sound which is modified in *pitch* by altering the aperture between the vocal cords (recurrent laryngeal branch of Xth cranial nerve) and in *timbre* by modifying the oropharyngeal cavity geometry (VII and IX). The vowel sounds are produced and modulated in this way. Fricatives require that the airstream be cut into long and short bursts and vibrated by the lips and tongue (VII and XII).

These movements are highly organized in speech and evidently have qualities of cortically controlled movements. *Vocalization* can be evoked by stimulation of the supplementary motor area above the cingulate sulcus or from the face area of the primary motor area of the cortex. No speech as such can be provoked by electrical stimulation of the human cortex. On the contrary, *speech arrest* is caused by stimulation of more extensive cortical areas and even spontaneous vocalization is arrested. These areas are Broca's and Wernicke's areas (*see* Chapter 12) and the superior speech cortex of the supplementary motor area of the hemisphere dominant for speech. It is probable that the stimulus interferes with the integrative aspects of speech and language functions rather than with the motor aspects of speech.

SUCKING, CHEWING AND BITING

These are coordinated movement patterns for intake of food. In the infant, or the adult with loss of cortical inhibitory control (commonly associated with dementia), the movements are reflex, stimulated by touching the lips or tongue (sucking) or oral mucosa (chewing). The trigeminal and glossopharyngeal afferent nerves relay polysynaptically in their appropriate medullary and pontine nuclei to the motor nuclei of VII (lower facial muscles), V (muscles of mastication) and XII (tongue) and muscles attached to the hyoid bone. In *sucking* the mouth is tightly closed, the soft palate occludes the posterior nasopharynx and negative pressure is produced in the buccal cavity by moving the tongue downwards and backwards. In *chewing* the mouth is also closed and the mandible raised and lowered with transverse grinding movements by the synergic action of the muscles of mastication.

Both of these activities are bilateral and cannot be performed unilaterally. They are reflex in the infant but rapidly come under voluntary control (for initiation and suppression). Chewing involves the same muscles as swallowing but the trigeminal innervated muscles of mastication predominate. Both sucking and chewing can accompany respiration, but breathing is inhibited as soon as a food bolus reaches the glottis during swallowing.

Fundamentally, mastication is rhythmical. A controlling area in the vicinity of the red nucleus, substantia nigra and central grey matter of the mid-brain is suggested by electrical stimulation of the *ventrolateral tegmentum* in the cat. It may be responsible for the automatic orobuccal dyskinesia seen in patients overdosed with dopaminergic drugs. There is some evidence that this area projects to the *superior olive* and to the *motor nuclei of the trigeminal, facial and hypoglossal nerves*, probably bilaterally.

Rhythmical alternation of muscles opening and closing the jaw probably uses a reciprocal, mutually inhibitory, control of motoneurones similar to that postulated for respiration and locomotion. Like both of these rhythmical movements, the same motoneurones can be commanded in a non-rhythmical way by corticobulbar neurones of the pyramidal tract. The cortical masticatory area is in *area 4* near the thumb area. This control, temporarily overriding rhythmical mastication, is used to evoke the powerful jaw closure of *biting*, predominantly trigeminal and always bilateral.

The bite is a remarkably precise movement, accurately adjusted in force and displacement according to the consistency of the food. The jaw-closing muscles are richly supplied with monosynaptic reflex arcs from the spindles (and probably also polysynaptic arcs) but the problem of servo-control versus programmed innervation is the same as that encountered with isometric contraction of limb muscles and discussion will be postponed until limb movements are examined (p. 240). The brisk stretch reflex gives the jaw postural stability during locomotion and keeps it from bouncing up and down to prevent uncontrolled contact of the teeth.

TASTING

The primary motor response to an acceptable taste stimulus (or its anticipation) is autonomic: salivation and secretomotor activity of the upper gut are stimulated. The tongue is pressed against the teeth and palate. The excess of saliva evokes the swallowing reflex. Afferent fibres in cranial nerves VII and IX enter the gustatory nucleus (an enlarged upper part of the solitary nucleus) and are relayed bilaterally via the thalamus to the insular cortex for taste sensation and to salivatory nuclei, and X and XII efferents. The nucleus ambiguus (X) inhibits the respiratory centres.

VOMITING

If the taste is unacceptable (as judged by the limbic system, modified by acquired behavioural patterns), swallowing is arrested, gut peristalsis reversed and a strong expiratory response with abdominal muscle contraction causes vomiting. The afferent side of the reflex may be from taste fibres in VII and IX nerves, or by olfactory nerve (II) fibres converging on a '*vomiting centre*' in the *area postrema* of the lower medulla oblongata. It is itself a chemoreceptor zone with dopaminergic receptors responsive to levodopa and dopaminergic substances such as apomorphine. Other afferent signals reaching this centre pass in the vagus, glossopharyngeal, vestibular and possibly the splanchnic nerves. It controls a motor output via the dorsomotor nucleus of the vagus and unidentified pathways to the abdominal wall and diaphragm.

SWALLOWING

If the taste of a substance in the mouth is acceptable, a chain of reflexes is initiated. Liquids will be swallowed if the fluid is passed back to a triggering zone in the posterior buccal cavity innervated by the glossopharyngeal nerve (IX). Taste along with tactile stimulation in the mouth (trigeminal nerve) initiates a chewing behavioural pattern followed by swallowing. Though both are reflex, the command to initiate them is under strong voluntary control, but unlike chewing the swallowing reflex cannot be voluntarily stopped once the fluid or food bolus has passed the posterior part of the pharynx. Oral automatisms elicited by olfaction and taste have corticofugal pathways from the insular and orbito-frontal cortex and may involve the amygdala.

Further reading

Bainton C.R., Kirkwood P.A. and Sears T.A. On the transmission of the stimulating effects of carbon dioxide to the muscles of respiration. *J. Physiol.* 1978; **280**: 249–72.

Cohen M.I. Neurogenesis of respiratory rhythm in the mammal. *Physiol. Rev.* 1979; **59**: 1105–73.

Dawes G.S. The central control of fetal breathing and skeletal muscle movements. *J. Physiol.* 1984; **346**: 1–18.

von Euler C. Central pattern generation during breathing. *Trends Neurosci.* 1980; **3**: 275–7.

Widdicombe J.G. Reflexes from the lungs in the control of breathing. In: Linden R.J. (ed.) *Recent Advances in Physiology*, 9. Edinburgh: Churchill Livingstone, 1974, pp. 239–78.

Wyman R.J. Neural generation of the breathing rhythm. *Ann. Rev. Physiol.* 1977; **39**: 417–48.

Chapter 21
Locomotion

In the early chordates, before the development of limbs, movements towards food or away from danger required coordinated activity of axial muscles at all segmental levels, with the leading segment dominant. Movements of the head and neck, and locomotion of animals with limbs, still show evidence of the primitive organization but the mechanism for the automatisms can be entered at various points, including an overriding corticofugal control. The primitive drive from the appetitive areas of the brain may be subjected to commands from cortical areas concerned with the exploration of extracorporeal space.

Movements of the trunk and head

There is remarkably little information in the major textbooks of physiology about the motor control of the axial musculature except for its disturbances due to lesions at the level of the basal ganglia or lower. There is a very extensive literature on the maintenance of posture and the reflexes controlling recovery of the displaced body and head, which is summarized in Chapter 17, but no authoritative account can be traced on exploratory or 'voluntary' movements of the axial musculature.

Segmental reflexes would suffice for a primitive animal moving in an irregular environment, but to find food or a sexual partner it must respond appropriately to signs recorded by distance receptors. The most primitive of these are olfaction and taste. At first acting reflexly through the ventral posteromedial nucleus of the thalamus, the phylogenetic development of the cerebral cortex with thalamocortical projection to the post-central gyrus (taste) and rhinencephalon (smell) introduced the possibility of contingent responses with exploratory behaviour. Later in evolution, vision has added precision to the goal-directed movements, but presumably incorporates the same effector mechanism, turning first the head and then the trunk to orientate towards a desirable target (Chapter 19). No elaborate trunk control system is required since the head–on–body reflexes previously described would suffice to control the trunk. The problem is, what controls the head?

Without prejudice to a later discussion on the roles of the cerebral cortex in overriding and bypassing the postural reflex mechanisms of the basal ganglia, it appears probable that the association areas of the cortex for smell, taste, vision and also hearing, have 'command' neurones which project to the striatum and to the cerebellar control of the bulbospinal motor centres for the axial muscles. Some of these corticofugal fibres may be identified with the corticopontine tracts lying posterior and anterior to the main corticospinal projection from area 4. They include the *temporopontine tract* (Turck's bundle) and the *frontopontine tract* (Arnold's bundle) which relay in the pontine nuclei to the vermis of the cerebellum. The *vermis* coordinates the outflow of the reticulospinal, vestibulospinal and other projection systems modulating muscle tone and in particular the orientation of the head on the trunk (*see* Chapter 23). Abnormal head posturing occurs in Bruns' syndrome, a form of ataxia with defective postural set of trunk muscles occasionally found with bilateral lesions of the frontal lobes and less commonly with parietal or temporal lesions.

The cerebral command of axial movements is bilateral. The site of crossing of the command or effector neurones is not known.

With the development of vision, the same motor system is brought under the command of neurones fixing the gaze on external targets (*see* Chapter 19). However, it is clear (by introspection) that the head and trunk can also be moved voluntarily, regardless of external cues. The limited range of movement is controlled (bilaterally) by command signals from a comparatively small area of the cortical motor strip. Penfield's stimulation studies in man indicate some representation of trunk movements near the convexity which presumably sends corticobulbar and corticospinal fibres under control of the somatic afferent system similar to those for limb movement. Nevertheless, the relative retention of whole body movements to command in apraxic patients has been considered to indicate that the temporopontine pathway remains very important in man, at least so far as auditory commands are concerned.

Gait

Walking with two hind limbs is essentially similar to quadrupedal locomotion. An important difference is the increased requirement to maintain equilibrium while the body weight is supported by a single limb. An automatism system for *stepping* resembles the system for respiration. It is linked with the mechanism for adjusting the position of the centre of gravity already described for maintaining or correcting body posture (Chapter 17). A useful bonus of this adaptation to bipedal gait is that gravitational force is used to assist the horizontal component of the thrust exerted by the lower limb muscles. A stepping mechanism in the spinal cord is coordinated with a higher level system for shifting the centre of gravity by an unidentified mesencephalic system.

INITIATION OF WALKING

It is believed that an intrinsic mechanism for stepping is inhibited until it receives derepressing signals from the *subthalamic area* of the diencephalon commanded by the cerebral cortex or behaviour-controlling parts of the hypothalamus, probably acting through or along with the *putamen*. It is responsible only for the initiation of locomotion as part of goal-directed behaviour, eg searching, hunting, defending. The subthalamic centre or the adjacent putamen initiates a body movement (p. 208) shifting the centre of gravity forwards and laterally over the head of one femur. The effect is as if the weight of the body were sliding down an inclined plane or moving on the rim of a wheel of which the supporting leg is a spoke. A newborn infant with an intact stepping mechanism does not begin to show stepping movements until the body is tilted forwards and rocked a little from side to side. An adult with severe Parkinsonism may be unable to start to walk until rocked in the same way, probably using a combination of vestibular and neck reflexes. A righting reflex (p. 169) then brings forward the unloaded lower limb and derepresses the stepping mechanism.

EQUILIBRIUM

Locomotion continues by a combination of four motor controls: (i) stepping movements; (ii) maintenance of equilibrium; (iii) reflex compensation for unevenness of the terrain; (iv) negotiation of obstacles. Only the last function, requiring the use of distance receptors such as vision and hearing, makes significant use of the cortex. Cortical command from the primary motor area (pyramidal tract) is used to change the direction and rate of gait. *Rate changes* are effected by increasing the power output of the muscles responsible for propulsion and the cycle time follows passively (*see below*). *Changes of direction* are achieved by turning the head and trunk and differentially modulating the interneurones and motoneurones distal to the stepping generators on each side of the cord so that movement is no longer symmetrical. The efferent pathways involved are the pyramidal tract, vestibulospinal (to extensor and abductor motoneurones) and reticulospinal (to flexor and adductor motoneurones). Linked balancing movements of the upper limbs are described below.

These postural adjustments involve the pallido-putaminal system by afferent feedback from vestibular and dorsal horn neurones, and are coordinated by the cerebellum (p. 229). In the absence of the latter, stepping is still possible but rhythm is less regular and the vestibular control deficient; the human subject staggers on walking. The cerebellar control is to the ipsilateral side of the spinal cord.

Corticofugal, basal gangliar, cerebellar, vestibulospinal and reticulospinal controls are all important in normal bipedal walking. The centre of gravity of the body rises and falls and shifts from side to side. The arms swing, and the trunk rotates. The pelvis moves forwards on the side of the swinging leg, while the ipsilateral shoulder does the reverse, keeping the head and eyes facing towards the direction for walking. All of these controls are modulatory and are not the primary drive for locomotion. Their roles are the same in principle as the accessory pathways in respiration described in Chapter 20. Like that function, they modulate a more fundamental system with a tonic (non-phasic) drive from brain stem level, a spinal cord generator of rhythmical movements, and a complicated segmental reflex system to compensate for irregularities of the ground, and all using final common paths consisting of motoneurones accessible to alternative commands such as voluntary movements which may be imposed at any phase of the stepping cycle.

MESENCEPHALIC LOCOMOTOR AREA

Although there is no satisfactory direct evidence in man, experiments on the cat indicate that, like respiration, a low level rhythm generator is driven by tonic impulses from the mid-brain bilaterally (the nucleus cuneiformis in the cat) which are inhibited by the diencephalon. It is described as a mesencephalic locomotor area in analogy with the 'pneumotactic centre' and is believed to influence the stepping mechanism in the cord via a tract with nuclei in the pons.

PONTINE RETICULOSPINAL FIBRES

These are not well defined anatomically as the axons are not myelinated. They differ from the faster conducting myelinated reticulospinal fibres described on p. 158 which facilitate motoneurones and interneurones in the cord but which bypass the spinal stepping generator. The unmyelinated fibres, on the contrary, depolarize the neurones of the stepping generator. They are noradrenergic and act on alpha-adrenergic receptors, raising their excitability to a level where the generator is activated by further command signals from cortex, basal ganglia or peripheral reflexes. The monoaminergic neurones are insufficient to start stepping movements independently. Conversely, stepping does not depend on afferent input from sensory receptors in the limbs as stepping is still possible after complete deafferentation of the lower limbs. In man, the very severe deafferentation of tabes dorsalis or sensory polyneuropathy makes the gait ataxic but walking remains possible. A severe unilateral pyramidal tract lesion (hemiplegia) may abolish goal-directed movements of the lower limb but walking is still possible, the circumducting gait being initiated by the body rocking manoeuvre.

BIPEDAL GAIT

The alternating bipedalism of adult human walking depends on supporting the body weight on at least one leg (with body weight shifted over it) while the other is swung forwards. The swing phase is, like expiration, relatively passive but can be voluntarily increased. The knee is flexed by inhibiting its extensors. (The consequent reduction of the effective length of the swinging leg lowers its moment of inertia. To increase the stride by extending the knee increases walking speed at metabolic cost.) The swing phase terminates when the heel strikes the ground and the forward propulsion of the body, due to its gravitational shifts and friction between heel and ground, moves the body's centre of gravity forward over and beyond the heel and on to its downward incline. This fall is checked by the limb abruptly switching to its support phase: the entire foot is placed on the ground, extensor muscles fix the limb at its maximum length, raising the centre of gravity of the body and at the same time providing a rigid 'spoke for the wheel'. The body again moves forwards. Thus the body is propelled forwards by the combined effect of the centre of gravity shifts and a little thrust against the ground.

It is not unreasonable to describe the support phase of gait as the propulsive phase, though in fact more work is done by lifting the body than by thrusting backwards. The thrust develops as the forward motion lifts the heel and allows the forefoot to push on the ground. Very little of this thrust comes from the knee flexors and plantiflexors of the foot (gastrocnemius-soleus). The main propulsive force is from the gluteal muscles which move the leg backwards with respect to the body, but the body forwards with respect to the foot on the ground provided there is adequate friction. (Skating requires certain acquired foot positions to obtain the necessary friction but exploits the gravitational part of locomotion.)

For the purposes of this book it is not necessary to analyse the finer details of human gait. Essentially the support phase (propulsive) utilizes the antigravity extensor muscles and the swing phase the flexors. But some muscles, notably those spanning two joints, are active in both phases and some only during the transition from support to swing or vice versa. One is reminded of the *'phase-spanning'* respiratory neurones, here directed to the motoneurones of discrete muscles. Their neural control cannot be 'hard wired' since the timing of muscular activity varies between subjects and even in the individual who can vary his walking pattern in detail, either by conscious decision or by reflex response to environmental requirements. The sequence of joint movements does not change with speed of locomotion but the muscle sequence does. (Note that electromyographic evidence does not give the full picture. The negative work of inactive muscle when it is stretched is not accounted for.) Ignoring the plasticity for the moment, it is now appropriate to examine the fundamental rhythm generator and its switches.

SPINAL STEPPING GENERATORS

Each limb has its own rhythm generator for stepping movements, normally interlocked but capable of independent rhythms. The descending command from the noradrenergic reticulospinal system activates a mechanism in the spinal cord interneuronal pool resembling the spinal generator postulated for respiratory movements (Chapter 20). Like the latter, the two components of the step cycle are not symmetrical, arguing against a simple system of alternating flexor and extensor motoneuronal discharge with mutual reciprocal inhibition.

Speed of locomotion is increased by recruitment of more motor units in the support-phase muscles (with very little alteration of firing frequencies). With increasing frequency of stepping the support phase becomes shorter but the swing phase is kept nearly constant. This does not necessarily imply that the swing phase is a passive recoil. Increased recruitment of phase spanning motor units is required to overcome the inertia at the transition from extension to flexion, but limb inertia is significant in swinging the leg forward when the body's centre of gravity is ahead of the hip joint.

The exact nature of the spinal organization of the stepping automatism is unknown. Four theories have been proposed.

(a) Chain-reflex hypothesis — Sherrington's analysis of spinal reflex activity led to the concept that most, if not all, movement is conducted by a chain of reflexes (Chapter 17). This concept remains attractive to paediatric neurologists and physiotherapists. If the newborn is placed with feet on a solid base and the body tilted forwards, a stepping movement is elicited. Unlike the adult, the distal lateral part of the foot touches the ground, evoking an *extensor thrust* (p. 160). Contact of the sole on the ground then evokes dorsiflexion of the hallux and spreading of the toes (*Babinski response*), but this is immediately suppressed by a *grasp reflex*. It may be true that contact and stretch reflexes contribute to the timing of stepping movements, but few would now accept that walking is entirely a chain of reflexes because stepping automatism remains after deafferentation.

(b) Reciprocal half-centre hypothesis — Sherrington's collaborator Graham Brown explained the rhythmical processes breathing, stepping and scratching by activity of antagonistic muscles, each driven by a 'half-centre' which inhibits the other by collateral branches. After some time *'fatigue'* would accumulate in one half centre (or accommodation, p. 10) leading to cessation of its activity and *release* of the other half centre. An important argument against the concept is the relative stability of the expiratory phase of respiration and the swing phase of gait despite alterations of total cycle time.

(c) Ring hypothesis — A ring circuit consisting of many successive neurones can be designed to determine the order of activation of various muscles of the step cycle and its

modulation by segmental reflexes, but it also fails to explain the disproportionate change in the durations of the swing and support phases when the speed of locomotion varies.

(d) *Pacemaker hypothesis* — In primitive nervous systems neurones can be identified which rhythmically fire bursts of action potentials like the pacemakers in the intrinsic nervous system of the heart. Coupled to a reciprocal inhibitory network this could account for a generator of autonomous rhythmical activity in agonist and antagonist muscles. Briefly, there is no evidence that this type of neurone exists in the mammalian spinal cord.

At present we do not know the exact mechanism of the stepping generators and specialists argue cogently for their favourite model. We do not even know the segmental level. Indeed, a distributed system with mesencephalic and spinal components is entirely feasible. In experimental animals, stepping can be induced by stimulation of the periaqueductal grey matter.

INTERLIMB COORDINATION

Regular walking on a smooth surface is done by shifting the weight from one leg to the other, alternating the support phase between each leg, rotating the limb girdle and neck, and swinging the arms. Arm swing, important to maintain balance and to add to the forward inertial movement, is an adaptation of quadrupedal gait. (The latter is still seen in the child before bipedal walking develops. The limbs move in typical *quadrupedal order*, showing diagonal coordination — left leg, left arm, right leg, right arm — but like four-legged animals, in a hurry the child brings both lower limbs forward together and both hands are then stretched out in a 'gallop' pattern.) Thus the interlimb coordination must allow for correct phasing of four limbs with the possibility of altering the pattern according to the speed of locomotion. This would be difficult to explain by simple interlimb reflexes.

Connections are postulated between independent stepping generators in the lumbosacral and cervical segments of the cord using propriospinal neurones and spino-bulbo-spinal and spino-cerebello-vestibulo-spinal reflexes.

The cells of the ventral spinocerebellar tract are phasically active during each step cycle, even after deafferentation. Diagonal coordination and transition from one gait phase to the other may involve linkage between the phase spanning units or certain phase switching reflexes.

SEGMENTAL REFLEXES IN WALKING

The regularity of walking could be accounted for if the swing phase were started and stopped by some position receptor related to flexion and extension of the hip. Indeed, there is some evidence that this exists. Receptors in the joint capsule (not sacrificed with hip prosthesis) either trigger the central generator or block the switch from extensor to flexor activity until the movement has progressed to a selected position. Like the Hering–Breuer and chest wall reflexes in respiration, this would only be invoked to alter the central rhythm when the drive (in this instance some method of signalling that the centre of gravity is too far forward) requires a longer gait or faster pace. No similar reflex control can be identified for the knee and ankle.

Load-compensating reflexes also regulate the contraction and relaxation of individual muscles when walking on uneven ground or when carrying extra loads. They are the same stretch and tension reflexes described under postural control (Chapter 17). They are overridden by *protective reflexes* which inhibit anti-gravity muscles and facilitate flexion withdrawal (causing the walker to stumble) but the *righting reflexes* immediately restore equilibrium.

Like the muscles of respiration, the motor innervation of the limbs during walking shows strict *alpha–gamma coactivation* (Chapters 9 and 23). This permits the spindle sensors to be active throughout the whole stepping cycle, maintaining the inflow of information on muscle length and tension to the cortex and cerebellum without which smoothly coordinated walking is impossible.

Running, dancing and diving

To increase the speed of walking, the stride is first increased by prolonging the support phase and retarding the transition from swing to support, ie the turnaround switches are reset, presumably by corticofugal control of the spinal generator. When the individual breaks into a run the gait becomes digitigrade (forefoot support) instead of plantigrade (heel first), with increased thrust from the plantiflex-ors. Increased elevation of the centre of gravity, and greater use of the latent energy of gravity by leaning further forward and swing-ing the arms further forward, seem to indicate increased vestibulospinal drive. In dancing, the forefoot thrust and body sway increasingly dominate and the alternation between the two limbs changes. In diving, the weight shift of body and arms and the forefoot thrust are so dominant that both legs push off together, like the gallop phase of the quadruped. Clearly the spinal rhythm generator is readily modified by higher level command signals, presumably from the cortex and using corticospinal fibres (not necessarily uniquely).

This is an example of how skilled movements are developed by 'increasing encephalization' of command signals acting through intrinsic spinal cord mechanisms by (i) inhibiting unrequired muscle activity and (ii) probably adding direct corticofugal signals injected into the system immediately before the 'final common path' of the lower motoneurones and at the first relay of the proprioceptive sensory input (Chapter 9). The requirement to incorporate information on gravitational and movement effects may account for the fact that the coordination of these higher controls has used the higher ganglia of the vestibular system, the cerebellum and striatum, during the course of evolution and the mesencephalic periaqueductal grey matter. The latter area organizes running movements associated with 'flight', or aggressive behaviour commanded by the posterior hypothalamus and transmitted through the pre-rubral field.

Further reading

Grillner S. Locomotion in vertebrates — central mechanisms and reflex interaction. *Physiol. Rev.* 1975; **55**: 274–304.

Shik M.L. and Orlovsky G.N. Neurophysiology of locomotor automatism. *Physiol. Rev.* 1976; **56**: 465–501.

Chapter 22

General principles of control of movement

Since the discovery that muscular movement resulted from stimulation of an area of cerebral cortex in front of the Rolandic (central) sulcus, it has been generally believed that a 'motor area' and its 'upper motor neurones' commanded 'lower motor neurones' in the brain stem nuclei and anterior horns of the spinal cord and that the timing and degree of innervation of the latter were 'co-ordinated' by the cerebellum. The role of the basal ganglia was uncertain. Some earlier writers considered the striatum to be a remnant of a primitive motor system rendered obsolete by phylogenetic development of the cortex and hence 'pre-pyramidal'. Others considered that it had an accessory or 'extrapyramidal' role in maintained posture, overridden by corticospinal (pyramidal) tract activity in voluntary movement. There is no doubt that the striatal system is important in reflex control of posture, and in particular in the righting reflexes described in Chapter 17. Equally, it is indisputable that the cerebellum is involved in the continuous correction of postural and voluntary movements, but recent research indicates that both structures are also involved in the *initiation* of voluntary movement.

A simple model would be that corticospinal efferent activity could use parallel routes, direct cortico-spinal, cortico-striato-reticulospinal, and cortico-ponto-cerebello-rubrospinal. This recently fashionable model, placing the motor area of the cortex in a master position for each efferent pathway, must be rejected because of electrophysiological data indicating that striatal and cerebellar activity actually precedes neuronal firing in the cortical motor area 4. It has also become apparent that motor patterns programmed in a pre-motor area of cortex, or afferent pathways from sensory areas of cortex or their association areas cannot directly trigger the motor area. These concepts are abandoned because of long latency between pre-motor and parietal activities and activation of the motor cortex.

We have already seen (Chapter 16) that slow cortical *movement related potentials* (Bereitschaftspotential and pre-motor positivity) occur bilaterally before a unilateral motor potential over an area of motor cortex appropriate to subsequent electromyographic activity in contralateral muscles. A currently favoured model is that goal-directed movement is planned in the various associative cortices and in the frontal lobe. (Denny-Brown recognized two major conflicting but balanced systems for grasping and avoiding under tactile and visual control.) These movements are (i) *pre-programmed* but (ii) *modified* during their course by proprioceptive feedback to the thalamus, either directly or indirectly via the cerebellum; (iii) *adjusted* to take account of bodily position in space by the striatum; and (iv) *goal-directed* by visual and tactile cortex. The new aspect of a currently favoured model is that the link between 'planning' cortex and motor area is threefold: (i) transcortical; (ii) via cortico-striate fibres from all areas of cortex (to caudate nucleus and putamen), relayed through the pallidum to the ventrolateral nucleus of thalamus and thence to area 4; and (iii) from association and frontal cortex to the cortex of the lateral cerebellum and back through ventrolateral thalamus to area 4 where all three inputs are integrated with the somatosensory transcortical influence. It is not surprising that there should be several hundred milliseconds between planning and execution of motor strip activity by the Betz cells. An alternative model proposed by one of us relegates the nigrostriatal-thalamo-cortical projection to a 'gating' function of the supplementary motor area postponing transcortical activation of area 4 until the postural muscle set is appropriate.

The further contribution of the cerebellum (in its intermediate zone) to the smooth graded execution of movement will be described later. It is now accepted that different parts of the cerebellum can be differentially involved in the planning and execution of movement. The same comment must now be made with respect to the corpus striatum. Though its mechanism remains uncertain, there can be little doubt that much of the difficulty has been due to attempts to describe a single function. Furthermore, a constant theme of this book has been that of 'distributed functions' and there is no reason to believe that planning and initiation of goal-directed movements are different in this respect. For reasons of timing of cell firing, the cerebellum has respectable claims for the movement planning centre, but we see no reason to regard it as unique in this respect, as claimed by some recent writers. These comments should be kept in mind when, for reasons of convenience, we describe separately some of the recognized connections and functions of the three important supraspinal areas for control of posture and movement: (i) the cerebral cortex; (ii) the basal ganglia; (iii) the cerebellum.

The elements of *postural control* have been described in Chapters 17–19. The spinal reflexes provided stabilization of posture by *feedback control*, but with the vestibular and righting reflexes we had moved into a category of postural adjustments appropriate to a wide variety of circumstances without fixed reference points except the vertical (vestibular) and a visual target. Stabilization of this type needs *feedforward control*, ie the link from primary receptors in muscles, neck and vestibular apparatus to the postural muscles must compute all space orientation signals and motor activity and then command the appropriate muscles accordingly. This computing function requires the integrating properties of polysynaptic convergent neuronal systems. These are the basal ganglia and the older vestibular part of the cerebellum (vermis). Without

wishing to attribute specific functions, it appears that the *thalamus-striatal system* is fundamentally for body-on-body and head-on-body stabilization and the *cerebellum* for adjustment of posture to stabilize retinal images. The phylogenetic development of the cerebral cortex has added more complicated functions and added an additional system of motor control.

Goal-directed movement

This term will be used to avoid semantic problems regarding 'voluntary' activity, since the type of movement involved appears to be identical whether the movement is willed or a conditional response. It is possible to contract a single muscle (or even a motor unit) with visual or auditory feedback, but training is usually required. In normal circumstances a movement involves a muscle synergy and also more or less adjustment of posture to provide a stable base.

ISOTONIC AND ISOMETRIC CONTRACTION

In the *movement synergy* for *isotonic contraction*, muscles act as (i) prime movers, (ii) antagonists, (iii) synergists, and these are all commanded by pyramidal tract signals. The associated postural adjustment is controlled reflexly by the basal ganglia. The reciprocal innervation of prime movers and antagonists is largely organized at spinal cord level since most of the corticospinal projection by the pyramidal tract is to the spinal interneurones (p. 239) but reciprocal innervation also occurs in the motor cortex. *Isometric contraction* differs in that antagonists do not relax. Indeed fine movements such as writing, adjusting a vernier etc., require strong antagonist contraction for the prime movers to work against. The control is visual or tactile rather than proprioceptive, involving at least the thalamus and probably the cortex.

Even isotonic movement (displacement of a constant load) is not a simple activity. Consider the movement of reaching out to touch an object. The limb starts in one *postural set* and ends in another. Between these points it may be moved slowly and 'carefully' or rapidly, by the shortest route with least articulatory constraint. The sequence of length control/ballistic movement/length control is the rule. The controlling mechanisms involved are not fully understood but it seems likely that postural control at the beginning and end (or throughout the 'ramp' displacement of the constantly controlled movement) is a function of the basal ganglia (but not necessarily initiated there). The putamen, acting through the anterior thalamus and supplementary motor area, may 'gate' the primary motor areas immediately after the postural set is switched.

BALLISTIC (OR SACCADIC) MOVEMENT

This is controlled by the pars intermedia of the cerebellum. Clinical experience with cerebellar lesions also indicates that the cerebellum is responsible for the timing of onset and cessation of activity of each muscle in a synergy, only possible at spinal cord level. It is clear that goal-directed movement involves cortex, striatum and cerebellum.

The greatest problem is to decide where movement is initiated. Recent evidence that neuronal firing in the striatum and cerebellum begins before it occurs in cortical area 4 is based on conditioned (trained) responses. It is impossible to deny the possibility that self-motivated movement may originate in the motor cortex. Otherwise the development of monosynaptic pyramidal tract neurones (from cortex direct to anterior horn cells) supplying distal limb muscles in the primates would confer little advantage. Nevertheless, at least in monkeys, the subcortical mechanism is perfect enough to function in the absence of its cortical pyramidal components, but it requires visual guidance. The defective factor is tactile orientation.

The crux of the matter is the localization of the *command neurones*. These are certainly not restricted to the cerebral cortex. The cat has an organization in its spinal cord for the alternating reciprocal movements of stepping and this can be activated from the mid-brain (p. 208). In the earlier discussion on reflexes (Chapter 17) it was shown how a hierarchy of postural and withdrawal reflexes is modified by inhibition of lower level reflexes in whole or in part. The clinical signs of basal ganglia disease are dominated by '*release phenomena*' (dystonia, dyskinesia) indicating that the normal activity of the basal ganglia involves powerful inhibition of brain stem and spinal reflex mechanisms. It is likely that inhibition is a major factor in the command function of the cortex: previous experimental work takes little account of this. The human infant makes mass movements of its limbs which become selective as the pyramidal tract matures. (A similar progression is seen when spastic hemiplegia resolves after a recoverable lesion of the pyramidal tract in the adult.) Certainly this could be due to recovery of topically organized excitatory neurones, but it is much more likely that the restored cerebral command is due to returning inhibition and this is also apparent in the reflex responses.

UPPER MOTOR NEURONE

The fibres originating in the so-called motor area of the cortex (*area 4, the pre-central gyrus*) constitute only a small proportion of the fibres of the *pyramidal tract*. Many arise in the post-central cortex and even in cortical areas where no movement can be excited by electrical stimulation. Many of the pyramidal tract fibres do not end on motoneurones or their immediate interneurones, but on the synapses of the afferent systems at different levels (Chapter 8). The possibilities for inhibition of all or part of reflex synergies are multifold and they are necessary if movement is to be commanded towards a goal in preference to undirected response to the massive barrage of impulses from the periphery, but the inhibition must permit, for instance, the grasping hand to start from many different postures and to reach it by as many trajectories as there are occasions to grasp. Oddly enough, what are commonly regarded as *skilled movements* are not of this type. By frequent repetition the skilled performer (musician, typist, sportsman or other) finds a personal best solution for the fastest and most economical pattern of movement which, once *learned*, can be carried out without a conscious direction and can be modified by sensory monitoring (such as auditory feedback in playing a stringed instrument). When the system is damaged by disease or physical constraints, the resourceful brain can formulate alternative motor strategies.

THE COMMAND FUNCTION

Mountcastle has pointed out that a distributed system, such as is being proposed for motor control, has many entries and exits and has access to outflow systems of the brain at many levels. It displays a redundancy of potential loci of command, and the command function may from time to time reside in different loci of the system, in particular that part possessing the most urgent and necessary information. The concept of command neurones for initiating and driving to completion a behavioural act under a specific *motivational drive* is referred to on p. 114.

Whereas the spinal and brain reflexes evoke motor responses to deep and surface stimuli, neurones of parietal areas 5 and 7 generate commands to pay attention to an object within the immediate extrapersonal space. The hand is reached towards it and the object then grasped and manipulated. Command neurones respond to both visual and somatosensory cues only when the animal (monkey) initiates a movement. Similar neurones in area 7 elicit saccadic movements of the eyes, frequently associated with a blink, but only during appropriate motivation (eg hunger). The command neurones are subordinate to 'volition' and 'motivation', presumably by unidentified control from frontal and limbic mechanisms.

It is already clear that 'voluntary movement' does not start in the so-called motor areas (which are many). Clinical tradition attributes a major command function in the above sense to the *'pre-motor' area 6*. The evidence for a programme synthesizer commanding area 4 has never been good and dates from a time when all pyramidal tract neurones were believed to originate in the motor strip of area 4.

For evidence about the initiator of movement we must look at those diseases which cause *akinesis* without paralysis. Recent writers on the subject have stressed the difficulty in initiating voluntary movement experienced by the patient with Parkinson's disease and nominated the striato-pallidum as an initiator of movement, entraining the motor cortex via

the thalamus. Others have suggested that the cerebellum is responsible. Neither view is satisfactory to a clinical neurologist. A more satisfactory starting point would be akinetic mutism, a disorder in which the conscious, sentient, non-paralysed individual is unable to make any voluntary movement except with the eyes — it has been described as a *global apraxia* sparing eye movements, blinking and swallowing. The various lesions causing it are are all related to the walls of the IIIrd ventricle (*peri-ependymal grey matter* and medial thalamic nuclei). No single locus has been identified, but a plausible suggestion is that the disorder is a disconnection syndrome from interruption of pathways from hippocampus to temporal cortex or from parolfactory and septal nuclei projecting to the cingulate cortex or hypothalamus and thence to the reticular formation (p. 139). (Some possible deefferenting lesions discussed in the literature fail to differentiate akinetic mutism from the 'locked in syndrome' which is due to a low or mid-pontine lesion of efferent tracts.) Disconnection between association cortices (including frontal) and hypothalamus seems plausible in most cases of diencephalic akinetic mutism.

HYPOTHALAMUS

The autonomic efferent functions of the hypothalamus are well known and will be described in Chapter 25. Somatic motor activity is limited to appetitive responses such as sexual functions and feeding behaviour. If the hypothalamus and its brain stem outflow are isolated from cortex, basal ganglia and the bulk of the thalamus, the phenomenon of 'sham rage' is observed in experimental animals. These movements are primitive and 'driven' by chemical changes in hypothalamic receptors until shut off by other 'satiety' neurones, but they differ in an important respect from the elaborate postural and defensive reflexes described in earlier chapters. The behaviour driven by the hypothalamus is *exploratory*, ready to be moulded by higher analytical and integrating systems into goal-directed movement. More versatile behavioural patterns require that the hypothalamus is inhibited by these higher structures, but it could still provide the essential gating mechanism for a purely somatic motor system in the basal ganglia.

Basal ganglia and the modulation of postural sets

The exact role of the corpus striatum (caudate nucleus, putamen and pallidum) and its related nuclei is not known and various models presented in contemporary literature are speculative. The following account is no more authoritative but is presented as a plausible interpretation of function based on the disorders seen in human disease and with experimental lesions in primates, notably the experiments and clinical insights of Denny-Brown. To understand the model it is necessary to outline the salient features of the anatomy, but we must emphasize that many details remain obscure (*Fig.* 22.1).

THE CORPUS STRIATUM

The corpus striatum has a receptive grey area, the striatum, lying radial to a motor nucleus, the pallidum. The striatum is divided anatomically into caudate nucleus and putamen by the white fibres of the internal capsule but they function as a single afferent area which projects to the efferent pallidum.

THE STRIATUM

The striatum receives two important afferent systems, from cortex and thalamus. The thalamostriate fibres arise from the centromedian-parafascicular nuclear complex of the thalamus and cross the internal capsule to the putamen and part of the body of the caudate nucleus. Intralaminar thalamic nuclei project to the remainder of the striatum. It therefore receives major afferents from the *integrated* spinothalamic, vestibular, 'panoramic visual' and the cerebellar input to the brain (Chapter 8) and also from the locus coeruleus arousal system (Chapter 15) but not directly from proprioceptive, vestibular or visual receptors.

These integrated proprioceptive, cutaneous and (predominantly) vestibular afferents are relayed via the pallidum to modulate the stereotyped spinal and brain stem reflexes in the more versatile *righting reactions* described

in Chapter 17, by appropriate facilitation or inhibition of competing extension and flexion reflexes. The control is of feedforward type (p. 213), to orientate the head and eyes in space in such a manner as to minimize input from the vestibular otoliths and to stabilize retinal images, particularly in the vertical plane.

A major part of the proprioceptive input must be via the sensory area 3 or possibly the paleo-spinothalamic fibres which relay in the reticular formation. The intralaminar nuclei also have intricate intrathalamic connections so they are well suited to present the corpus striatum with a coordinated picture of eye–head–body relations for orientation and control of axial muscles. For this purpose the striatum projects to the pallidum.

PALLIDUM

When *the pallidum* and lower connections are intact but the striatum is damaged, there is presumably pallidal release. Profound ipsilateral hypotonia with abrupt postural lapses (*chorea*) results in man, suggesting that the pallidum has a role in *inhibiting vestibular and spinal postural reflexes*. When the pallidum is severely damaged, these reflexes are released, causing rigidity and alternating postures (*athetosis*).

A major outflow from the pallidum is to the ventrolateral nucleus of the *thalamus* and thence to cortical area 6 (the supplementary motor area and pre-motor area) and by the ventro-anterior nucleus of the thalamus to the *frontal cortex*. Studies on Parkinson's disease suggest that the pallido-thalamo-cortical projections are gate-controlling for area 4 goal-directed responses, timing these in association with postural sets. The pallidum also has polysynaptic projections to the spinal and bulbar motoneurones via the tegmentum and efferent *reticular formation*. The major action on lower level reflexes is selective inhibition, as judged by the effects of pallidal lesions in man. Lost regulatory functions are (i) inadequacy of righting responses, (ii) defective vertical gaze and eye-centering response to objects in the periphery of the visual field (Chapter 19), (iii) disordered modulation of gait by vertical and horizontal stripes in the visual field. These losses are accompanied by release of postural

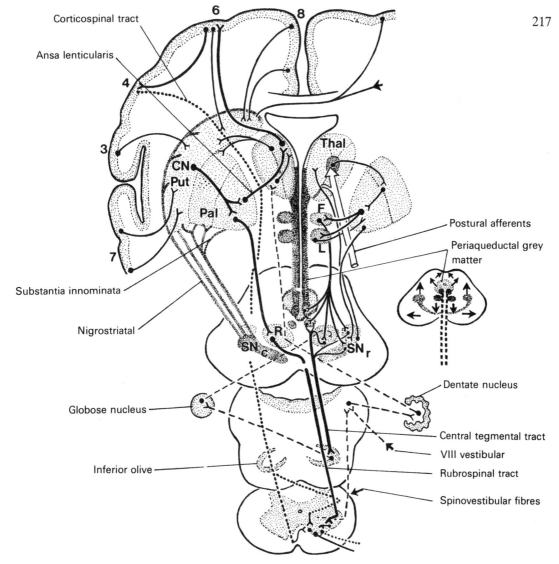

Corticospinal tract
Ansa lenticularis
6 **8**
4
3
CN **Thal**
Put
Pal **F**
L
7
Substantia innominata
Nigrostriatal
Postural afferents
Periaqueductal grey matter
R
SN_c **SN_r**
Dentate nucleus
Central tegmental tract
Globose nucleus
VIII vestibular
Rubrospinal tract
Inferior olive
Spinovestibular fibres

Fig. 22.1. The extrapyramidal motor system. The central grey matter in the walls of the ventral part of IIIrd ventricle and its continuation in the periaqueductal grey matter is involved in the initiation of movement at mesencephalic level. Its driving of the pontomedullary efferent reticular nuclei, and of the upper nuclei of the medial longitudinal bundle (inset and *Fig.* 19.1 – – –) is controlled by the paleostriatum (*right*). This receives integrated spinal and vestibular signals (*open arrow*) from the intralaminar and centromedian nuclei of thalamus to the lateral segment of the pallidum and is relayed through the medial part to subthalamic nuclei of Luys and Forel. The former (L) has feedback to the pallidum which inhibits ballistic movement, the latter (F) exerts inhibitory control on a group of tegmental nuclei — the red nucleus (R), substantia nigra pars reticulata (SNr) and dorsal and ventrolateral tegmental nuclei. These adjust tonic postural commands for head and trunk position. (*Inset:* lateral movement from SNr, neck flexion from dorsal and extension from ventrolateral tegmental nuclei, and neck rotation from the nuclei of the medial longitudinal bundle.) Each of these nuclei relays to the inferior olive of the medulla by the central tegmental bundle. The inferior olive projects to the opposite globose nucleus of cerebellum which projects back to the red nucleus on the original side (- - - -). The red nucleus facilitates flexor muscles, the tegmentum facilitates extensor muscles reciprocally (? tremorgenic).

The neostriatum is represented *left*. The nigrostriatal pathway from substantia nigra pars compacta (SNc) is probably a diffuse dopaminergic inhibitory control of the caudate nucleus (CN) and substantia innominata. The main topographic input to caudate/putamen is from all cortical areas except the visual. It inhibits the paleostriatum but may facilitate part of the red nucleus. Its main outflow, the ansa lenticularis to the anterior nucleus of thalamus, is relayed to the supplementary motor areas 6 and 8 which gate the corticospinal tract (· · · ·) to the contralateral spinal cord. The neostriatum inhibits the paleostriatal postural set and permits corticospinal driving of motoneurones. The supplementary motor area also receives cerebellar control from the contralateral dentate nucleus and an adjacent area of thalamus (not convergent), adding spinovestibular influences.

reflexes, both length and tension types, causing rigidity, lengthening reactions and, possibly, alternating tremor. The other features of *Parkinson's syndrome* with respect to voluntary movement are discussed below.

In addition to the large thalamostriatal connection described above in the context of righting reflexes (and important controlling fibres received from the substantia nigra), the receptive part of the corpus striatum receives fibres from most areas of the neocortex, some as direct *corticostriatal fibres*, others as collaterals of the pyramidal tract fibres. Although no part of the striatum is entirely controlled by a single cortical area there is, in general, a topographic organization. It is mainly ipsilateral, but bilateral corticostriate fibres probably arise from the supplementary motor and sensory areas. There is practically no direct input from the visual cortex.

The afferent fibres excite the otherwise inactive striatal cells (evoked inhibition is rare and probably via interneurones) which project both excitatory and inhibitory factors to the substantia nigra and pallidum, as just described — the basis of a *switch or selection system* similar to that seen in the anterior horn of the spinal grey matter. In barbiturate anaesthesia the inhibitory drive persists and the facilitatory one is lost. The inhibitory transmitter in striato-pallidal neurones is believed to be GABA. The output of the switch is applied through the pallidum to the *tegmental nuclei* and, most importantly, to the *ventral anterior and lateral nuclei of the thalamus* and onwards to the *supplementary motor area*. It is now doubted that there is convergence of output pathways of the basal ganglia (and of the substantia nigra if certain nigrothalamic projections are of independent significance) and of the cerebellum with overlapping, but not necessarily convergent, projection to the motor cortex as recently advocated.

This switching action is a fundamental function of the pallidum and its related nuclei. However it is organized, it changes the musculature from one postural 'set' to another, necessary for the righting reflexes of walking (leg swing as well as arm swing) (p. 208). Since movement, defined above, involves dissolution of one *postural set* and transition to another, it is clear that there will be difficulty in initiating

voluntary movement when pallidal control is absent, but resetting could still be open to alternative control. The Parkinsonism patient who is unable to initiate normal controlled limb movements can carry out ballistic/saccadic movements if startled by an urgent visual stimulus (kinesie paradoxale) or emotionally aroused. The disorder of motor control affects axial muscles more than limbs, proximal limb muscles more than distal, and upper limbs more than lower.

Denny-Brown considered that in addition to suppressing proprioceptive reflex activity, the corpus striatum *facilitates tactile motor activity* (grasping and avoiding) of cortical area 7 and the *visual pursuit* activity of frontal eye fields (area 7). Indeed, as the major pallidofugal outflow through the ansa lenticularis to the ventrolateral nucleus of the thalamus is relayed indirectly to the motor cortex, it would appear that the striatal control over a lower motor system dominated by peripheral afferent and vestibular input is essential for the tactile and visual directed exploratory movements which are made possibly by the cortical analysers. It is not surprising that the basal ganglia begin to discharge before the motor cortex in voluntary movement. Kornhuber has described the corpus striatum as a *generator* of progressive 'ramp' movement, in competition with a ballistic (rapid alternating) and end-point holding movement generated by the cerebellum. We prefer to regard the basal ganglia as permissive or channel-directing switches or '*gate controls*' of a primitive slowly progressive type of movement, originally food seeking (p. 127), with transfer to tactile guided movements which have priority over proprioceptive reflexes except for major displacements of the centre of gravity. Corticospinal and lower motoneurones are both put at the disposal of the cortex.

SUBTHALAMIC NUCLEUS OF LUYS

Fibres from the lateral segment of the pallidum project across the internal capsule to the small *subthalamic nucleus* and are relayed back to both segments of the pallidum (*Fig. 22.1*). The normal function of this feedback system is unknown, but interruption of the arc releases violent ballistic movements of the proximal segments of ipsilateral limbs (*hemiballismus*; hemichorea). Apparently the glycinergic efferents of the subthalamic nucleus inhibit some pallidal activity which is related to abrupt displacement of limbs, possibly an 'off-switch' terminating the ballistic phase of limb movement when the new postural set should be established.

It is unreasonable to regard the cerebellum as the sole generator of ballistic movement. In the rat, an output using GABA neurones has been identified to the entopeduncular nucleus. Its homologue in man is the *internal part of the pallidum*. It projects to the lateral habenula which has a role in head–eye movements (Chapter 19).

SUBSTANTIA NIGRA

Lying dorsal to the cerebral peduncle, the substantia nigra extends the length of the mid-brain. It receives fine catecholamine-secreting neurones from the head of the caudate nucleus and the putamen, and GABA-secreting neurones from the pallidum. It sends out two distinct types of efferent neurones.

The non-pigmented cells of the *pars reticulata* synthesize GABA. Some, if not all, send nigrothalamic fibres to the lateral and anterior ventral nuclei and to the dorsomedial nucleus of the *thalamus* where they are relayed to the frontal eye field. They may be disordered in the oculogyric crises of some types of Parkinsonism. The main function of this system is unknown and it may have nothing to do with motor control. (The postencephalitic Parkinsonism in which oculogyric crises are most common has characteristic disturbances of sleep rhythms and of interpersonal behaviour.)

The large melanin pigmented cells of the *pars compacta* project dopamine-secreting nigrostriatal fibres which end in both the *striatum and the pallidum* — the main source of the striatal dopamine which is depleted in Parkinsonism. Topographic organization of these fibres to and from the substantia nigra suggests a closed feedback loop modulating the striatal input to the pallidum. When this loop is defective there are major defects of voluntary movement as well as the postural disturbances described above. The human subject has difficulty in initiating movements, carries them out slowly and cannot change easily from one motor pattern to another, not only with respect to postural set, but with regard to movements regarded as 'cortical'. The detailed orientation of the hand in response to contact is impaired and the normal balance between exploratory and avoiding movements is lost. Parkinson's disease prevents a patient from carrying out two concurrent voluntary motor acts.

The importance of the pallido-thalamic-cortex-pyramidal tract route to the spinal motoneurones is further shown by the fact that cortical ablation abolishes chorea and athetosis, and pyramidal tract section immediately abolishes the tremor of Parkinsonism. A suggestion that *tremor* is a release of a latent primitive alternating pattern responsible for fin movement in fishes may seem far-fetched, but *release of the alternating brain stem automatisms* of chewing and respiration are common in Parkinsonism, to the detriment of speech production. In normal speech the basal ganglia arrest respiration and chewing until appropriate, or until overridden by the respiratory drive (Chapter 20). In striatal disease (chorea) they are inappropriately inhibited. (Anaesthetists might reflect that concentration on chemical control of the respiratory rhythm may have caused relative neglect of the neurological mechanisms.)

TEGMENTAL NUCLEI

Very little is known about the pallidofugal fibres through the field of Forel to the *mid-brain tegmentum*, completing a feedback loop driven by the vestibular nuclei (p. 173). They appear to be involved in controlling torsional movements of the trunk and neck (p. 206). Disorders there have been blamed for torsional dystonia, dystonia musculorum deformans and isolated *dystonias* (spasmodic torticollis, blepharospasm, oromandibular dystonia and possibly writer's cramp). Like the vestibular nuclei, the right and left tegmental nuclei appear to be in balance.

The tardive dyskinesias associated with the use of neuroleptic drugs are believed to be due to functional overactivity of extrapyramidal mechanisms mediated by dopamine (and diminished by dopamine antagonists or depleters such as tetrabenazine). The exact site of the synapses involved is unknown. The functional disorder could be overproduction of dopamine, denervation sensitivity of dopamine receptors, or destruction of inhibitory neurones.

OLIVARY NUCLEI

Projections from the pallidum and *red nucleus* descend by the central tegmental bundle to the *inferior olivary nucleus* of the medulla and are relayed across the midline via the inferior cerebellar peduncle to the cerebellar cortex. These are presumably for integration of extrapyramidal and pyramidal motor activities but whether in pre-programming movement or in its ongoing control (or both) is not known.

PALLIDO-RETICULO-SPINAL PROJECTIONS

The pallidum and its subsidiary nuclei do not project directly to the spinal cord but probably modulate the reticulospinal system by chains of short neurones in the central grey core. Clearly, the pallidum is an integrating centre for movement patterns with a small outflow to tegmental and lower brain stem centres controlling the trunk, a cerebellar input and a major outflow to the thalamus from which it is relayed back to the cortex. If this were all, it would be a regulating centre for the righting reflexes reacting to an input from the thalamus, but we are now to discuss a corticostriatal input which has developed later in evolutionary development.

CORTICOSTRIATAL AFFERENTS

The earliest of these to evolve must have been afferents from the archipallium, the oldest cortical structure typified by the hippocampal formation and the rhinencephalon (Chapter 14). Fibres from the olfactory bulb go to the amygdaloid complex, a specialized part of the tail of the caudate nucleus which is involved in motor and visceral responses to appetite functions. The primitive drives of hunger and thirst depend on chemoreceptors in the hypothalamus (Chapter 25) and the first 'distance receptors', appropriate for an aquatic environment, are similar (smell, taste). They

had to direct a limbless body towards food. It is plausible that head–trunk movements were evolved by olfactory brain-pallidal-tegmental homologues. The *claustrum*, lying between the insular cortex and the striatum, may be involved in appetitive behavioural responses, but its deep connections have not been identified.

CORTICAL INHIBITION OF THE STRIATUM

With the development of the neopallium, cross-modality linkages (p. 110) with tactile and visual association areas developed by corticofugal projections from all areas of cerebral cortex to the striatum. As with the lower levels of extrapyramidal control, it seems that they inhibit the instinctive behavioural responses and righting reflexes until *appropriate segments* of these are disinhibited by the motor command systems of the hypothalamus and cortex. The corticostriate connections select from a repertoire designed to move the central axis towards food and to correct the position of the displaced body, but this provides the necessary postural base for the type of movement the cortex is interested in. In this respect, most if not all of the *corticostriatal control is inhibitory to the pallidum*. There was formerly a vogue for recognizing 'suppressor areas' of the cortex with extrapyramidal functions. The strong inhibition attributed to these areas was over-valued, but some inhibition of postural sets is certainly necessary for goal-directed movement. It is the concept of specific suppressor areas which has been abandoned, not the inhibitory property which is generalized in the cortex.

With increasing encephalization of motor function, for discrete goal-directed movement of limbs and eyes, the drive to the amygdala (p. 128) is paralleled by a pallidofugal outflow via the thalamus to the cortex and this has become a major pathway for directing movement, taking the diencephalic motor stimulus to *secondary* motor command areas in the cortex which are gated by the various association areas of the receptive cortex, a distributed cortical motor system which could, in principle, be entered by cortically initiated signals. Some of these efferent neurones can only be identified by appropriate sensory inputs. Observation is simple with respect to the eye movements which follow visual and vestibular stimulation (Chapter 19) but it is more difficult for limb movements which are responsive to all known afferent signals.

Praxis

Vocalization (vowel sounds involving activation of muscles of the abdomen, larynx, pharynx and tongue) occurs from electrical excitation of a number of cortical areas in man. They include the primary motor area of the pre-central gyrus, some parts of the post-central gyrus and the supplementary motor area. Ongoing speech is arrested by electrical stimulation of these areas in the conscious subject, with aphasic phenomena if the left hemisphere is stimulated. Stimulation of the inferior frontal lobe, parietal area and temporal lobe of the speech-dominant hemisphere produces temporary confusion of words.

Speech is never evoked by cortical stimulation. In the same way, movement of the limbs can be evoked from primary and supplementary motor areas, but it is never a skilled ('praxic') movement pattern. Like speech, these patterns require to be formulated by receptive association areas of cortex (Chapter 24).

We have already described some of this corticofugal outflow going from all areas to the striatum to inhibit selectively the gross motor patterns triggered at diencephalic level. More direct control has been evolved by fibres from the cortex to the cerebellum via the pontine nuclei and, in a late evolutionary stage, by a specialized output from the Rolandic area via the internal capsule and pyramids of the brain stem, the corticospinal or pyramidal tract. Since the pyramidal tract is increasingly regarded as a 'final common path' for programmed movement, its description will be postponed until the cerebellar mechanism has been reviewed.

Further reading

DeLong M.R. and Georgopoulos A.P. Physiology of the basal ganglia — a brief overview. In: Chase T.N., Wexler N.S. and Barbeau A. (ed.) *Advances in Neurology*, vol. 23: *Huntington's Disease*, 1979, pp. 137–53.

Denny-Brown D. *The Cerebral Control of Movement*. Liverpool: Liverpool University Press, 1966.

Evarts E.V. Changing concepts of central control of movement. *Canad. J. Physiol. Pharmacol.* 1975; **53**: 191–201.

Hassler R. Striatal control of locomotion, intentional actions and of integrating and perceptive activity. *J. Neurol. Sci.* 1978; **36**: 187–224.

Kornhuber H.H. Motor functions of cerebellum and basal ganglia: the cerebellocortical saccadic (ballistic) clock, the cerebellonuclear hold regulator, and the basal ganglia ramp (voluntary speed smooth movement) generator. *Kybernetic* 1971; **8**: 157–62.

Martin J.P. *The Basal Ganglia and Posture*. London: Pitman Medical, 1967.

Chapter 23

Cerebellum: a comparator and regulator

The cerebellum is a 'little brain' only in respect to its volume. The surface area and cellular content of its cortex are little inferior to those of the cerebrum. Indeed, its manner of function is essentially the same and an understanding of cerebellar mechanisms illuminates the mechanisms of the cerebral cortex.

The cerebral cortex, tonically activated by the ascending reticular system, selectively inhibits the basal ganglia righting reflexes and puts the bulbospinal motor system under the command of the telereceptors. A later evolutionary development has encephalized the exteroceptive, and to a lesser extent the proprioceptive input of the thalamus and elaborated cross-modality linkages, with storage of abstracted 'symbols'. In the human cerebrum this later development has provided a substrate for intellectual functions and a discriminative exteroceptor sensory analysis which is put to the service of a motor system with late evolved interneurones, the pyramidal tract, bypassing the basal ganglia.

The cerebellar cortex, tonically activated by the vestibular nuclei as well as by the reticular formation, inhibits the vestibulospinal and reticulospinal outflow to the spinal cord interneurone and motoneurone pool. The most 'primitive' parts, the archicerebellum (vestibular cerebellum) and paleocerebellum (spinocerebellum) provide cross-modality linkages between the vestibular and proprioceptive senses required for postural maintenance (extensor reflexes) and the cutaneous receptors activating flexor reflexes. A later evolutionary development, the neocerebellum (pontocerebellum), has added an input from the encephalized sensory systems and their new motor controls. The cross-modality linkages are principally used to provide controlling signals modulating or gating the pyramidal and basal ganglia systems.

Like the cerebral cortex, the cerebellar cortex abstracts and stores 'symbols', but the memory and learning is for acquired patterns of motor behaviour instead of for sensory patterns. Thus the cerebellum is not obligatory for production of reflex or cerebral commanded movement, but neither of these is fully coordinated without it. For this reason, the cerebellum has come to be regarded as the coordinating centre of the brain. Clearly it is not the only part of the nervous system with this function, only the most specialized one. When it is destroyed by a lesion, the cross-modality linkages and inhibition/facilitation functions of the cerebral cortex and bulbospinal systems are sufficient to provide almost complete compensation.

In the same way as a sensory pattern can be 'recognized' regardless of size and orientation, a practised motor performance can be reproduced with a unique postural set of the muscles, or even with different muscles, eg signing one's name with pen on paper or with chalk on a blackboard, or playing a musical instrument held in a novel position. The sequence and force of muscular contractions cannot be pre-programmed but the impact on the environment certainly is. The nervous system analyses a unique environment and reacts to it uniquely to produce a standardized effect. Sensors activating servomotors with feedback control can do this. The cerebellum has developed as a servo-control system for the muscles of the limbs, but it retains some of its 'primitive' postural control functions since even a voluntary movement starts and ends with posture. The new facilities are to provide *feedforward control* for ballistic movements driven by commands from distance receptors, and a misalignment detector for *feedback control* of 'measured' movements, comparing actual movement with that required by the command neurones in the cerebral cortex and elsewhere. The latter function needs a recurrent input from length and tension detectors in muscle, and joint and skin sensors, but in addition it requires corollary discharge from the motor command areas of the cerebral cortex and basal ganglia.

Detection of misalignment between intrafusal and extrafusal muscle fibres is used to regulate muscle length as a segmental reflex and the sensitivity of this system is biased by the fusimotor (gamma) motoneurones (p. 92). The cerebellum is involved in some of the 'long loop' reflexes and in alteration of the ratio between alpha and gamma motoneurone innervation to the muscles (p. 240). It is a *second order misalignment detector* with regional as well as segmental functions and its decision on misalignment depends on the motor problem demanded by the cerebral cortex. It is not just a length stability problem, though a compensating device is necessary so that muscle length is maintained appropriate to the required displacement even if a load is suddenly applied or removed. We stress the word 'appropriate' since this requires an integration of the whole motor activity of the organism in the context of a changing internal and external environment plus *expected* changes computed by the frontal lobes. It is necessary for all stabilizing reflexes (spinal, brain stem, pallidal and cortical) to have their gains continuously updated and optimized. It is also desirable that repetition of a task should lead to progressive improvement without stereotyping (like the difference between a skilled pianist and a mechanical pianola).

The cells of the flocculus *compare* visual and vestibular signals and modify the output of the vestibular nuclei to the extraocular muscles. The major functions of the cerebellar hemispheres are to compare the afferent data from vestibular, muscle, joint and skin receptors with the immediate or learned requirements of the motor driving systems and to *correct misalignment by modulating the gain of spinal and long-loop reflex arcs* to the muscles. Unlike the motor area of the cerebral cortex

which regulates *power* by controlling motor unit recruitment, the cerebellum adjusts gain mainly by altering *firing rates* and *timing of motor unit discharge*. (This is not surprising since most of its control is effected by altering gamma motoneurone bias.) These gain controls and timing patterns are 'learned' by the memory system of the cerebellum and there is evidence that after a cerebellar lesion human subjects may fail to improve their performance by repetition.

Elementary control circuits of cerebellum

It must be acknowledged that the functions of the cerebellum are not fully understood. A reasonable model can be constructed by reducing the input–output connections to simple mechanisms based on their appearance during evolution and then speculating on the effect of cross-linking these in a similar manner to that proposed for the cerebral cortex. Only fractions of the primitive functions have survived in the primate cerebellum, but some clues to these are to be found in the functional defects observed after lesions, experimental or pathological.

VESTIBULO-CEREBELLAR ARCS

The cerebellum was developed in primitive fish for the processing of information derived from the lateral line receptors and their specialized development in the vestibules of the inner ear. In both of these, ciliated hair cells respond to the pressure or velocity of water, with a directional response according to the direction of displacement of the cilia (and to acceleration, because of the inertia of the labyrinthine fluid). Each of these organs has an efferent nervous supply which inhibits the receptor and also its reflex drive to trunk and limb extensor muscles (Chapter 18). It has been shown that each vestibular apparatus inhibits the extensor tonus of the contralateral labyrinth on its ipsilateral limbs and on the system for controlling conjugate eye movements (Chapter 19).

This inhibitory control is applied by a long-loop reflex arc from the vestibular nuclei of the brain stem through the archicerebellum ('vestibulocerebellum') (*Fig. 23.1*). In man it is the *flocculonodular lobe* and the *anterior*

224

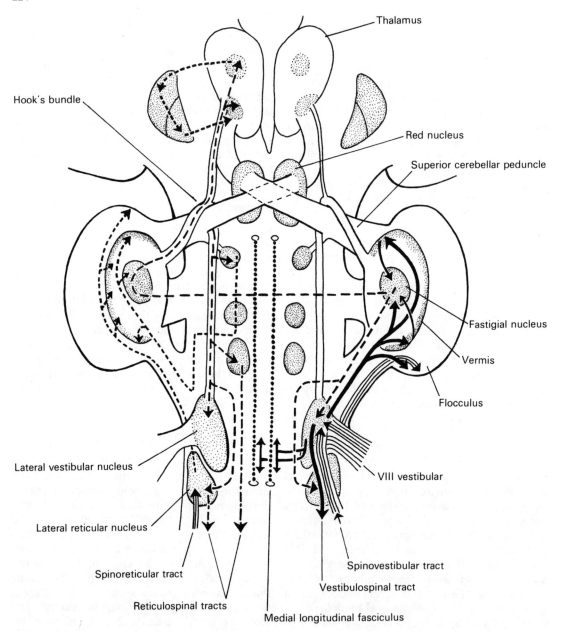

Thalamus

Hook's bundle

Red nucleus

Superior cerebellar peduncle

Fastigial nucleus

Vermis

Flocculus

VIII vestibular

Lateral vestibular nucleus

Lateral reticular nucleus

Spinovestibular tract

Spinoreticular tract

Vestibulospinal tract

Reticulospinal tracts

Medial longitudinal fasciculus

Fig. 23.1. *The 'vestibular' cerebellum. Lower right*: vestibular nerve and spinovestibular fibres (≡) converging on the lateral vestibular nucleus. Some first order vestibular neurones pass directly to the cortex of the floccular area of the cerebellum. (The diagram also shows the descending vestibulospinal tract) and bilateral connections to the medial longitudinal fasciculus illustrated in *Fig.* 18.1.) Second order vesitbulo-cerebellar neurones pass directly to the fastigial nucleus and indirectly through the cortex of the vermis. Efferent fibres decussate in the vermis (– – – –), emerge by the contralateral superior peduncle, looping round it in Hook's bundle and descend to the efferent part of the vestibular nucleus. Some fibres do not decussate but pass back to the ipsilateral vestibular nucleus, coordinating the vestibular control of eyes, head and trunk. Both cerebello-vestibular paths also synapse with reticular nuclei of the medulla which have their own cerebellar areas and reticulospinal outflow (–·–·–). Note also an upward projection (*upper left*, ----) carrying integrated vestibular and spinal proproiceptive signals to the central nuclei of the thalamus where they enter the thalamostriatal control circuits.

vermis. First, second and third order neurones relay from the vestibular ganglion and vestibular nuclei through the brachium restiforme (inferior cerebellar peduncle) to the cortex of the flocculonodular lobe and anterior vermis as *mossy fibres* activating the *Purkinje cells* of these areas. These send inhibitory impulses via the *fastigial nucleus* (in the cerebellar vermis) which projects bilaterally to the vestibulospinal outflows and to the efferent reticular formation. In the vestibular nuclei they converge with spinovestibular afferents.

The powerful *extensor inhibition* of this circuit is shown in carnivores by a strong extensor rigidity which is released when the cerebellum is ablated. This is not present in man or indeed in the higher animals which have developed their flexion movements for manipulative functions, especially the forelimb projection from the anterior vermis.

Man does retain the cerebellar control over the vestibular drive on conjugate eye movements, effected via the medial longitudinal bundles (Chapter 19), though this appears to be less important than in lower animals. Unilateral ablation of the vestibulocerebellum or its outflow (ipsilaterally through the inferior and contralaterally through the superior cerebellar peduncle, *Fig. 23.1*) causes imbalance between the vestibular nuclei of each side, with *nystagmus* as a 'release phenomenon'. After a period of time a new balance is restored. For the same reason a sensation of loss of *equilibrium* occurs, with falling to the side of the lesion, and this also tends to adapt (more rapidly for static than for kinetic vestibular function). This type of conjugate nystagmus is sometimes seen with acute flocculonodular lesions but rarely with chronic lesions in which the adaptation occurs *pari passu*. There is no vertigo. The only type of nystagmus considered specific for cerebellar disease is *rebound nystagmus*, a type of gaze paretic nystagmus that either disappears or reverses direction while the gaze position is held. When the eyes are returned to the mid position there is another burst of nystagmus in the direction of the return saccade. *Ataxia of the eye muscles* may be found, with true incoordination of the extraocular muscles of both eyes: the more common phasic nystagmus is a well-coordinated movement (p. 181).

SPINOCEREBELLAR ARCS

The early phylogenetic development of the supravestibular grey matter into a cerebellum is associated with integration of vestibular and spinal cord afferent impulses required for posture (Chapter 18). It was an important evolutionary step as one of the first uses of the principle of cross-modality linkage, later so effectively exploited by the cerebral cortex.

Unlike the vestibular input, there are no known examples of primary afferent neurones of spinal nerves passing directly to the cerebellum. Second order afferent neurones relay ipsilaterally from Clarke's column of cells in lamina VII at the base of the dorsal horn of the spinal grey matter as the *dorsal spinocerebellar tract* (DSCT) (*Fig. 23.2*). A cervical cord equivalent is termed the 'cuneocerebellar tract'. The afferent fibres relay proprioceptive (Ia, Ib, II) impulses from muscle receptors and joints and group III afferent impulses from skin, muscles and joints by the restiform body (inferior cerebellar peduncle) ipsilaterally to the paleocerebellum ('spinocerebellum'), which is the anterior vermis, pyramis, uvula and paraflocculus, ie the *vermis and intermediate zone* of the cerebellum, hindlimbs posteriorly and forelimbs anteriorly.

Some second order neurones pass from the interneuronal area of the spinal cord grey matter by the laterally situated *ventral spinocerebellar tract* (VSCT) of Gowers, both crossed and uncrossed. It ascends through the medulla to the upper pons, then bends dorsolaterally over the root of the trigeminal nerve to enter the cerebellum by its superior peduncle (brachium conjunctivum) to end in the anterior vermis. It is believed to be concerned only with hindlimb and lower trunk afferents but a forelimb equivalent has recently been identified in the cat. The type of sensory information carried is much more restricted than in the dorsal tract, almost exclusively from type Ib afferents of the Golgi tendon organs, recording muscle tension from a wider receptive field. It has been suggested that this tract may signal interaction between contraction of each muscle and the resistance to movement of the limb as a whole. A major part of the VSCT fibres crossing in the spinal cord re-cross in the vermis. A component from the

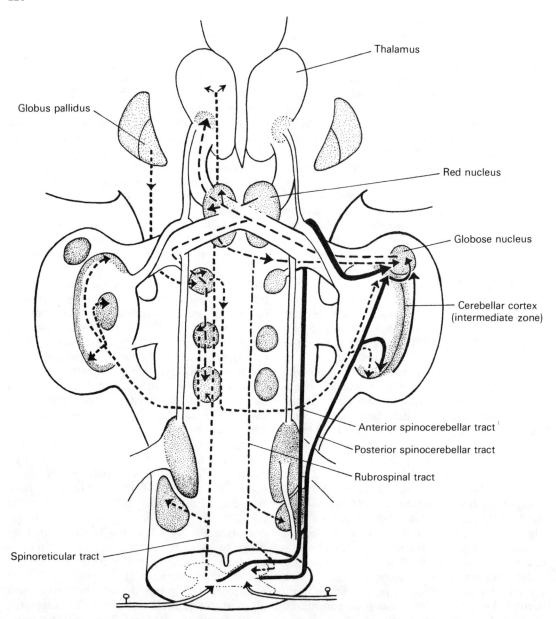

Fig. 23.2. *The 'spinal' cerebellum.* The lower part of the diagram shows the uncrossed posterior and mainly crossed anterior spinocerebellar tracts ascending to the intermediate zone of the cerebellum by the inferior and superior peduncles to the globose nucleus directly and via the cerebellar cortex. This area also receives important inputs from the contralateral reticular formation of the pons (· · · · ·) (also receiving spinal and pallidal influences) and from the contralateral red nucleus which is a main target of the efferent fibres from the globose nucleus. The red nucleus sends a decussated rubrospinal tract (–·–·) to upper parts of the spinal cord, for head and trunk flexion (and to a lesser extent limb flexion). Some cerebellofugal fibres from this area probably continue through the contralateral red nucleus to the thalamus (----) (*upper left*).

upper limbs remains ipsilateral. Linkage between them by vermis cortex neurones may correlate the patterns of muscle contraction of both fore and hind limbs which are necessary for walking (p. 210).

Third order neurones carrying spinal nerve impulses to the cerebellum are, by definition, relayed again before entering the cerebellum. This exposes the ascending impulses to some of the effects already described for converging neurones — viz. integration, 'sharpening' and 'gating' by contingent signals from other parts of the nervous system. There is little detailed knowledge about this important aspect of signal processing before presentation to the cerebellum but some important relays are known and some functions tentatively suggested.

SPINO-RETICULO-CEREBELLAR (SRC) FIBRES (FIG. 23.2)

These carry impulses relayed in the dorsal horn from group III afferents with a wider receptive field than those relaying to the DSCT. They have no specific modality and their wide receptive field may embrace three or four limbs. It has been suggested that they convey information concerning the levels of interneuronal activity in the spinal cord.

The same problem of lack of local sign and of modality specificity applies with even greater force to the *spino-olivo-cerebellar paths* (*Fig.* 23.3) (there are four of them ascending in the ventral, dorsolateral and lateral funiculi of the spinal cord). Some fibres are crossed, others ipsilateral, or cross and recross, and some have intermediate relays in the dorsal column nuclei. Their functions, obviously interrelating all limbs, may be deduced from some features common to all of them. Like the SRC path, the receptive fields are large and vaguely delimited, but the type of signal relayed and the site of delivery are quite different. All the spinal pathways relaying into the inferior cerebellar peduncle from the *inferior olivary nucleus* (*Fig.* 23.3) are activated by afferents (from skin, muscle and joints) of the groups II and III types *which also activate the flexion withdrawal reflexes* and inhibit extensor muscles (Chapter 17). They all

project to narrow sagittal strips in the anterior lobe of the corpus cerebelli. To summarize, a diffuse non-specific 'protective' afferent bombardment is funnelled to a topographically discrete area of the cerebellar cortex which is also receiving somatotopic second order neurones from the limbs.

This area of cerebellar cortex, *the intermediate zone* parallel to the vermis, sends efferent fibres to the *globose nucleus*. It projects through the superior peduncle to the contralateral *red nucleus* (*Fig.* 23.2) which relays back to the original side of the cord. The rubrospinal tract facilitates flexion muscles: in man this is largely restricted to the upper limbs. A proportion of cerebellar efferent fibres continue to the ventrolateral and non-specific nuclei of the *thalamus*. The *globose nucleus* output exerts a tonic facilitation on the cerebral cortex and on the flexion musculature which the *Purkinje cells* of the intermediate zone *inhibit* in response to stimuli from the flexor reflex afferents of skin and muscle (in that order of significance).

BRAKE CONTROL

These long loop reflexes through the intermediate cerebellum and/or cerebral cortex may be supposed to provide a 'brake' for flexion responses in a similar manner to the vermis-fastigial loops for extension responses. Removal of the brake allows a limb segment to swing too far in response to a tendon tap before it is arrested by a flexor stretch reflex. The jerk becomes pendular. A similar 'brake failure' disrupts goal-directed movements requiring accurate position control of extensor and flexor muscles, with oscillation of the limb extremity about the desired trajectory — so-called 'intention tremor'.

CEREBRO-CEREBELLAR ARCS

It is implicit in this statement that the cerebellar inhibitory machine is incorporated into the mechanism of goal-directed or voluntary movement. This is an important evolutionary development associated with relative decline of the role of the cerebellum in vestibular reflex control. The contralateral sensori-motor

228

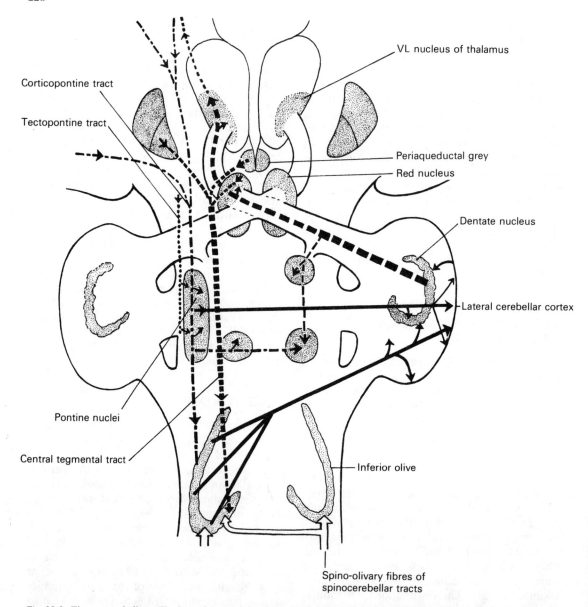

Fig. 23.3. *The neocerebellum.* The lateral zone of the cerebellar hemisphere receives signals from the cerebral cortex and the inferior olive (mossy fibres) and integrates them with spinocerebellar fibres (climbing fibres, *Fig.* 23.4). The latter are not shown in this diagram above their input to the inferior olives (*open arrows, bottom*). The inferior olivary nucleus integrates ascending spinal cord signals with two major descending bundles. These are the central tegmental tract (**- - -**) from the diencephalic and periaqueductal grey matter, the pallidum, substantia nigra and red nucleus and from sensori-motor areas of the cerebral cortex (–·–·). Most of the cerebral cortex and the tectum (····) also send parapyramidal corticopontine and tectopontine tracts to the pontine nuclei which relay the large pontocerebellar projection (——) through the middle cerebellar peduncle to the dentate nucleus directly or via the lateral cerebellar cortex. The dentate nucleus efferents (■ ■ ■) pass mainly to the contralateral VL thalamus. Some uncrossed fibres (---) also pass to medial reticular nuclei in the pons involved in motor automatisms. The dentato-rubro-olivary-dentate connections form a circuit: damage to this loop causes palatal nystagmus and one type of myoclonus.

cortex, caudate nucleus and periaqueductal grey matter send important contributions through the central tegmental tract to accessory nuclei of the *inferior olive* (*Fig.* 23.3). This is an important nuclear area for integration of cortical, extrapyramidal and spinal afferent signals from the limbs with re-entry of motor command signals *through the thalamus to the pyramidal tract*, amplifying inhibitory control derived from limb receptors.

The functional role of the diencephalic input must remain speculative, but the direct command from near the presumed site of initiation of voluntary movement (p. 215) may be noted. Monkeys trained to follow a target activate their visual cortex and cerebellum about the same time, and both before the motor cortex — ie the *lateral cerebellum* is not simply a monitor of the spinal cord record of limb movement (that is a function of the medial cerebellum) or even of corollary discharge of the pyramidal tract. It appears to be at least one, possibly the major, route from posterior cerebral cortex command neurones to the motor cortex, entraining memory stores of motor patterns by exciting them in the circumstances of contemporary body and limb position and then recruiting the appropriate pyramidal tract repertoire. This role of the cerebellar cortex as a *comparator between the cerebral command and the spinal feedback* is continued throughout the movement. It has been suggested that pyramidal collaterals to the cerebellum permit comparison of the misalignment between the commanded movement and its execution.

In man, the largest and most complex development of the cerebellum is the *lateral zone* of the corpus cerebelli, the neocerebellum ('pontocerebellum') (*Fig.* 23.3). It receives a considerable projection from the olivocerebellar fibres just described and these are integrated with pontocerebellar fibres entering by the middle cerebellar peduncle (brachium pontis). This is the most massive input to the cerebellum from the cerebral cortex. All parts of the cerebral cortex contribute fibres to the *corticopontine tracts*. They descend with the pyramidal tract to the ipsilateral pons but separate out in the cerebral peduncle.

The fibres from the distance receptor analysers (occipital and temporal lobes) descend laterally in the peduncle, relay in the lateralmost part of the pontine nuclei along with fibres from the colliculi, and are distributed to the vermis bilaterally for coordination of eye, head and trunk movements (Chapter 19). In the cat, the visual cortex neurones to the pontine nuclei are activated only by moving objects. The cerebellum does not 'hear or see', but is informed of auditory and visual cues from moving targets in the distant environment.

The parietal lobe projection is more medial in the cerebral peduncle and the pontine relay immediately crosses the basis pontis to enter the middle cerebellar peduncle for distribution to the intermediate and lateral zones of the contralateral cerebellar hemisphere. It is a particularly dense projection to the cerebellum from that area of the brain with 'command cells' for exploratory movement of limbs in extracorporeal space — a late development of an 'old' sensory function (Chapter 8) — the 'skilled' movements.

Medial to the corticospinal (pyramidal) tract in the cerebral peduncle is a large descending path from the frontal lobe to the pontine nuclei. It is also relayed to the whole corpus cerebelli. Thus the cerebrum sends signals into the cerebellum where they are more elaborately integrated with each other and with spinocerebellar inputs than is possible with the olivocerebellar paleocerebellum. Nevertheless, although inputs and outputs differ in distribution, the cerebellar machine is fundamentally the same for archi-, paleo- and neocerebellum and this will be described below.

The lateral zone of the cerebellar hemisphere sends efferent fibres to the *dentate (lateral) nucleus*, which is inhibited by the cortical *Purkinje cells* when these are satisfied that the difference between command and execution is minimal — ie the movement is arrested when it has reached its goal. This model immediately raises the question, what activity of the dentate nucleus is inhibited by the Purkinje cells? It projects through the superior cerebellar peduncle (*Fig.* 23.3), a large bundle of fibres which immediately cross in the mid-brain, plunging through the contralateral red nucleus, to which it contributes. They end in the ventrolateral nucleus of the thalamus in association with the main outflow from the corpus striatum. Both are integrated there and pass to the *sensorimotor area of the cerebral cortex*.

Kornhuber's model of two function generators 'driving' the motor cortex is plausible. He suggests that the striatum is a 'ramp generator' and the cerebellum a 'ballistic generator'. His clinical reasons for this formulation are not convincing and other writers consider that ballistic movement is generated in the basal ganglia (p. 218). We regard this dichotomy as too simplistic and consider that both types of movement are entrained and regulated by both areas. The difference is in the type of gating control — the basal ganglia for righting reflexes and postural set, the cerebellum for overruling the demands of postural control in favour first of protective behaviour and later of goal-directed movement.

Goal-directed, or intentional, movements remain possible after ablation of the cerebellum unilaterally. A study of the input–output connections of the cerebellum shows that the main input from the spinal nerves and labyrinth is ipsilateral, and the input–output connections with the cerebral hemisphere and striatum are contralateral, ie each side of the cerebellum receives signals from and controls motor signals directed to the lower motor neurones of the same side of the body. Despite some bilateral connections, the cerebellar hemisphere is largely ipsilateral in its sphere of interest: the vermis is bilateral. Thus a lateral cerebellar lesion or a brachium conjunctivum lesion causes loss of coordination of movement (*ataxia*) and disorders of muscle tone in ipsilateral limbs.

The loss of dentate nucleus facilitation of the motor cortex is seen as *asthenia* and increased fatiguability of movements. The major defect is *asynergia*, a lack of capacity to time and grade the motor drive to muscles required to work as a synergy (p. 235). The movement is completed but it is decomposed, not closely regulated to the required muscle length (*dysmetria*) and underdamped by lack of braking (overshoot, *intention tremor*), particularly when a movement is required to stop suddenly at a chosen point and then immediately to reverse (*dysdiadochokinesis*). Misalignment

between cortical demand and spinal monitored effect causes excessive deviation to the directed side of a movement which is deprived of visual control (*past pointing* and compass gait). Asynergia of motor control of speech causes *dysarthria*. (There are different types, dysphonic and articulatory.)

This syndrome of the neocerebellum is, of course, commonly added to those of the paleo- and archicerebellum involving defects of gait, trunk posture, eye–head movement and stretch reflexes. These are all disconnection syndromes. There is no known clinical syndrome associated with spontaneous overactivity of the cerebellar cortex. Its function is entirely inhibitory of the interaction between the input and output of the rest of the nervous system. It does this via the intracerebellar nuclei and some release manifestation might be anticipated if the Purkinje cells are inactive.

It appears that the *intracerebellar nuclei* are signal-triggered by direct excitatory input from the various afferent sources already described as going towards the cerebellar cortex (*Figs 23.1–3*). Some of this input is by collaterals but direct inputs from spinal, olivary and pontine projections are also present. These nuclei therefore have a *tonic activity which is modulated by the cerebellar cortex*. Their cells can be both inhibited and disinhibited. When disinhibited they tonically activate the whole cerebral cortex (with associated EEG responses) as well as the efferent vestibular, reticular, rubral and pyramidal spinal projections. *Selective inhibition* by the cerebellar cortex coordinates motor activity. Electrical stimulation of this inhibitory control is being explored as a possible treatment for epilepsy.

MYOCLONUS

The dentate nucleus, which is the intracerebellar nucleus for the lateral zone of the cerebellum, is triggered from both pontocerebellar and olivocerebellar inputs. One particular type of focal epilepsy (*myoclonus*) occurs when there is disconnection within a loop involving the central tegmental tract, inferior olive, contralateral dentate nucleus and back to the red nucleus of the original side (*Fig. 23.3*). Involuntary twitching of the soft palate (palatal myoclonus or 'nystagmus') continues during sleep and does not interfere with speaking, chewing or swallowing. On the contrary, voluntary movement seems to inhibit the myoclonic twitches.

Other types of myoclonus involving the face and limbs and associated with olivo-cerebellodentate disorders are stimulus-related. The site of the responsible lesion is difficult to determine as the disease process commonly involves wide areas of the cerebellar and striatal connections. The abrupt motor discharge may be pyramidal, striatal or segmental and related to photic, acoustic, proprioceptive or exteroceptive stimuli. The flexor motoneurones (which are facilitated by the red nucleus) are most readily recruited and none of the efferent paths, including transcortical connections, are obligatory. Cortical spike and slow wave discharges in the EEG, resembling responses evoked by abrupt visual, acoustic or somatic stimuli (Chapter 16) occur *in parallel* and synchronously with the myoclonic jerks but are not essential for their appearance. There is a breakdown of the normal reciprocal innervation between agonists and antagonists.

Stimulus-related myoclonus tends to disappear in the first stage of sleep or just before awakening. A relation to consciousness is present in myoclonic epilepsy, a 'petit mal variant' with three per second polyspike and slow wave discharges appearing bilaterally synchronously in the EEG. The myoclonic jerk may be preceded or followed by lapse of muscle tone and akinesia. If there is a single disorder of control, it is not at the level of cerebral cortex, thalamus, basal ganglia or reticular formation, but rather at the system which modulates their excitability, the cerebellum.

The effect of disease can be temporarily simulated by drugs such as metrazol and (in some animals) chloralose and occasionally by anaesthetics. A permanent stimulus-related myoclonic state may be caused by cerebral anoxia, sufficient to destroy the Purkinje cells of the cerebellar cortex. Conversely, an increased firing rate of Purkinje cells aroused by phenytoin may be important in its anticonvulsive action. Chronic phenytoin overdosage, which destroys Purkinje cells, may cause

increased epileptic seizures. Disinhibition of the intracerebellar nuclei may well be the factor common to all types of myoclonus. The great desynchronizing inhibitory system of the cerebellum does not even appear in Penfield's diagrams of the motor control system relevant to epilepsy. There is no doubt that the cerebellum through its fastigial and globose nuclei inhibits epileptic activity. It is quite another matter to attribute epilepsy to dysfunction of the cerebellum, but the possibility must be considered.

It is now appropriate to examine the mechanism of the cerebellar cortex for integration of spinal, diencephalic and association cortex inputs for the higher control of the intracerebellar nuclei of the three cerebellar zones which orchestrate all the motor systems and, probably, also for modulation of the intensity of afferent bombardment of the cerebral cortex and the major convergence point in the thalamus.

Cerebellar cortex

A striking feature of the cerebellar cortex is that its neuronal structure is essentially the same in all three zones. Only the input and output connections differ. In this context they will be described as afferent and efferent neurones though it has already been shown that a high proportion of the neurones afferent to the cerebellar cortex are second order efferents from the cerebral cortex.

There are three afferent systems: (i) climbing fibres; (ii) mossy fibres; (iii) a diffusely projected afferent system from the locus coeruleus of the brain stem. The connections and functions of the latter system are still obscure but probably for general noradrenergic modulation (Chapter 3).

The climbing fibre afferents are the olivo-cerebellar fibres described above (p. 227). Each climbing fibre arborizes with the dendritic tree of a single Purkinje cell in the cerebellar cortex 'like a vine climbing through the branches of a tree', making synaptic contact with the 300 or so spines of its dendrites. It therefore causes powerful 'all-or-none' excitation of the single Purkinje cell, causing a high frequency discharge which

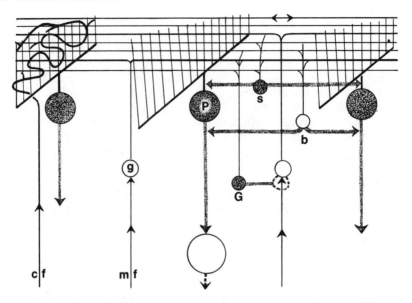

Fig. 23.4. *Cerebellar cortex.* The Purkinje cells (P) project inhibitory commands to a deep cerebellar nucleus from which cerebellofugal neurones arise (– – –). The dendritic tree of each Purkinje cell has multiple synaptic connections with a single ascending climbing fibre (cf) from the inferior olive (*Fig.* 23.3) and multiple connections from parallel fibres which synapse with many Purkinje cells. The parallel fibres, running orthogonal to the plane of the P dendritic tree are the terminal axons of granular cells (g) and transmit in both directions. The granular cells receive excitatory mossy fibres (mf) ascending by the spinocerebellar tracts. The granule cell input to the Purkinje cell dendrites is under inhibitory control by Golgi cells (G) acting on a glomerular structure at the dendrites of the granule cells and activated by parallel fibres from the mossy cells. The parallel fibres also activate inhibitory interneurones to groups of Purkinje cells at the inputs of their main dendrites (stellate cells, s) and at their axon hillocks (basket cells, b).

declines slowly and irregularly. It is possible that this is a gate control which makes the cerebellar input discontinuous. (A sampling process would compensate for the delay inevitable in continuous feedback control of vision-directed movement and permit feed-forward, predictive, movement based on target velocity.)

The mossy fibre afferents convey impulses directly from the dorsal horns by the two direct spinocerebellar pathways (p. 225). Their conduction time is about 10 ms shorter than the spino-olivo-cerebellar pathway to the climbing fibres but their inhibitory synaptic potential develops slowly and is maximal after the climbing fibres sample the excitatory–inhibitory pattern evoked by the mossy fibre component. Unlike the climbing fibres they do not terminate directly on Purkinje cells but on small interneurones, the *granule cells* immediately under the Purkinje cell layer. These extremely numerous cells (calculated as 90 per cent of all the cells in the brain) spread the afferent signal to other interneurones (Golgi, basket and stellate cells) and by remarkably orientated axons — the *parallel fibres* of the molecular layer — which run parallel to each other. The dendritic trees of the Purkinje cells are orientated at right-angles to the parallel fibres which run through their branches and make synaptic contact with their receptors. Thus each mossy fibre contributes to the depolarization of numerous Purkinje cells, and each Purkinje cell is influenced by many parallel fibres.

A single Purkinje cell may receive 100 000 parallel fibres but only one climbing fibre. The mossy fibre–granule cell system is continuously active, modulating the spontaneous activity of the Purkinje cells according to the whole environmental input to the cerebellum. The climbing fibres add brief bursts of repetitive discharges to the Purkinje cells immediately after their collaterals have stimulated the intracerebellar nuclei. As the Purkinje cells transmit strong inhibiting impulses to these nuclei (dentate and others), the tonic output of the deep nuclei is immediately chopped.

These outputs to the motor centres are specially suited to inducing ballistic contractions during the inhibition of postural tone. There is evidence that each climbing fibre regulates the synchronous movements of *groups of muscles*. The cerebellum is more concerned with limb segments than with individual muscles.

INTERNEURONES OF THE CEREBELLUM

The mossy fibre (direct spinocerebellar) input is modified by *interneurones* to convert some of its influence to inhibit Purkinje cells as well as to facilitate them. In the deepest layer of the cerebellar cortex, the granule-cell layer, there are *Golgi cells* which receive mossy fibre and granule cell–parallel fibre impulses. They have a specialized synaptic connection, the *cerebellar glomeruli* consisting of Golgi cell axons surrounding granule cell dendrites which are wrapped around a swelling in a mossy fibre. This suggests a gating device to select the mossy fibre input to the Purkinje cell layer, possibly activated by climbing fibre branches to the Golgi cells.

The climbing fibres and parallel fibres also excite some of the interneurones in the Purkinje cell layer, the *basket cells*, which are inhibited by Purkinje collaterals and in turn inhibit Purkinje cells. The *stellate cells* of the parallel fibre layer convert some of its facilitation into inhibition of the Purkinje cells. A study of *Fig.* 23.4 will show that these connections are less complicated than would appear from a written description.

All three types of interneurones are inhibitory but they influence the Purkinje cells at different points, at the granule cell (Golgi), at the Purkinje dendrites (stellate) and at its soma (basket cells). The complete system provides adequate machinery for 'sharpening' and focusing the input to the Purkinje fibres so that the inhibitory command which they exert on the intracerebellar nuclei is much more selective than would appear at first sight. At the same time they regulate the threshold of excitability of granule and Purkinje cells. This is undoubtedly of functional importance as the Purkinje cells have a much wider dynamic range of frequency than most neurones in the central nervous system. Where other neuronal systems depend largely on recruitment to signal intensity, the comparatively small number of Purkinje cells use a frequency code.

This provides an exceedingly rapid and versatile *brake control* on all the motor systems to which the cerebellar efferents project. It is difficult to accept a popular formulation of the cerebellum as an activator of voluntary movement. Furthermore, it is necessary to regard the cerebellum as the ultimate of a series of regulatory loops at four levels — spinal grey matter, vestibular, striatal and cortical. When the cerebellum is removed bilaterally, a very acceptable 'compensation' is achieved by the other long loops. Incomplete and, especially, unilateral cerebellar lesions are less well compensated in many disease states. The organism is better with no cerebellum than with a damaged one.

ALPHA–GAMMA LINKAGE

The cerebellum certainly does not project directly to the lower motoneurones or even to the motoneurone pools of single muscles. Nevertheless, its control of motor driving centres is not entirely at brain stem and higher levels. A very important regulation of motoneurone excitability is effected by modifying the alpha–gamma linkage (Chapter 24). Granit and his colleagues have concluded that the anterior lobe of the cerebellum controls a neural switch directing motor excitation (reflex or goal directed) into the alpha or gamma route together or separately. The route from cerebellum to fusimotor neurones is not known but the link with the alpha motoneurone is clearly a flexible one, probably at spinal interneurone level. Like the vestibular nuclei, the cerebellum modifies its own (spindle) input. If the ignition mechanism of a fusimotor servo-loop (Chapter 24) is accepted, the cerebellum may after all have a role to play in initiating voluntary movement, but it is not obligatory. Its comparator and timing functions work as gate controls, not as generators.

This model is essentially the same as Robinson's model for the control of visual saccades (Chapter 19). It may be a basic model for all motor control systems.

Further reading

Eccles J.C. The cerebellum as a computer: patterns in space and time. *J. Physiol.* 1973; **229**: 1–32.

Eccles J.C., Ito M. and Szentágothai J. *The Cerebellum as a Neural Machine*. Berlin: Springer-Verlag, 1967.

Oscarsson O. Functional organization of the spino- and cuneo-cerebellar tracts. *Physiol. Rev.* 1965; **45**: 495–522.

Chapter 24

Goal-directed movement

The limbs may be used to touch and grasp or to evade an object detected by distance receptors, or to search for one 'modelled' by the integrative areas of the cerebral cortex. The fore limbs are particularly adapted for this purpose with the development of an anatomy permitting a variety of grips and exploratory palpatory movements. Command neurones can be identified in the association areas of the cortex and in the frontal lobes anterior to the so-called 'motor areas'. The command is conditional in nature and is considered by Mountcastle to depend for action upon the outcome of a matching function between the neural signals of the nature of objects — quality, location, novelty — and those of central drive states integrated with a continually updated image of the position of the body, head and eyes relative to the environment and the gravitational field, in fact to the cerebral mechanisms for directed attention and consciousness (Chapter 15).

Goal-directed movement, whether from a conditional response or 'voluntary', starts and ends from a posture regulated by thalamo-striatal reflexes (Chapter 22). The striatum is also involved in the control system for initiating voluntary movements. Between the start and finish of the movement a limb may be moved ballistically or by slow modification of posture. The ballistic part is probably controlled and may be driven by the cerebellum (p. 230). A *movement synergy* requires appropriately timed and recruited activation of prime mover agonist muscles, inhibition of antagonists, with synergic muscle activation to provide a firm base, and adjustment of body posture to maintain equilibrium. The cerebellum is certainly necessary for the best adjust-ment of these functions. What then remains for the cerebral cortex?

Clinical neurologists, following Sherrington, have considered that the 'motor areas' of the cortex control movement synergies, sending '*upper motor neurones*' to appropriate bulbo-spinal *lower motor neurones*, each innervating a discrete group of skeletal muscle fibres. The lower motoneurone, its axon and its unique group of muscle fibres constitute a *motor unit* and groups of motor neurones ending in a common muscle constitute a spinal or bulbar 'centre' for that muscle. Thus the *cortex controls movements* and the *cord controls muscles* through motoneurones which are accessible to different upper neurones and also to segmental (reflex) and basal ganglia inputs (the Sherring-tonian concept of a '*final common path*').

The original concept requires modification with the recognition that 'tonic' and 'phasic' types of muscular contraction commonly use motor units specialized for one or other type of activity. Tokizane and others have investigated the possibility that the cortex drives only phasic units and the lower postural systems drive the tonic units. Experimental findings could be adequately accounted for by evidence that the cortically driven movements are relatively less subject to segmental reflex control, but the exact status of the higher control of the two types of unit remains debatable and it is unlikely that any goal-directed movement is devoid of reflex modification. It is possible that they are differentially controlled, the tonic units being served from areas of cortex which have been given the confusing name 'extra-pyramidal', since their corticofugal fibres are not in the classic pyramidal tract.

Possibly reflecting evolutionary develop-ment, the link from receptive and integrative cortices to the motor areas is made at a number of levels — cortex–thalamus–cortex; cortico-cortical by arcuate fibres in the white matter of the cerebrum; and by intracortical connections. All of these pathways convey afferent cortex command signals to the 'motor areas of the cortex'.

Motor outflow from the cortex

This heading was selected to emphasize that the so-called motor areas do not initiate movement. In a sense the corticofugal neurones are interneurones between the afferent cortex and the spinal centres. Corticofugal fibres with large axons and few synapses are more easily stimulated electrically than small fibres with multisynaptic connections to the lower neurones. The use of terms such as 'primary', 'secondary' and 'supplementary' implies a value judgement out of place in examining the function of the nervous system. We will discuss them in reverse order as this provides better understanding of how motor control has evolved.

SUPPLEMENTARY MOTOR AREAS

On the medial surface of the frontal lobe in man, Penfield and his collaborators found a small area (about 10 mm diameter) from which bilaterally synergic movements could be evoked by electrical stimulation. It is believed to be homologous with callosomarginal and cingulate areas in primates from which tonic movements can be evoked. (Movements evoked by stronger stimulation of other areas are probably induced by Mountcastle's 'command' neurones, p. 114.) This area is probably in the efferent pathway for tactile-orientated limb movements such as the grasp reflex and forced grasping (p. 166). An epileptic seizure originating in one supplementary motor area starts with turning of the head away from the side of the lesion, and elevation of the contralateral hand as though the patient was trying to turn to look at his upraised hand. The ipsilateral hand is extended and pronated, trunk rigid and legs either flexed or extended in a tonic posture. Consciousness may be retained. Phasic movements including speech are arrested. The efferent pathway from the

supplementary motor area(s) is probably a corticorubral projection, relaying via the rubro-spinal tracts of both sides, and to the striatum (*Fig.* 22.1). No somatotopical pattern has been demonstrated. Possible gate-control of the primary motor area is discussed in Chapter 22.

SECONDARY MOTOR AREA

A secondary motor area in man is believed, from stimulation studies, to be situated along the upper border of the Sylvian fissure, projecting ipsilaterally to the face and limbs, and bilaterally to ocular and masticatory muscles. It is strictly a sensori-motor area and is, spatially at least, the same as the sensory area SmII described in Chapter 8. Its output is more somatopically organized than the diffuse output from the supplementary motor area and has presumably evolved later. Its projections are not well defined but include a somatotopical projection to the pontine nuclei and corticospinal projections to the sensory relay nuclei of the thalamus and dorsal column (p. 80). These would make movement more precise by inhibiting unwanted parts of mass responses. (A possible inhibitory role of the supplementary motor areas is conjectural. It may be related to suppression of 'primitive' motor responses after childhood.)

The second motor area is a major contributor of corticostriatal fibres to the neostriatum which relay back to the cortex via the thalamus, to reach the spinal cord by the primary motor area's pyramidal tract (p. 216). At an earlier evolutionary stage an onward projection to the subthalamus and mid-brain reticular formation may have been more important. The reticulospinal tract facilitates tonic motor neurones, but in man it is not normally adequate for raising the lower motor neurones to firing threshold. Its possible role in the tonic phase of a generalized epileptic convulsion is also speculative.

PRIMARY MOTOR AREA

This cortical motor area has been left to last to emphasize that it is not the primary generator of movements as is so widely believed, but rather a later evolved communication from thalamus (receiving sensory, striatal and cerebellar signals), from integrative cortex (including frontal lobe) and from the appetite-driven limbic systems (Chapter 14) to the lower motor neurones, bypassing the homoeostatic controls and at the same time inhibiting them in whole or in part. It adds a new dimension of flexibility and speed under more or less direct command from the experiential cortex but is not the exclusive corticofugal outflow to the bulbospinal centres for muscle activation.

The cortical grey matter, in *area 4*, the central or Rolandic area, is an agranular cortex characterized by the presence of giant cells of Betz in layer V. Layers II and IV (receptive layers) are poorly developed, but this area of cortex is not entirely efferent in function. Its sensory functions, described in Chapter 8, represent overlap of neurones and do not necessarily indicate direct sensory to motor connections. Nor is area 4 the exclusive origin of the pyramidal tract which also receives fibres from cortical areas in front of area 4 (area 6) and posterior to it (areas 3, 1 and 2). Furthermore, these areas project by corticostriatal, corticobulbar and corticoreticular projections as well as by the direct corticospinal tract (pyramidal tract). An important difference is that stimulation of area 4 evokes *phasic* movements on the opposite side of the body. (The corticopontine fibres to bulbar and trunk muscles may be distributed bilaterally though predominantly to the opposite side of the body.)

PURPOSIVE MOVEMENTS

Movements evoked by electrical stimulation are not 'skilled' serial movements. This degree of organization is imposed by the association cortices commanding goal-directed movement. Disconnections from these areas do not paralyse the patient but lead to a range of *apraxias* according to the sensory modality deprived of its command function (Chapter 22). It was formerly believed that a 'pre-motor area' (area 6a) at the anterior margin of the motor strip was intercalated between association areas and area 4. There is little support for this concept.

The areas of grey matter allocated to movement of different body regions, though arranged somatotopically, are not proportional to the size of the region or its muscles but rather to their capacity to perform controlled phasic movements. A similar disparity of cortical areas for sensation was shown to be related to the density of sensory innervation at the periphery and the receptive area of sensory units (p. 84). In the same way the cortical 'representation' of a movement is related to the number of lower motor units used in the movement. The muscles responsible for the most delicate movements (intrinsic muscles of the hands, lips, tongue and extraocular muscles) have motor units with a small number of muscle fibres compared with the motor units of proximal limb muscles.

LABILITY OF THE CORTICAL MAP

Based on limited electrical stimulation studies, a cortical map has been tentatively outlined by Penfield. It is well known in association with a homunculus showing in cartoon form how the human body might look if its parts were distributed and had the relative sizes of the cortical areas evoking movement of these parts. The marked predominance of the areas controlling lips, tongue, thumb and other fingers is clear from the cartoon (*Fig.* 24.1). However, this map should only be considered as a helpful guide for a surgeon. It is not exactly repeated from one individual to another, and indeed repeated stimulation may evoke different movements.

The most important factors causing this apparent instability of the motor points are that foci of different (upper) motoneurones overlap, and their response to near threshold stimulation depends on (i) the immediately preceding *history of stimulation* or suppression, and (ii) the position of the limb (ie proprioceptive feedback). No doubt in normal life *directed attention* is also important. In monkeys the activity of some of the pyramidal tract neurones is altered by the 'intention' or 'motor set' of the animal concerning a subsequent learned reaction. The apparent instability represents fluctuations of confluent excitatory and inhibitory synaptic potentials. There is no reason to believe that one cell can activate a face or thumb muscle at different times — at present the connections from a particular motor cortical point to specific lower motoneurone pools seem to be fixed.

PYRAMIDAL TRACT

The corticofugal fibres projecting to the brain stem and cord are the axons of large pyramidal cells in layer V of the primary motor area and adjacent areas described above. The giant cells of Betz constitute only a very small proportion of them. Conversely, not all pyramidal-shaped cells contribute to the corticospinal tract, especially those fibres from the fringe of the motor strip that pass separately through the centrum ovale and internal capsule to the cerebral peduncle, lying medial and lateral to the pyramidal tract fibres. The former relay in the *pontine nuclei* to the cerebellum via the contralateral middle cerebellar peduncle, probably for coordinating purposes (p. 229).

The main outflow from area 4 is called the *pyramidal tract* as, having descended through internal capsule and cerebral peduncle, it descends through the pyramid of the medulla oblongata (*Fig. 24.1*). It decussates at a variable position in the lower medulla. Some fibres pass to the motor cranial nerve nuclei bilaterally, but mainly make crossed connections to the hypoglossal nucleus (XII), nucleus of the accessory nerve (XI) and the parts of the facial nucleus (VII) concerned with the lower parts of the muscles of facial expression.

After giving off corticobulbar fibres, the pyramidal tract, having crossed in the medulla, continues caudally through the lateral white column of the spinal cord (*lateral corticospinal tract*). A small proportion of fibres do not cross

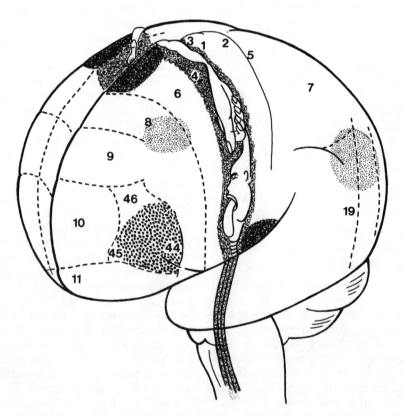

Fig. 24.1. *Motor areas of the cerebral cortex.* The corticospinal tract descending to the medullary pyramid (decussating lower in the medulla) is shown (*shaded*) arising from cortical area 4 (MsI) with the movement homunculus. Two secondary motor areas are shown (*dark grey*) at the upper Sylvian bank (SmII) and at vertex of area 6 spreading to medial cortex adjacent to the foot area of MsI. This supplementary motor area may include the pre-motor area 6. The frontal and parieto-occipital eye fields (*stippled*) are not sharply defined, and there are motor command units in area 7 for manual exploration, probably projecting to MsI. On the left hemisphere speech is controlled by Broca's area (*dots*). Stimulation of this and other (afferent) speech areas evokes speech arrest. Vocalization is evoked by stimulation at the lower end of area 4.

in the medulla but continue as the *ventral corticospinal tract* in the ventral funiculus of the cord along the anterior fissure, as far as the thoracic segments. Most corticospinal fibres decussate either in the medulla or near the termination in the ventral tract, but a few fibres are believed to remain uncrossed. (This makes it difficult to interpret the significance of retained or returning movement after apparently complete lesions of one corticospinal tract.)

The pyramidal tract fibres have a wide spectrum of diameter from large, rapidly conducting to small, myelinated and unmyelinated slow fibres, so a volley of discharges which is synchronized at cortical level is no longer synchronized at the lower motoneurones. In addition, some fibres project monosynaptically, others polysynaptically to the anterior horn cell pool. Thus, as well as providing a rapid pathway for motor commands routed through the cortex, these are spread in time to give a relatively prolonged depolarizing pressure (40 ms or more) to the anterior horn cells. It appears that increased cortical discharge results in increased *recruitment* of the lower motoneurone pool rather than regulation of motoneurone frequency. The cortex is concerned with *force* and is a relatively crude activator of muscles unless contraction is regulated by brain stem and segmental inputs, in exactly the same way as we have already discussed for respiration and automatic stepping. It is not the speed of the pyramidal tract or a fine adjustment of motor unit firing rates that account for its role in performing delicate movement. This is due to the provision of a direct route from goal-seeking areas of cortex which is capable of overriding all other motor controls based on automatisms and reflexes.

A corticospinal tract depolarizing pressure which is insufficient to evoke motoneurone firing may be quite sufficient to *facilitate* spinal reflex arcs, especially the polysynaptic arcs which go mainly to *flexor motoneurones*. As this facilitation subsides, there are sequential waves of inhibition and renewed facilitation. A pyramidal tract volley also *inhibits* some reflexes, especially the monosynaptic and oligosynaptic postural reflexes which go mainly to *extensor motoneurones*. The inhibition may be used to refine motor commands selectively.

The progressive economy of movement of the infant, or of the adult learning a new skill, suggests that this function is important. It may be applied at the solitary cells of the dorsal horn and the small cells of the external basilar region of the cord grey matter. Inhibition at this level also *allows postural reflexes to dominate over the protective reflexes* unless the noxious stimulus is severe. Thus, in the developing infant the withdrawal reflex is suppressed and replaced by supportive reactions when the pyramidal tract becomes myelinated and the child begins to stand. At the same time mass limb movements become refined and goal-directed grasp followed by ability to manipulate becomes apparent. Conversely, a *lesion of the pyramidal tract* abolishes skilled movements, raises the threshold for movement (and these are more automatic, like stepping, than goal-directed), releases associated movements, disinhibits stretch reflexes and increases anti-gravity tone, but allows protective plantar reflexes (Babinski response) to become dominant.

The 'motor' fibres of the corticospinal tract are probably different from the inhibitory fibres. It is possible to have paresis with extensor (dorsiflexor) plantar responses without spasticity (occlusion of medial striate artery). It is relatively common to have dissociation between 'spastic' stretch reflexes and the dorsiflexor toe response. Lower animals less dependent on control by association cortex may have surprisingly little apparent loss of locomotion but still show the reflex changes and impaired placing reactions to visual or contact stimuli when tested appropriately, especially for learned responses to a discrimination task.

During recovery from a pyramidal tract lesion, the human subject may recover a *prehensile grip*, followed by capacity for individual finger movement, but among the last to recover (and only with resolving lesions) is the *pincer or precision grip* used in picking up small objects. This movement is best developed in the human owing to the anatomical relationship of the thumb to the other fingers (it is adducted in a plane at right-angles to the palm of the hand). Without it the hand can still be used for many manipulative functions but never with normal skill. The muscles involved are among those believed to be supplied by motoneurones receiving a *monosynaptic input from the pyramidal tract*, probably only present in higher primates.

Denny-Brown summed up his experiments on primates with the aphorism that the pyramidal tract is concerned with those spatial adjustments that accurately adapt the movement to the spatial attributes of the stimulus. Thus grasping is adapted to the shape of the thing to be grasped, whether a particle of food, a pin, or a surface. The hand is first directed to the surface by visuomotor control.

Integration of motor drives

It is a common fallacy that the cerebellum is *the* coordinator of somatomotor activity. It is true that it is an important coordinator of motor control systems but the ultimate driving pressures on the lower motoneurone are integrated by its soma adding algebraically the excitatory and inhibitory synaptic potentials converging on it. Pyramidal tract neurones also contribute synaptic potential to other efferent neuronal systems by *collateral branches*. Within the cortex many pyramidal neurones send back recurrent collaterals to neighbouring pyramidal cells, both inhibitory and excitatory, a provision for synchronization and for 'focusing' by surround inhibition (Chapter 4), no doubt in part responsible for the motor point 'instability' described above.

Other collaterals of pyramidal tract neurones terminate either recurrently on cortical cells projecting to the red nucleus or, in passage, directly on the red nucleus, both excitatory and inhibitory. Collaterals to the striatum and reticulospinal systems have been identified and many authors consider that such 'extrapyramidal' relays account for the inhibitory control on postural reflexes exerted by the pyramidal tract. Their disinhibition by a pyramidal tract lesion may account for *spasticity* since the hyperreflexia of that condition does not occur if the pyramidal tract is sectioned at the pyramid of the medulla (a flaccid paresis resulting).

THE FUSIMOTOR SYSTEM

Some of the cortical neurones project by one or a few synapses to the *small (gamma) moto-*neurones of the anterior horns which also receive major inputs from the pontine and medullary reticular formation. These cells send slowly conducting fibres to the *intrafusal muscle fibres* of most skeletal muscles and their contraction alters the bias of stretch receptors in the muscle, signalled by fast conducting Ia neurones monosynaptically to the alpha motoneurones supplying the extrafusal (power) muscle fibres of the same motor unit, and polysynaptically to other units (Chapter 9). A theory that this may be a necessary preliminary to alpha motoneurone discharge (a 'follow-up servo') is not supported by most experiments, which indicate either simultaneous *alpha–gamma coactivation*, or alpha leading gamma. The functional importance of this linkage, eg as a 'follow-through servo', is still a matter of dispute, but it is generally agreed that the spindle activation smooths muscular contraction despite load variations. It may be necessary for controlling the distribution of tonic impulses to antagonist muscles. In the introduction to this section on movement control a simplified schema of motor synergy was given in which it was implied that antagonists to the prime movers must be inhibited. In fact, in some of the most delicate movements (eg writing, drawing, using tools, playing a musical instrument), the precision movement requires small displacements by the prime movers against *graded resistance* by antagonists.

THE DENDRITIC TREE OF THE ALPHA MOTONEURONE

This is the ultimate integrator of motor signals. Directly or indirectly, all somatomotor systems and segmental reflex inputs converge on the synaptic area of the alpha motoneurone. Probably no single input is sufficient to excite the motoneurone. The dendrites summate the excitatory and inhibitory potentials at these 'final common paths' (apparently separately for tonic and phasic motoneurones). The pyramidal tract adds the last contribution to a pool of synapses which are already facilitated or inhibited by influences determined by posture, surface contact, appetites, arousal and expectation.

During REM sleep vigorous phasic firing occurs in pyramidal tract neurones but the lower motoneurones remain below threshold because of inhibitory impulses from the medial vestibular nuclei. Even segmental reflex driving of the lower motoneurone varies according to the arousal state and set (*Jendrassik* effect). The addition of the pyramidal tract is to put this preset system at the disposal of command neurones elsewhere in the cortex. The resulting movement need never be the same twice running, since the force and displacement are monitored continuously by peripheral receptors feeding back rapidly to the afferent areas of the cortex. Plasticity is built in.

The function of these *long-loop reflexes* is currently arousing a lot of research interest. They probably regulate the *displacement*, and all that is required of the primary motor area is to recruit sufficient motoneurones to provide the required *force*. Long-loop adjustment (comparing current limb position with *intended* position) does seem to occur in 'ramp' movements. But a ballistic movement is pre-programmed and must run its full course without the possibility of modification. It is driven by a high frequency burst of motoneurone firing. Alteration of force by changing the firing frequency of motoneurones is otherwise relatively insignificant. *The major regulation is by recruitment* of motor units. Once recruited, a unit rapidly adopts its preferred working frequency and this does not increase much as effort is increased.

RECRUITMENT: THE SIZE PRINCIPLE

Observation on man and other animals has shown a remarkable consistency in the order of recruitment of motor units of a muscle, regardless of the type of activation — reflex, postural tone or voluntary movement. Henneman has shown that the recruitment order matches the size order of the motoneurones, small neurones being recruited before large. The plasticity of cortical control of movement makes it very unlikely that this is due to 'hard wiring' of corticomotoneuronal connections. An alternative explanation is that the *synaptic density* (number of synaptic terminals, irrespective of origin, per unit area of total cell membrane) is the important determinant of the synaptic potential amplitude. Given a relatively even or random distribution of terminals from descending neurones of all types, the synaptic density would be highest in those cells with the smallest post-synaptic membrane. Obviously many other factors would be relevant, including average conductance per terminal, geometry of the synapse, and intrinsic properties of the motoneurone membrane, but the synaptic density would govern recruitment order in general, with some latitude for modification in unusual circumstances.

Increased drive from any source, cortex, basal ganglia, brain stem or segmental, would recruit units from what Sherrington described as the *subliminal pool of motoneurones* in a relatively invariant order. Localized increase of subthreshold depolarizing drive ('altered set') could, however, bring some motoneurones nearer firing threshold and so alter the apparent recruitment order when voluntary command is added. This seems to happen when a muscle is used as a synergist rather than as a prime mover, or if additional reflex driving is added by continuous stimulation of the skin. Subliminal changes of this type could account for the ability of some trained subjects to activate selected motor units by volition. Units with higher force thresholds cannot be activated in isolation under any conditions.

The *mechanical action* produced by the muscle fibres of the motor units is not rigidly quantized in the same sense as the motor unit recruitment. It depends on (i) the type of muscle fibre; (ii) dynamic factors such as muscle fibre length; (iii) the history of unit activation which can produce mechanical potentiation or fatigue. It is therefore necessary for the central nervous system to monitor the result of muscle activation by feedback from muscle and joint receptors or observation by vision etc., or else to use an estimated *effort*. The latter seems to be the only practical solution for fully ballistic movements.

Effort

The existence of a property described as effort is assumed from subjective experience of a '*sense of effort*', which is used to judge the muscular force required in a voluntary task which does not depend upon sensory feedback from the limbs or eyes. More conscious effort to start a voluntary movement is required if the skin over a digit is anaesthetized. Its nature is unknown but it has been suggested that it is an appreciation by afferent cortex of activity in recurrent axon collaterals of corticofugal and other neurones. The matter is of some importance since this *efference copy* or *corollary discharge* could be compared with a similar *afference copy* from receptors at some misalignment detector using the same principle of coincidence detection described on p. 45. Precision movement could then be guided by minimizing the misalignment as in many mechanical servo systems. A function of this type may be present in the cerebellum (p. 223).

Accurate assessment of effort would be an ideal method for producing fast precision movements. It is noticeable that this principle is used for learned movement in sport and musical performance. Initial learning is by repeated slow performance of tasks, placing digits or limbs in sensory monitored positions, but the acquired skill is then transferred to rapid ballistic movements with adjustment of effort rather than of position. The *learned skill* then becomes 'subconscious' and attention can be directed to the target. Sudden perturbations of the pre-programmed movement are compensated for by very rapid segmental reflexes followed within 25 ms by 'long-loop transcortical reflexes' controlling the corticospinal neurones which summate convergent afferent information just as effectively as the alpha motoneurones. In the human, the interruption of a motor programme is only possible if the subject is consciously prepared to oppose the interrupting force. It is not automatic, and ballistic movements cannot be modified at all.

Types of motor units

The classic Sherringtonian view of the alpha motoneurone as a 'final common pathway' carries the implication that phasic and tonic functions depend on how the alpha motoneurone is employed by the higher nervous system and peripheral reflex arcs. In the past 30 years opinion has favoured a subdivision of alpha motoneurones into clearly separable groups typified by '*tonic*' and '*phasic*' categories. Tokizane and other Japenese workers considered that motoneurones could be

differentiated by their firing patterns and that the motor cortex controlled mainly the phasic neurones, but they later concluded that the functional characteristics were imposed by the afferent input into the motoneurones. Systematic surveys of the electrophysiological properties of motoneurones show a wide spectrum of characteristics which relate to the contractile properties of the muscle fibres innervated by each motor unit (*Fig. 24.2*). Thus the question of functional specification versus source of recruitment remains controversial.

Each alpha motoneurone controls a group of muscle fibres which it activates in an all-or-none manner, some with few muscle fibres (eg extraocular muscles), others with many (eg quadriceps). They are distributed widely throughout one muscle so that fibres of many units overlap territorially. Twitch characteristics and resistance to fatigue correlate with histochemical type based on enzyme content and type of metabolism (aerobic or anaerobic). Two major types recognized by histopathologists (and sufficient for clinical purposes) are only the extremes of a range of fibre types which can be roughly correlated with Burke's *functional types*: type FF (fast twitch, fatiguable); type FR (fast twitch, resistant to fatigue); type S (slow twitch); and some with intermediate properties. Evidence that these characteristics are related to corresponding fast conduction and slow conduction of their motor nerve fibres points to a parallel functional specificity of alpha motoneurones.

TETANUS

The twitch duration of a muscle fibre determines at what firing frequency the twitches will be fused into a *tetanus*, a maintained contraction. Driving of the motoneurone faster than its *tetanic fusion frequency* will not increase its motor effect. Even for fast twitch fibres, the fusion frequency is very much lower than a motoneurone is capable of firing. At the start of a muscular contraction high firing rates (up to 90/s) are common, but the motoneurone almost immediately adopts its most economical firing rate. Indeed, studies on human isometric contraction indicate that the steady firing rate of motoneurones is commonly about 6–8/s,

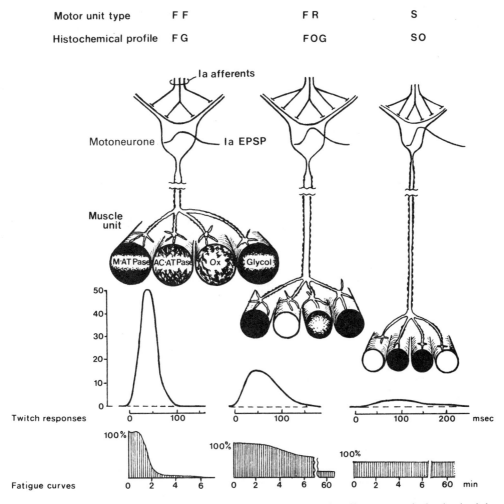

| Motor unit type | F F | F R | S |
| Histochemical profile | F G | FOG | SO |

Fig. 24.2. Motor units may differ according to the size of a motoneurone, the afferent synaptic density (and thus the amplitude and time course of the EPSP), the conduction velocity of its axon, amount of terminal branching and the histochemical profile of its muscle fibres. These factors cause differences in the twitch responses and fatiguability to repeated stimulation. The diagram (from cat) indicates a rough differentiation into fast twitch/fatiguable (FF), fast twitch/fatigue resistant (FR) and slow twitch (S) motor unit types. The shading of the fibres represents relative staining intensities for the histochemical stains. A unit contains only one type of muscle fibre.

which is well below the tetanic fusion frequency even for slow twitch fibres. This is due to an efficient rate-limiting regulatory control. Rates are much higher in ballistic movements (up to 140/s), but firing is then in bursts to start the movement. Even with this type of movement it is clear that recruitment of motoneurones is more important than firing frequency as a regulator of muscle force.

Human electromyographic studies suggest that the total number of motor units available to a particular muscle is the same regardless of personal muscle strength. Differences in maximum force are due mainly to differences in the diameter of the muscle fibres or in the number of muscle fibres per motor unit or both. Since firing frequency is relatively unimportant for isometric or slow contraction, the relative number of motor units recruited is clearly related to the *integrated EMG voltage*. However, brief 'double discharges' may increase the force output very considerably. The force output is also increased by rheological factors such as 'stiffness' of the actively contracting muscle and *post-tetanic potentiation* of its contractile force.

Accepting these advantages of occasional rapid firing, there is clearly a general tendency to fire at low rates, indicating an efficient regulatory control. Temporary increase in force can be obtained, at the cost of smoothing, by synchronizing the motor units, as in fatigue and shivering. In normal circumstances, it is more advantageous to desynchronize motor unit firing, obtaining the advantages of smooth contraction of the muscle as a whole, although individual units are at less than tetanic fusion frequency. The action potentials of the muscle fibres recorded by EMG show an *interference pattern* until fatigue leads to the synchronized firing of the *Piper rhythm*. Desynchronization at subtetanic rates is the normal state. What regulates this?

CONTROL OF FIRING RATE AND DESYN-CHRONIZATION OF MOTONEURONES

Progressive depolarization of the membrane of the motoneurone's soma (by synaptic transmitter or by transmembrane electrical stimulation) progressively raises the discharge frequency of the cell.

With stronger depolarizing pressures, the slope relating impulse frequency to transmembrane current rises abruptly at a particular point (primary and secondary firing ranges of Kernell). This phenomenon also occurs in many central neurones and is attributed to rapidly augmenting inactivation of the generative mechanism for the action 'spike', blocking excessive excitation. It is associated with a change in the *after-hyperpolarization*, which corresponds to the *subnormal state* and *refractory period* (Chapter 1). The stronger the synaptic or injected current, the sooner is the subnormal state counteracted and replaced by adequate depolarization for eliciting the next spike. The 'secondary range' of high firing rate is available at the *onset of a required movement*, to evoke a rapid rise in the rate of contraction of the muscle fibres. This may be all that is required for a ballistic movement. For *maintained contraction* the slower 'primary' firing range is adequate and delays the time of onset of adaptation, but the main physiological value of the primary firing range

is that the smaller depolarization pressure required is better suited for modulation by algebraic summation of EPSPs and IPSPs. Thus the refractory period, instead of being a handicap, is important in keeping the neuronal firing frequency within the range of linear response to small changes in any synaptic input — essential for the cell to act as an integrator. This is of limited importance for the initiation of burst discharges but quite essential for continuing control functions.

INHIBITION

Inhibition by pre-synaptic and post-synaptic controls is described in Chapter 4. A tonic post-synaptic inhibition, via specialized interneurones, is important in the stabilization of the motoneurone.

A particularly important inhibitory interneurone in the anterior horns, the *Renshaw interneurone*, is activated by a recurrent collateral of each alpha motoneurone, leaving the parent axon soon after the axon hillock, within the grey matter (*Fig.* 24.3). It is more

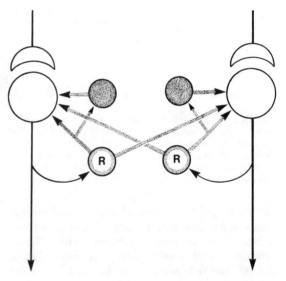

Fig. 24.3. *The Renshaw loop*. Two alpha motoneurones are shown with integrated synaptic inputs. A collateral from the efferent axon excites a special inhibitory (Renshaw, R) cell which suppresses its own and also neighbouring motoneurones. It may also excite a motoneurone by disinhibition. (Possible connections inhibiting inhibitory interneurones are shown. The interneurones are also subject to descending neurones.)

common and more powerful than a similar feedback loop to facilitatory interneurones but both are present, supposedly for stabilizing the firing frequency of alpha motoneurones (by feedback to the cell from which the collateral originated) and for *desynchronizing* or suppressing the firing of any closely adjacent motoneurones which have weakly supported discharges (aiding 'motor contrast'). The control is most apparent on the small tonic alpha motoneurones, less on larger phasic neurones, and only slightly on gamma fusimotor neurones (which do not have their own recurrent inhibition). Thus *phasic responses tend to inhibit tonic ones*.

Segmental reflex control of movement

Chapter 17 describes a range of reflexes for the maintenance and restoration of posture. There is little doubt that the facilitatory and inhibitory actions on the motoneurone derived from sensors in the muscle, tendon, joints and skin are used to modulate movement commanded from higher centres through the corticospinal and other descending tracts, for such functions as *load compensation*, to permit isometric contraction with varying loads, or smooth shortening or lengthening of isotonically contracting muscles. (The physiology of muscle contraction *while being passively extended* is not fully understood, though it must have functional importance.) To maintain the value of the muscle spindle as an internal measuring instrument even while the muscle is shortening, the spindle is stretched by simultaneous contraction of its intrafusal muscle fibres driven by gamma and beta motoneurones (Chapter 9). In all known circumstances in man (fast and ballistic movements cannot be investigated) there is simultaneous *alpha and gamma coactivation* (alpha–gamma linkage). Critics point out that this conclusion is based, in man, on intraneural recording by fine wire electrodes incapable of distinguishing between spindle Ia afferent impulses and the Ib afferent impulses from tendon organs which must be activated by any muscle generating tension.

It is possible that the alpha–gamma linkage may be broken in disease. In the cat the link can be broken by a lesion, or temporarily interrupted by cooling, of the *anterior lobe of the cerebellum*. A possible selective role of chlorpromazine and mephenesin in abolishing gamma motoneurone activity is no longer advocated to account for their lissive action in spasticity. (They have strong depressant action on polysynaptic reflexes, like general anaesthetics.)

Because of the strong stabilization of firing rate, the principal method for adjusting muscle length and tension by the segmental reflexes is by recruiting or de-recruiting from the subliminal fringe motoneurone pool by contributing EPSPs and IPSPs at appropriate synapses (overriding the hierarchy of the size principle). The firing rates remain remarkably constant.

The long-loop reflexes (p. 277, p. 241) are additional load compensation reflexes which are integrated with vestibular signals. The regulated factor may be *stiffness* of muscle rather than length or tension. These reflexes are facilitated by *expectation* of the stimulus though they have a shorter latency (15–55 ms) than the voluntary reaction time (about 70 ms).

A synchronized twitch superimposed on a submaximal contraction is followed by a *silent period* in the asynchronous firing due to a number of factors including the refractory period (p. 10), Renshaw inhibition, spindle unloading (p. 90), and a lengthening reaction (p. 162).

Autonomic associations of goal-directed behaviour

Motor behavioural patterns are modified by expectation, previous experience and motivation. The limbic and mesencephalic drive involves hypothalamic and autonomic discharges associated with the skeletomotor responses. The following chapters will outline some of these factors.

Further reading

Allen G.I. and Tsukahara N. Cerebrocerebellar communication systems. *Physiol. Rev.* 1974; **54**: 957–1006.

De Luca C.J., Le Fever R.S., McCue M.P. et al. Behaviour of human motor units in different muscles during linearly varying contractions. *J. Physiol.* 1982; **329**: 113–28.

Denny-Brown D. *The Cerebral Control of Movement*. Liverpool: Liverpool University Press, 1966.

Granit R. *The Basis of Motor Control*. London: Academic Press, 1970.

Henneman E., Somjen G. and Carpenter D.O. Functional significance of cell size in spinal motoneurons. *J. Neurophysiol.* 1965; **23**: 560–80.

Mountcastle V.B., Lynch A. Georgopoulos A. et al. Posterior parietal association cortex of the monkey: command functions for operations within extra-personal space. *J. Neurophysiol.* 1975; **38**: 871–908.

Nathan P.W. and Smith M.C. Long descending tracts in man. I. Review of present knowledge. *Brain* 1955; **78**: 248–303.

Phillips C.G. Cortical localization and 'sensorimotor processes' at the 'middle level' in primates — Hughlings Jackson Lecture. *Proc. R. Soc. Med.* 1973; **66**: 987–1002.

Phillips C.G. and Porter R. *Corticospinal Neurones. Their Role in Movement*. London: Academic Press, 1977.

PART 5   Regulation of the Internal Environment

Chapter 25
Homoeostasis and general responses to stress

The plan of this book, to outline distributed functional subsystems within the central nervous system, is the justification for the title of this chapter instead of the more conventional anatomical title — the *hypothalamus*. Much of the confusion about 'the function' of the hypothalamus and its clinical disorders is explained by unsuccessful attempts to attribute specific functions to various 'centres'. This is not appropriate for an area with important integrative functions receiving multiple inputs from the brain stem via the mesencephalon, mainly visceral, olfactory and taste afferents, and also from the frontal lobe and the septal and amygdaloid command neurones described in Chapter 14 (*see Fig.* 14.1), the retina, important tonic regulating noradrenergic and serotoninergic fibres via the medial forebrain bundle (p. 29), and having its own chemoreceptors monitoring the state of the internal milieu.

The many outputs of the hypothalamus feed back to these sources via the brain stem regulating centres for the autonomic nervous system (*see* Chapter 26), the hypophyseal and adrenal endocrine system, the limbic areas, frontal lobe, thalamus and somatic motor controls of the reticular formation. Involvement of hypothalamic zones in sleep and arousal have been described in Chapter 15, and in memory in Chapter 13. It is questionable whether the mammillary nuclei should be included with the homoeostatic nuclei of the hypothalamus, though anatomically the mammillary bodies and their fibre tracts are important constituents.

This massive convergence and divergence of neurones makes it difficult to identify the locus of effects associated with macroelectrode stimulation or with ablation. Indeed it is sus-pected, with good reason, that these procedures may involve fibre tracts such as the medial forebrain bundle rather than nuclei. In view of this uncertainty, it is prudent to regard clinical syndromes as regional rather than attributing each to a specific nucleus. Nevertheless, analysis of syndromes according to the anterior/posterior or periventricular/medial/lateral situation in the hypothalamus must be related to local specialization of functions.

The hypothalamus is to the non-myelinated nervous system what the thalamus and basal ganglia are to the myelinated. With the paleocortex it is a microcosm of the cerebral hemisphere, some would say a prototype, but more bilateral in its influence. Unilateral destructive lesions are asymptomatic. Clinical symptoms are either 'epileptic' or from outflow pathway lesions. Goal-directed behavioural sequences for feeding, drinking, sexual behaviour, aggression, locomotion etc are organized at mid-brain or lower levels, but the hypothalamus and other forebrain areas modify and regulate their expression via the medial forebrain bundle.

The analogy with the 'new brain' is worth pursuing a little further as it provides insight into the functional organization of the 'old brain'. In earlier chapters a hierarchy of segmental and long-loop reflexes for posture and protection, with reciprocal control, was described. It was explained that lower level reflexes were selectively facilitated or inhibited at basal ganglia level for versatile righting responses integrating polymodal inputs including vision and these were further refined by cortical integration to provide goal-seeking and, eventually, motivated behaviours. The hypothalamus is the homologue of the somatic righting reflexes control system — balancing the output of lower level hormonal, autonomic and somatic efferent systems and controlled by goal-seeking cortex and paleocortex with ultimate *frontal lobe control.*

The problems for the experimentalist are essentially the same as with the basal ganglia. Brain stem autonomic functions continue after destruction of the hypothalamus and 'release' signs are prominent. On the other hand, the behavioural studies of the experimental psychologists cannot isolate the hypothalamus from its higher driving and controlling circuits. When the *lateral hypothalamus* is stimulated electrically the behavioural response depends on the contemporary features of the external environment. That response will reappear with subsequent stimulation but it is not permanent and the response can be displaced by other environmental inputs. There is no prepotent or dominant behavioural tendency. The relevance of this to *imprinting* (p. 117) in immature animals will be obvious. In the mature animal hypothalamic stimulation seems to elicit and energize the dominant response for the contemporary situation.

REWARD SYSTEMS

The general category of response appears to differ according to whether an electrical stimulus is applied anteriorly or posteriorly in the hypothalamus of experimental animals, including the higher primates. Experiments with self-stimulation suggest that there are areas evoking 'rewards or punishments' which, with the limbic system, are interpreted as pleasure or discomfort (? pain). *Rewarding* or pleasant effects are elicited from the lateral septal area, certain portions of the amygdala, parts of the hippocampus, the lateral hypothalamus and the medial forebrain bundle (Chapter 14). The posterior part of the lateral hypothalamus (in front of the mammillary body) is particularly implicated. An *aversive* or quasi pain-avoiding behaviour is evoked by stimulation of the more anteriorly situated ventromedial nucleus of the hypothalamus but also from the central grey matter of the mid-brain, parts of the medial thalamus and the medial lemniscus. Other areas of the hypothalamus produce ambivalent responses.

It is certainly premature to talk of reward and punishment centres in the hypothalamus. An alternative interpretation is selective stimulation of the noradrenergic and serotoninergic modulatory systems conducted mainly in the *medial forebrain bundle* from the brain stem to the forebrain (p. 29). A working hypothesis that the pleasure system is activated by noradrenergic and the punishment system by serotoninergic projections is a rationale for some pharmacological attacks on psychiatric disorders. It is further proposed that the efferent control from the limbic cortex to somatic and autonomic motor nuclei passes through the *periventricular grey matter* of the hypothalamus where it is exposed to inhibitory control by cholinergic corticofugal fibres. Confirmation of this interpretation of self-stimulated reward areas would be important as it would remove the necessity to identify physiological inputs into unidentified 'centres'. It would, however, be premature to reject the possibility that the responses are variants of 'satiety/hunger' and homoeostat functions.

APPETITE AND SATIETY

Localized bilateral lesions in the hypothalamus involving the ventromedial nucleus of the tuber cinereum are associated with a voracious appetite (bulimia), with increased feeding (hyperphagia) leading to obesity. Bilateral destruction of the lateral hypothalamic nuclei abolishes the desire for food (anorexia) with loss of feeding (aphagia) leading to severe weight loss.

The striking constancy of the *body weight* has been attributed to a 'target setting' function of the hypothalamus and further examples of this will be described below. It is conceivable that neurones could be connected to detect imbalance between opposing receptor systems and that these could be connected reciprocally to the septal-amygdaloid nuclei as discussed in Chapter 14, and this might reasonably be a distributed system. There is no incontrovertible evidence. The type of stimulation required is unknown but could be related either to heat regulation (the thermostat hypothesis) or to regulation of the blood sugar (glucostat hypothesis). Variations of blood sugar level are associated with appropriate reciprocal changes in the electrical activity of *ventromedial ('satiety')* and *far-lateral hypotha-lamus ('feeding centre')*. For long-term regula-tion a similar 'lipostatic' mechanism has been proposed. The efferent mechanism would be hormonal from the pituitary gland and the sympathetico-adrenomedullary system, and in-volve a blood sugar regulating area in the floor of the IVth ventricle in the region of the dorsal nucleus of the vagus. Gastrointestinal function is regulated as described below.

In man, food intake (for preservation of the self) is not directly related to requirements of body heat, energy output or body weight. After infancy it develops a diurnal rhythm and is strongly influenced by learned behaviour, clearly supra-hypothalamic. Sexual appetite and behaviour (for preservation of the species) is even more supra-hypothalamic, but its efferent mechanisms, hormonal, autonomic and somatomotor, are similar (Chapter 14). Conversely, the regulated level of body core temperature is relatively independent of higher control and so it is the most suitable system for examining the basic mechanisms of 'target-setting' in the hypothalamus (Chapter 7).

CIRCADIAN AND LONG-TERM RHYTHMS

The existence of 'biological clocks' which regulate more or less rhythmical changes of body temperature, weight, blood chemistry, state of arousal and other parameters is now well accepted, though the nature and sites of the oscillators are matters of debate. Variation of neuroendocrine secretions may be circadian (eg ACTH), menstrual (eg gonadotrophins), seasonal (possibly growth hormone) or in comparatively short cycles (eg sleep–wake) and one rhythm may be superimposed on another (eg release of growth hormone during non-REM sleep, p. 142).

These fundamental rhythms are distorted by interaction between one activity and another. Furthermore, a cycle can become entrained by external stimuli. An important example of this is the effect of light on the set-points of some hypothalamic-regulated functions. Stimulation of the retinae by daylight activates a retino-hypothalamic projection to the suprachiasma-tic nucleus of the hypothalamus (*Fig.* 25.1). The *suprachiasmatic nucleus* projects to the ventromedial, dorsomedial and arcuate nuclei

of the hypothalamus to modulate the release of gonadotrophic hormones (and possibly ACTH and growth hormone), a fact known to the poultry industry. It is not identified as a distinct nucleus in man but intensive care staff should be aware of the requirements of the human subject for regular periods of darkness (and possibly of quietness).

The suprachiasmatic control is modulated by *serotonin* ascending from the raphe nuclei. The retinohypothalamic projection to the sup-rachiasmatic nucleus is also relayed through the medial forebrain bundle and the mesencephalic reticular formation, the lateral cell column of the upper thoracic spinal cord and the superior cervical sympathetic ganglion to the *pineal gland*. The pineal gland lies outside the blood–brain barrier (*Fig.* 25.1). The *noradrenaline* released there stimulates beta-adrenergic receptors which regulate synthesis of a serotonin-related hormone, *melatonin*. Environmental light entrains the endogenous cycle of secretion. The metabol-ism of this indole hormone is very responsive to noradrenaline and to stress. Although the functions of melatonin (or the other identified hormones in the pineal gland) are unknown, this discovery is an important pointer to the regulation of hypothalamic hormones by sen-sory stimulation and by noradrenergic and serotoninergic secretions since the enzymic basis of the pineal response has been identi-fied.

The pineal mechanism just described is an example of a general principle of the nervous system. Light waves act on rhodopsin-like pigment in the retina to evoke ganglion cell stimulation which is then relayed by normal neurotransmitter mechanisms to β_1-adrenergic receptors in an effector organ. There (with the intermediary of cAMP) the activity of a regulating enzyme is increased, leading to synthesis of a hormone which is secreted into the bloodstream. The pineal gland is supplied from the superior cerebellar and posterior choroidal arteries.

CONTROL OF FEEDING

Adrenergic stimulation of the hypothalamus elicits the feeding response. It has been claimed that noradrenaline initiates eating by

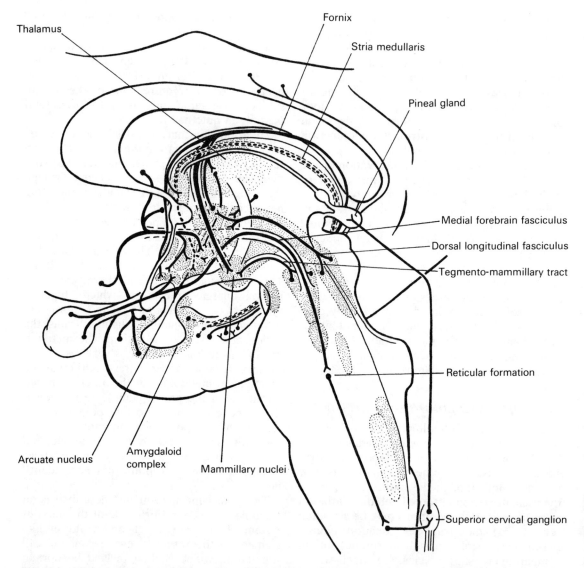

Fig. 25.1. Afferents to the hypothalamus. The medial forebrain bundle collects afferent fibres from preoptic areas including the orbitofrontal cortex and septal nuclei. The amygdaloid complex projects to the arcuate nucleus through the hippocampal formation and stria terminalis ($\cdots$). The mid-brain projects to the posterior hypothalamus by the dorsal longitudinal fasciculus and tegmento-mammillary tract, and a dopaminergic system (*see Fig. 3.3*). The hippocampus–fornix system includes projections to septum and anterior hypothalamus but its main contribution to the mammillary nucleus is relayed into the thalamus. The retina sends neurones to the supraoptic nucleus. The medial longitudinal bundle projects to pontomedullary reticular formation and ultimately the sympathetic nerve fibres of the upper thoracic cord. Extra-spinal sympathetic fibres ascend from the superior cervical ganglion to the pineal gland, which is therefore indirectly under optic control.

stimulating α-adrenergic receptors in the ventromedial nucleus which in turn inhibit lateral hypothalamic neurones and that eating is suppressed by β-adrenergic receptors in the lateral nucleus which inhibit the ventromedial nucleus through a brain stem relay. As adrenaline is more α-agonist than noradrenaline, it is possible that this is a role for the adrenaline-releasing bundle from the lateral tegmental nucleus to the hypothalamus (*Fig.*

25.1), but its role has yet to be defined. The role of adrenergic stimulation is uncertain since the anorexic effect of amphetamine is attributed by other workers to excitation of α-adrenergic receptors signalling satiety. The differential actions of α and β receptors make it impossible to assess earlier pharmacological studies. Growth hormone and prolactin release is stimulated by *endorphins*. Despite the incomplete evidence, it is clear that the hypothalamus does use well-recognized neural transmitter mechanisms. It shares with the respiratory and vasomotor control areas of the medulla the property of having receptors for temperature (p. 73) and for some chemicals.

CONTROL OF DRINKING

Cholinergic stimulation of the hypothalamus elicits the drinking response. The first hypothalamic receptors to be identified were believed to be *osmoreceptors* in the *preoptic anterior hypothalamus* which detect small changes in the osmolality of blood perfusing the hypothalamus. It is possible that dehydrated cells release a precursor of angiotensin II and that receptors for this peptide mediate the response. Whatever the immediate mechanism, small increases in the osmolality cause intravascular release of an antidiuretic hormone (*vasopressin*) from the *supraoptic and paraventricular nuclei* after transport within the neurones to the median eminence of the IIIrd ventricle (*see Fig.* 14.1) and *neurohypophysis*, where it is released into the blood to reduce renal excretion of water. Thirst satiety occurs and drinking behaviour is suppressed. Release of vasopressin is also inhibited by glucocorticoids, contributing to the water retention of steroid therapy.

Failure of this mechanism limits renal conservation of water and causes excessive thirst (diabetes insipidus). Small decreases in blood osmolality prevent release of vasopressin, but the water diuresis is also limited by an antagonist reflex action on the renal vasculature due to non-osmotic stimuli such as decreased blood pressure in carotid baroreceptors and hypovolaemia detected by central and peripheral *volume receptors* (Chapter 27). Inappropriate secretion of vasopressin occurs with cerebral injury and other causes but

recognition may be delayed if fluid is being added to the vascular compartment. The decreased thirst (adipsia) is then obscured, but hypernatraemia is found. The possibility that some clinical states of hypo- or hypernatraemia are due to alteration of the 'set point' of the osmoreceptors is still speculative since an imposed water load still results in excretion of urine of low specific gravity.

Steroid sensitive neurones are present in the brain, and especially in localized areas of the hypothalamus, for oestrogen and corticosterone. It is probable that these are inhibitory for neurones regulating releasing hormones trophic to the gonads and adrenal cortex, permitting feedback control of blood levels of the hormones they secrete. The nature of receptors which stimulate release hormones, as in stress, is uncertain. They are probably aminergic.

SUPRA-HYPOTHALAMIC AND BRAIN STEM CONTROLS

The preoptic region is involved in the neural control of gonadotropin secretion. Projections from the amygdala pass through the stria terminalis (p. 129) to many parts of the hypothalamic and mammillary nuclei, particularly the periventricular (arcuate) nucleus (*Fig.* 25.1). The septal nuclei project similarly by the medial forebrain bundle. Additional extra-hypothalamic control comes from the substantia nigra. The dopaminergic projections are mainly to the *median eminence*. The mesencephalic and pontine raphe nuclei project serotoninergic neurones. The complexity of the important monoamine projections to the hypothalamic nuclei has still to be elucidated. The overlap of monoaminergic neurones restricts dissection by pharmacological methods and also limits the possibility of selective chemotherapy.

It is impossible to provide a simple and meaningful flow diagram of the interconnections of hypothalamic and preoptic nuclei but it may be clinically valuable to identify major sites of action of the monoaminergic projections. *Noradrenaline* is rather widely distributed (arcuate and paraventricular nuclei, periventricular and perifornical regions, and the median eminence). *Dopamine* is mainly directed to the median eminence. *Serotonin* is the important input to the suprachiasmatic nucleus ('the biological clock'). Free serotoninegic nerve endings in the ependyma of the IIIrd ventricle liberate serotonin into the CSF. It originates in the raphe nuclei and its functional significance is unknown, but it could be the 'hypnogenic substance' sometimes reported as present in the CSF.

The limited range of neurotransmitters or modulators must involve loss of local sign, consistent with the concept of general integration and regulation functions for the hypothalamus, though gating signals could select from a number of outputs. The main condensations of the grey matter of the medial hypothalamus which are recognized as nuclei can be correlated with some known functions concerned with the control of the internal milieu and general metabolism of the body through long acting and short acting widely diffused efferent systems, the neuroendocrines and the autonomic nervous system respectively. These are 'final common paths' available for a range of regulatory functions and not abolished by destructive lesions of the hypothalamus.

EFFERENT NUCLEI OF THE HYPOTHALAMUS

For the present purpose the hypothalamus will be regarded as the regulating area at the base of the brain extending from the preoptic region into the tegmentum of the mid-brain. Anatomically this includes the nuclei of the *mammillary bodies*. These are important intercalated neurones in the hippocampal-thalamic circuits involved in memory functions (Chapter 13), but the mammillary nuclei have no identified homoeostatic functions despite the presence of major afferent and efferent connections with the dorsal and deep tegmental nuclei, the *mammillary peduncle* (*Fig.* 14.1). Conversely, the *pineal body*, though anatomically remote, is a functional part of the neuroendocrine system.

The grey matter between the preoptic area and the diencephalic–mesencephalic junction may be subdivided on functional grounds. For some purposes, notably the regulation of the autonomic system and consciousness, it is best to divide the mass into anterior and posterior

regions. For others, and especially the neuroendocrine functions, a radial subdivision is more appropriate as differences can be observed from stimulation or lesions in three areas — lateral, medial and periventricular (lining the inferior part of the IIIrd ventricle). Thus the Hess school of physiologists recognize an anterior '*trophotropic*' region organizing the neurogenic basis of rest and recuperation (sleep and parasympathetic discharge) and a posterior '*ergotropic*' region organizing the neurogenic basis for autonomic activity associated with alertness, food seeking, fight and flight. The behaviourist school, interested in the limbic system imbalance of the hypothalamic regulators, stress the radial subdivision with the medial zone registering satiety and inhibiting food, water and sex-seeking activities and the lateral zone activating them, a distinction which is helpful in understanding clinical syndromes.

The *ventromedial nucleus* of the hypothalamus has been implicated in behavioural mechanisms, including evidence of satiety for food, water and procreation. It regulates the production of *releasing factors* for certain hormones including growth hormone, insulin, glucagon, thyrotropin, corticotropin and gonadotropins.

The *arcuate nucleus*, in the tuberal region near the entrance to the infundibular recess, projects by the tuberoinfundibular tract to the median eminence and stalk of the pituitary gland and conveys dopaminergic fibres to cells that release hormones to the hypophyseal portal system.

The *median eminence* has axons secreting every known neurotransmitter and neuropeptide, including angiotensin II and peptide-releasing factors for luteinizing hormone, thyrotropin and somatostatin. These peptides are named for their first identified actions and are used for other neuroregulatory functions (Chapter 3), but a major part of this special concentration of peptides is secreted into a portal vascular system connecting the median eminence with the *adenohypophysis* through the infundibular stalk of the pituitary (*Fig.* 25.3). They influence the anterior pituitary gland in at least three ways: (i) by stimulating the hormone-producing cells; (ii) by acting as neurotransmitters at axoaxonic contacts; (iii)

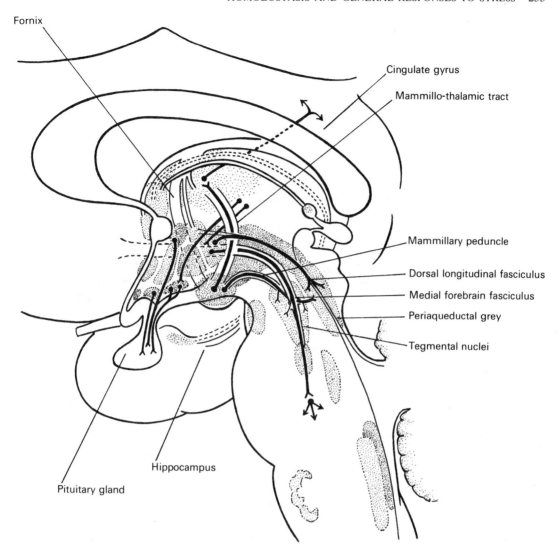

Fig. 25.2. Efferents from the hypothalamus. The nuclei of the median eminence, supraoptic and arcuate nuclei project to the pituitary gland directly or by a portal vascular system (*Figs.* 25.3–4). The mammillary nuclei connect the olfactory brain and hippocampus with the limbic cortex through the fornix and mammillo-thalamic bundle of Vicq d'Azyr to the anterior thalamus. The mammillary peduncle also projects back to the dorsal and deep tegmental nuclei involved in head movement. Posterior hypothalamic nuclei also project caudally to the pontomedullary reticular formation through the medial longitudinal bundle, and through the dorsal longitudinal fasciculus to the periaqueductal grey matter. These are important connections for initiating appetite-directed movement.

by acting on specialized glial cells (*tanycytes*), which are considered to control secretion of substances from the median eminence — ie some peptides are hormone-regulatory rather than hormone-releasing. It is at this site that the monoamine dopamine inhibits prolactin secretion. (Dopamine agonists, including bro-mocriptine, are used therapeutically for this purpose.) Conversely, enkephalins (and mor-phine) stimulate the release of prolactin. The remote effects of drugs are increasingly impor-tant. Prolactin levels in the blood rise consider-ably during and after a major epileptic seizure.

It is beyond the scope of this book to pursue

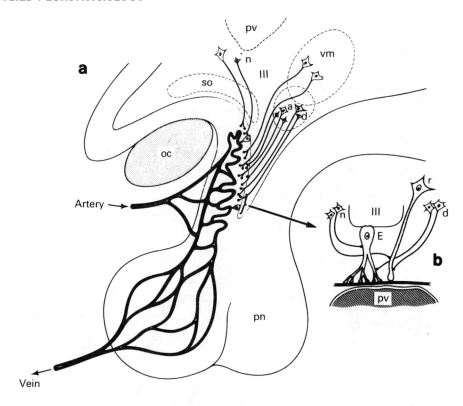

Fig. 25.3. *Neurosecretory and ependymal elements in the median eminence. a,* Some peptidergic and aminergic tracts which terminate in the median eminence. Dopaminergic systems (d), particularly in the arcuate nucleus (a), appear to be related to pituitary FSH activity. Noradrenergic systems (n) may be concerned in LH activity (pn, pars nervosa of pituitary body). *b,* The main elements in the median eminence. It has been suggested that aminergic systems (n and d) may affect the action of specialized ependymal cells (E) and releasing factor cells (r) either by direct contact of by diffusion. me, median eminence; oc, optic chiasma, pv, paraventricular nucleus; so, supraoptic nucleus, vm, ventromedial nucleus.

the functions of the anterior pituitary hormones after they have been secreted into the blood.

SUPRAOPTIC AND PARAVENTRICULAR NUCLEI

Another part of 'the diencephalic gland' is this pair of nuclei in which large nerve cells produce granules or protein 'colloid' released into blood vessels at their terminals in the posterior part of the pituitary gland, the *neurohypophysis* (which includes the pituitary stalk). Their efferent fibres run medially in a common bundle, the supraopticohypophyseal tract, through the median eminence (infundibulum) (*Fig.* 25.4). Secretions already identi-

fied are two nonapeptides *vasopressin* (antidiuretic hormone) and *oxytocin*, and their associated proteins, the *neurophysins*, which may be 'carriers' of the hormones. One is released by oestrogen and another by nicotine. Oxytocin is specially concentrated in the dorsal region of the supraoptic nucleus.

The anti-diuretic, vasoconstrictor and uterine stimulating effects of these peptides are only the most obvious of their actions. The APUD cells (amine content and/or Amine Precursor Uptake and Decarboxylation cells of A. G. E. Pearse) occur in many tissues of neuroectodermal origin, including cells in the gut, and peptides which they secrete have neurotransmitter or modulatory ('paracrine' rather than endocrine) functions (Chapter 3).

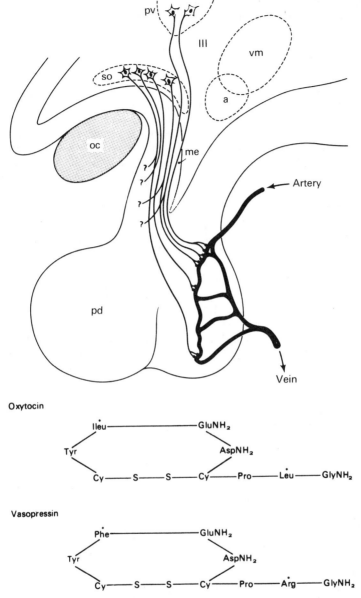

Fig. 25.4. The neurohypophysis. The supraoptic nucleus (so) and paraventricular nucleus (pv) neurones produce vasopressin and oxytocin which are discharged into vessels in the posterior lobe (pars nervosa) of the pituitary (and possibly into portal vessels of the median eminence). (Lettering as *Fig.* 25.3.)

Fortunately entry of peptides from the systemic circulation into the brain is limited by the blood–brain barrier and enzymic inactivation is rapid.

The antidiuretic action of vasopressin is briefly referred to on p. 25. Oxytocin stim-ulates the uterus in late pregnancy and evokes the milk-ejection reflex in suckling. Its function at other times, and in the male, is obscure. Secretion of both these peptide hormones is evoked centrally by acetylcholine and nicotine and blocked by anticholinergic drugs and by emotional stress. A noradrenaline depression of their secretion is blocked by α-adrenergic blocking agents.

Control of the autonomic system

The short-term regulation of homoeostasis, particularly the control of body temperature, distribution of oxygen, intake and excretion of food and water, and sexual functions, is effected by the autonomic nervous system. It is a push–pull system with a balanced state for homoeostasis in the resting animal but unbalanced during sleep and feeding at one extreme and alerted reaction against the environment on the other. Whereas the endocrine system affects all target cells indiscriminately, the autonomic motor system, being neuronal to the point of control, is selective. Upper neurone control may activate some of the lower neurones and not others, according to the requirements. The hypothalamus regulates *autonomic sets* in a manner analogous to the basal ganglia control of postural sets and does not exclude lower level drives of the efferent system: only the major sets have been recognized. A predominantly parasympathetic discharge and somnolence or sleep with increased heat dispersal occur with anterior hypothalamic stimulation. Conversely, stimulation of the posterior hypothalamus is alerting and evokes a predominantly sympathetic discharge, shivering and heat conservation. Both states have somatomotor changes appropriate to the proposed 'purpose' of these responses, presumably mediated through the mesencephalic reticular formation. The regulation of body temperature is paramount. These differences are most evident between anterior and posterior hypothalamic stimulations. This need not imply two distinct 'centres' but rather reciprocal gradients. The Hess nomenclature is convenient, though not universally accepted.

TROPHOTROPIC REACTION

Stimulation of the *anterior hypothalamus* of laboratory animals evokes visceral and somatomotor responses appropriate to sleep or feeding. The bulbar vasodepressor mechanism is activated. Blood vessels of the skin and splanchnic bed dilate and blood is shunted from the muscles. Heart rate is decreased, systole shortened and diastole relatively prolonged. The blood pressure falls. Respiration is slowed and the bronchioles constrict slightly, reducing dead space. Salivary and gastrointestinal secretion increases, peristalsis increases but sphincters relax slightly. Urine output is increased and bladder reflexes disinhibited. The internal sphincter may relax slightly (a combination which may cause enuresis which is responsive to amphetamine or arousal). Driving of the Edinger–Westphal nuclei constricts the pupils and sleep is promoted if the brain stem arousal system is not active (Chapter 15). Skeletal muscle tone is reduced.

ERGOTROPIC REACTION

Stimulation of the *posterior hypothalamus* elicits continuing visceral and somatic responses appropriate to the alert state with preparation for rapid muscular activity. The splanchnic vessels constrict but the skeletal muscle, coronary and pulmonary arterioles dilate. Heart rate and force increase and the blood pressure rises. The spleen contracts, causing increased circulating red cell mass. The constricted renal vessels reduce urine excretion. The slight constriction of cerebral vessels is compensated, as described in Chapter 27. The bronchi relax, inspiration is prolonged and breathing is faster (Chapter 20). Gastrointestinal secretions are reduced, peristalsis diminished. The cardiac sphincter of the stomach and the rectal sphincter contract. The urinary bladder relaxes and the tone of its internal sphincter increases, to store more urine. Liver glycogen is mobilized. The pupils of the eyes dilate, skeletal muscle tone is increased and muscles become less fatiguable. Vigilance is increased and sense organ sensitivity increased. All of these are sympathomimetic effects. An apparent paradox is that the skin sweats and may be pale (fright, anxiety) or flushed (anger, fight), cholinergic effects of the sympathetic system but with adrenergic primary neurones (Chapter 26).

These parasympathomimetic and sympathomimetic responses are not mutually exclusive. Both discharges occur together or serially in the reactions associated with strong emotion, in sexual orgasm and in epileptic fits. Splanchnic vasoconstriction associated with gastric secretion and hypermotility cause acute gastrointestinal ulceration (Cushing's neurogenic ulcers) and even rupture of the oesophagus in frightened overstressed patients, even in an intensive care ward.

Alternative use of lower level efferent neurones by 'upper' neurones occurs with this motor system, as with the pyramidal tract motor system.

Efferent fibres from the hypothalamus (*see* Fig. 25.2) pass through the tegmentum of the mesencephalon by the lower part of the *medial forebrain bundle* to the superior central nucleus, ventral tegmental nuclei and the central grey matter. A further connection, the *dorsal longitudinal fasciculus*, projects from the medial and periventricular part of the hypothalamus to the tectum and central grey matter. These pathways probably recruit the somato-

motor responses associated with hypothalamus evoked behaviour. The pathway(s) connecting the autonomic control areas to the appropriate nuclei in the medulla and spinal cord are unknown but probably involve the reticular formation and the superior colliculus for onward relay to the bulbar autonomic centres described in the next chapter.

Autonomic responses may be evoked by stimulation of certain areas of the neocortex. It is strange that these are relatively discrete and not a coordinated response, such as the hypothalamic stimulation evokes. Examples are vasomotor changes (cortical areas 4,6), cardiac acceleration (various areas), pupillary constriction (area 19), pupillary dilatation (area 8), sweat secretion and piloerection (area 6), and gastrointestinal secretion or motor changes (posterior orbital and insular cortex).

Further reading

Knowles F. Endocrine activity in the central nervous system. In: Bellairs R. and Gray E.G. (ed.) *Essays on the Nervous System.* London: Oxford University Press, 1974, pp. 431–50.

Lebovitz H.E. and Feldman J.M. Neurologic aspects of hyperpituitary and hypopituitary states. In: Goldensohn E.S. and Appel S.H. (ed.) *Scientific Approaches to Clinical Neurology*, Vol. II. Philadelphia: Lea and Febiger, 1977, pp. 1849–70.

McHugh P.R. Endocrine control and the hypothalamus. In: Goldensohn E.S. and Appel S.H. (ed.) *Scientific Approaches to Clinical Neurology*, Vol. II. Philadelphia: Lea and Febiger, 1977, pp. 1786–800.

Chapter 26
The autonomic nervous system

The hypothalamus, as discussed in the preceding chapter, acts as the central controller and integrator of many of the physiological homoeostatic processes that enable the individual to adapt to changes in his external environment. The maintenance of this internal homoeostasis involves patterns of behaviour which, for example, enable the individual to defend himself (flight or fight), which ensure the propagation of the species (sexual behaviour) and which allow him to compensate for extremes in environmental temperature (sweating, shivering, use of clothes and design of houses). The autonomic nervous system is the means by which the hypothalamus effects, usually reflexly, the numerous mechanisms involved in this control of the internal environment (arterial pressure, gastrointestinal motility, bladder function etc.).

As its name implies, the autonomic — or involuntary or visceral — nervous system behaves differently from the somatic nervous system in that, by and large, it is not subject to voluntary control. However, in effect the system is neither completely autonomous, nor is it entirely involuntary. It does not function in total independence of the somatic nervous system: the two systems are integrated centrally, and their actions often interlinked (for example, the somatic and autonomic mechanisms required by 'flight' or 'fight').

For the clinician there are good reasons for dividing the efferent portion of the autonomic nervous system into two functionally separate parts: the sympathetic, with its thoracolumbar outflow, and the parasympathetic, with its cranial and sacral origins. As well as being anatomically discrete, these two subdivisions of the autonomic nervous system subserve different — and at times antagonistic —

functions, and generally speaking utilize different transmitter substances. For those reasons, we will consider the two components of the system separately although, as will become clear later, the functional balance between the two may be of more importance clinically than the degree of activity in one or other component.

Autonomic activity is largely dependent on the 'feedback' of information from the skin, special senses (eye, ear, taste), gastrointestinal tract (presence of food in the stomach, handling of the bowel), respiratory system (intubation of the trachea), cardiovascular system (baroreceptors, volume receptors) and so on. Unfortunately, the afferent portion of the autonomic nervous system cannot be classified so clearly into its component parts as the efferent portion.

FUNCTIONAL ANATOMY OF THE AUTONOMIC NERVOUS SYSTEM

An appreciation of the basic anatomical lay-out of the autonomic nervous system is not unimportant to the anaesthetist, since it helps to demonstrate visually which nerves supply which organs (*Fig.* 26.1), and at what anatomical level it would be possible to effect blockade of a particular function. For example, to achieve effective blockade of the sympathetic supply to the intestines extradural blockade would have to be sufficiently extensive to include all nerve roots between L2 and T5. Looked at another way, decreases in systemic arterial pressure are less frequent and/or less marked when extradural or intrathecal blockade is confined to the lower thoracic and lumbar roots.

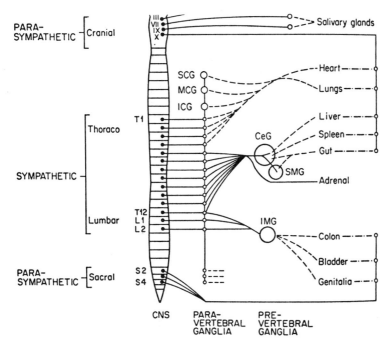

Fig. 26.1. Schematic representation of the peripheral autonomic nervous system: sympathetic and parasympathetic divisions are shown. Preganglionic fibres are represented as solid lines, postganglionic as broken lines.

SYMPATHETIC (THORACOLUMBAR) OUTFLOW

The sympathetic and the parasympathetic subdivisions of the autonomic nervous system possess both preganglionic and postganglionic neurones. The *preganglionic neurones* of the sympathetic nervous system are located in the intermediolateral nuclei of the thoracolumbar (T1–L2) portion of the spinal cord (*Fig.* 26.2). The axons arising in these cholinergic neurones emerge from the spinal cord via the anterior roots, form the white (largely myelinated) rami communicantes and then pass to the paravertebral sympathetic trunk, where they may synapse with a postganglionic neurone at the same segmental level, ascend or descend in the sympathetic chain before synapsing with a postganglionic neurone at a different segmental level, or pass through the sympathetic trunk to relay on postganglionic neurones in ganglia near the viscera. Those preganglionic fibres that form synapses in the *sympathetic ganglion* tend to do so with more than one adrenergic neurone. Thus, the number of fibres emerging

from a sympathetic ganglion is greater than the number of fibres entering it — so accounting, to some extent, for the more diffuse and divergent activity of the sympathetic component of the autonomic nervous system. Many of the *postganglionic fibres* pass back from the sympathetic chain into the spinal nerves via grey rami communicantes. Approximaely eight per cent of the fibres in the average skeletal nerve are sympathetic fibres (C fibres) passing to blood vessels, sweat glands, the piloerector muscles of the hairs, viscera etc.

The *cervical ganglia* lie anterior to the transverse processes of the vertebrae: the superior cervical ganglion anterior to C1–C4, the middle (C5–C6) and the inferior (C7–C8), which is usually fused with the first thoracic ganglion to form the stellate ganglion. Fibres supplying structures in the head originate from neurones in the superior cervical ganglia. Preganglionic fibres to the abdominal and pelvic viscera pass through the *paravertebral* (chain) *ganglia* without relay, form the superior, middle and inferior splanchnic nerves and terminate in one of the intra-abdominal (pre-

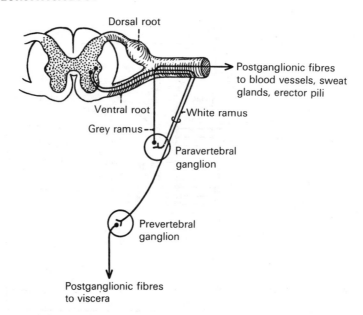

Fig. 26.2. Distribution of sympathetic outflow: paravertebral and prevertebral ganglia are represented.

vertebral) plexuses (coeliac, renal). Postganglionic fibres originating in these *prevertebral* (collateral) *ganglia* pass distally with the branches of the aorta to supply the relevant viscera. Above the diaphragm, all the preganglionic fibres synapse in the ganglia of the sympathetic chain.

The preganglionic sympathetic nerves to the adrenal medullae pass from the mediolateral horn of the spinal cord, through the sympathetic chain (without synapsing), through the splanchnic nerves and, finally, to the *adrenal medulla*. They end there by relaying directly with the cells that secrete the adrenaline (or noradrenaline). Embryologically, these secretory cells are derived from nervous tissue, and are analogous to postganglionic neurones.

PARASYMPATHETIC (CRANIOSACRAL) OUTFLOW

The functional anatomy of the parasympathetic component of the autonomic nervous system is illustrated in *Fig.* 26.1. It consists of two divisions: the *cranial*, with its preganglionic neurones located in the brain stem in the nuclei of the IIIrd, Vth, VIIth, Xth and XIth cranial nerves, and the *sacral*, with its preganglionic neurones in the sacral portion of the spinal cord (usually S2–S4). Of these the outflow via the *vagus nerves* is by far the largest and the most widely distributed with supply to heart, lungs, oesophagus, stomach, small intestine, liver, gallbladder, pancreas, upper portion of the ureters and the proximal half of the colon.

Like the sympathetic system, the parasympathetic system has preganglionic and postganglionic neurones. However, except in the case of a few cranial parasympathetic fibres, the preganglionic fibres pass without interruption, or relay to the target organ. The postganglionic neurones are located in the wall of the organ, and short (1 mm up to a few cm) postganglionic fibres pass from these and are distributed in the substance of the organ (pp. 282 and 290). A further (third) division of the autonomic nervous system — the *enteric nervous system* — has been proposed on account of the relative independence of the gastrointestinal tract from the rest of the autonomic nervous system. However, we have chosen to follow the classical (two division) pattern in our discussion of the physiology of the autonomic nervous system.

Now that the basic morphological divisions of the autonomic nervous system have been detailed, we will consider the functional divisions (sympathetic, parasympathetic) of the system; for simplicity, we will consider them separately.

SYMPATHETIC NERVOUS SYSTEM

The term 'sympathetic' was used originally to describe all visceral nerves. However, in 1886, Gaskell demonstrated that there were gaps in the autonomic outflow in the cranial and sacral regions and some 20 years later in 1905 Langley showed that the thoracolumbar segment differed pharmacologically from the craniosacral part — and designated them the 'orthosympathetic' system and the 'parasympathetic' system, respectively.

The sympathetic (or adrenergic) nervous system can be considered as being composed of two (or possibly more) systems which release from their nerve terminals a number of substances (dopamine, noradrenaline, adrenaline) common to all. For the purposes of this book it is probably adequate to subdivide the sympathetic nervous system into central (brain and brain stem) and peripheral (spinal) systems.

Central sympathetic nervous system

The central organization of the autonomic nervous system resembles that in the somatic nervous system in that it is composed of reflex arcs and segmental pathways which are interrelated functionally at different levels within the brain and brain stem. However, in addition to such locally integrative mechanisms there are numerous 'centres' which promote interchange between the autonomic system, somatic efferent and afferent pathways, receptor systems and higher functions (emotion, anger, mental activity).

Within the brain stem groups of neurones ('centres') have identifiable functions subserving, classically, cardiovascular function, respiratory function and control of the bladder. However, there are in addition areas in the medulla which, when stimulated, will induce coughing, sneezing, swallowing, salivation and vomiting. Many of these so-called centres lie within the reticular activating system, and the reticulospinal tract is thought to be one of the principal pathways by which autonomic activity

in the spinal cord can be influenced by these brain stem 'centres' (Chapters 4 and 20).

As alluded to earlier, the autonomic nervous system is not entirely involuntary: there is ample evidence that the cerebral cortex can influence autonomic function. Indeed, the presence of reasonably discrete autonomic areas within the cerebral cortex has been established. As might be expected, most of such cortical control is mediated via the hypothalamus. However, there is evidence that some mechanism exists whereby the cortex can influence autonomic activity and the sympathetic system in particular, without passing information via the hypothalamus. The insular–opercular area is probably involved.

As far as the sympathetic component of the autonomic nervous system *per se* is concerned, the most important central connections relate to the hypothalamus, the nuclei of the tractus solitarius and the dorsal and ventral (noradrenergic) 'bundles' of fibres which link the central and peripheral parts of the sympathetic nervous system (Chapters 3 and 25). These various nuclei and pathways are related primarily to the control of arterial pressure and will be considered in detail later (p. 277). However, it seems appropriate to introduce certain general considerations at this point. First, and not unexpectedly, those areas in the brain that appear to be involved most closely in the control of arterial pressure contain many catecholaminergic cell bodies or nerve terminals. For example, higher catecholamine concentrations have been measured in the nuclei of the solitary tract and the dorsal nucleus of the vagus than in other medullary nuclei. Both noradrenaline- and adrenaline-containing neurones have been identified — observations supportive of a central (as well as a peripheral) role for these neurotransmitters (Chapter 3). Secondly, as at the periphery, the central effects of noradrenaline and adrenaline result from the activation of α- and β-adrenoceptors. Certainly, both of the principal types of adrenoceptor (α and β) have been identified in brain. More recent investigations have, however, demonstrated the presence of both α_1 and α_2 adrenoceptors in preparations of neural membranes. Of these, the α_2 sub-group appears to be of particular importance in the control of autonomic function. Thirdly, it has

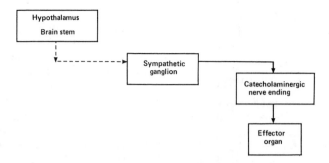

Fig. 26.3. Schematic representation of the major component parts of the peripheral sympathetic nervous system. Preganglionic fibres are represented by the broken line; postganglionic by the solid line.

been demonstrated that the catecholamines are not the only substances involved in neurotransmission within the central part of the sympathetic nervous system. For many years it has been claimed that acetylcholine and gamma-aminobutyric acid influence arterial pressure and heart rate by central mechanisms: 5-hydroxytryptamine may influence efferent sympathetic activity. More recently, it has been suggested that a number of peptides (substance P, angiotensin II, enkephalin, endogenous opioids) play some role in the central modulation of sympathetic function. Indeed, it has been proposed that there could be an angiotensin II which is endogenous to brain. Fourthly, while it is assumed quite naturally that the central component of the sympathetic nervous system can modulate and modify the peripheral the converse may also be true: the two components are not only interrelated but are also interdependent.

Peripheral sympathetic nervous system

Of the two divisions of the sympathetic nervous system, the peripheral component is that with which the anaesthetist is more familiar. It can be divided into a number of component parts (*Fig.* 26.3): however, not all will be considered in detail. This should not be taken to imply that the other components are less important physiologically: merely that their modulation has less immediate relevance to clinical practice.

THE SYMPATHETIC GANGLION

Within the ganglia numerous points of contact exist between the nerve endings of the preganglionic group of neurones and the cell bodies of the postganglionic neurones. Thus, the propagation of impulses from the central nervous system is interrupted by this synapse. It seems likely that fibres that form synapses within the ganglion are excitatory — the arrival of an impulse increasing the discharges from the postganglionic neurone. Although only one transmitter substance (*acetylcholine*) is released by action potentials in the preganglionic fibres, a number of sympathetic ganglia contain two varieties of postganglionic fibres. For example, sweat glands and the blood vessels in muscle are innervated by postganglionic fibres quite different from those that innervate the blood vessels in the skin or the piloerector muscles. Thus, the relay, within the ganglion, between the central nervous system and the peripheral organs, provides for the dual (cholinergic, adrenergic) innervation at the periphery.

Acetylcholine is synthesized in the terminal endings of the preganglionic cholinergic nerve fibres. Most of this synthesis occurs in the axoplasm, and the acetylcholine is then transported to the interior of the vesicles. At rest, small amounts (quanta) of transmitter are released spontaneously from the pre-synaptic nerve endings. On stimulation, a number of quanta are released, to react with receptor substances in the effector cells, before being broken down into acetate ion and choline by the enzyme acetylcholinesterase. Thus, the pattern of the mechanism is similar to that which occurs at the neuromuscular junction, a more detailed description of which has been presented in Chapter 2.

In high concentrations acetylcholine can occupy the postganglionic receptor for a prolonged period and block the onward transmission of impulses by maintaining the depolarization of the receptor. Many autonomic ganglia, particularly those in the prevertebral plexuses, contain peptides which may be transmitters or modulators of transmission. For example, *substance P* is present in fibres thought to function in reflex arcs associated with the transmission of visceral pain, and some noradrenergic fibres passing from ganglion cells to the intestine contain *somatostatin-like* immunoreactivity.

POSTGANGLIONIC SYMPATHETIC NERVES

The postganglionic sympathetic nerve consists of a cell body, a long axon and an extensively branched nerve terminal (*Fig.* 26.4). The cell bodies vary greatly in diameter (15–60 µm), have several long or short dendritic processes and adrenergic vesicles can be demonstrated in the substance of the cell body by specific fixation and staining techniques. Each adrenergic neurone has one axon which extends to the effector organ: 'long adrenergic neurones' innervating heart, blood vessels and glands and 'short adrenergic neurones' supplying some of the internal reproductive organs

in both sexes. These latter neurones respond differently to certain drugs (and utilize different transmitter mechanisms) when compared with the more typical adrenergic neurones (the 'long adrenergic neurones') which have their cell bodies located in the paravertebral ganglia. The length, and degree of branching of the terminal, varicose part of the adrenergic neurone varies widely between species, and between organs in any individual species. For the purposes of this discussion, however, it is probably sufficient to note that the branching is extensive (the total length of the terminal ramifications in the rat iris has been estimated to be 10 cm), that the varicosities are present in large numbers (250–300 varicosities per millimetre) and that the varicosities lie in close proximity to receptor sites. As a result, each adrenergic neurone can innervate several cells — this arrangement being consistent with the diffuse responses to stimulation of the sympathetic nervous system in contrast to the more localized responses which are characteristic of parasympathetic stimulation.

The terminal varicosities contain neurotubules, neurofilaments, mitochondria and, most significantly, the *dense core (granular) vesicles* which are believed to be the sites of the synthesis (possibly) and the storage of the adrenergic transmitter — *noradrenaline.* Although granular vesicles may be formed locally in the nerve terminal, the majority are synthesized in the Golgi apparatus of the cell body and then transported by axonal flow (Chapter 3) to the terminal varicosity. Two types of dense core vesicles have been described: the majority have a mean diameter of about 45 nm (small dense core vesicles) with a smaller proportion (5 per cent) of large dense core vesicles (approximate diameter 70 nm). The dense core vesicles are decreased in size and number following treatment with drugs (eg reserpine) which deplete the store of noradrenaline, increase in size and number when incubated with noradrenaline and are, therefore, believed to correspond to the sites of noradrenaline storage. In the vesicles, noradrenaline is bound with ATP, Ca^{2+}, and the proteins chromagranin A and dopamine-β-hydroxylase. Vesicular storage allows a large amount of transmitter to be stored in a biologically inactive form, and is the means by which the noradrenaline is protected from

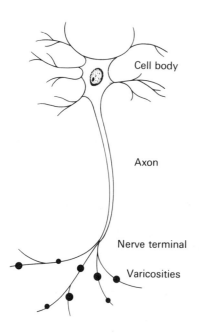

Cell body

Axon

Nerve terminal

Varicosities

Fig. 26.4. Schematic representation of a postganglionic sympathetic nerve.

enzymic breakdown (by monoamine oxidase) in the cytoplasm. The larger vesicles appear to act as a large stable store (pool) of noradrenaline which is rarely saturated, and which can be replenished readily by local synthesis from *tyrosine* and by the binding of cytoplasmic noradrenaline. Noradrenaline is transferred from this store to the smaller readily available store in the small dense core vesicles from which it is released on the arrival of a nerve impulse. However, this latter store also has the capability of synthesizing noradrenaline from its precursors and of replenishing its contents by binding cytoplasmic noradrenaline.

SYNTHESIS OF NEUROTRANSMITTERS

Noradrenaline is synthesized from the essential amino acid *L-tyrosine*, by a series of enzyme-controlled steps (*Fig.* 26.5), in adrenergic neurones, and in adrenal and extra-adrenal *chromaffin cells*. Synthesis of noradrenaline occurs in all parts of the adrenergic neurone — the cell body, the axon and the varicosities. However, the actual amount of noradrenaline synthesized in the cell body represents a very small proportion of that stored peripherally. This suggests that the main function of those adrenergic vesicles that originate in the cell

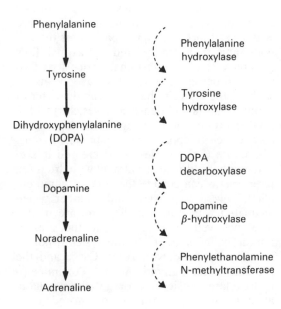

Fig. 26.5. Biosynthesis of catecholamines.

body is to supply the terminal varicosities with the machinery capable of *local synthesis and storage* of noradrenaline. Tyrosine is transported from the circulation into the varicosity of the nerve terminal (*Fig.* 26.6a). The enzyme *tyrosine hydroxylase* converts the tyrosine into *dihydroxyphenylalanine* (DOPA). This is the enzyme-dependent, rate-limiting step at which the synthetic pathway can be controlled, either by the presence of an increase in the concentration of circulating noradrenaline or by drugs that inhibit specifically the enzyme (eg L-DOPA). DOPA is then decarboxylated to *dopamine* which is transported from the cytoplasm of the varicosity to the storage vesicles in which the dopamine is converted to noradrenaline by *dopamine β-hydroxylase*.

In postganglionic sympathetic fibres, the synthetic pathway stops with *noradrenaline*. However, in the adrenal medulla (and other extra-renal chromaffin tissue) an additional enzyme, phenylethanolamine N-methyl transferase, methylates a variable (depending on species) percentage of the noradrenaline to *adrenaline*. In the chromaffin cells, the catecholamines act as *hormones* — they are released into the bloodstream and act as chemical messengers 'to all the cells equipped with receptors able to decode the message'. Obviously, as far as the adrenergic neurone is concerned (p. 269), the message only reaches those excitable units innervated by the neurone. In addition, it should be remembered that, in certain neuronal pathways in the central nervous system (as well as in some instances at the periphery) adrenaline and dopamine are the neurotransmitters and the synthetic pathway either stops at dopamine or proceeds to adrenaline (*see* Chapter 3).

Regulation of the biosynthesis of noradrenaline is achieved by two mechanisms: a fast regulatory mechanism and a slow regulatory mechanism. The former occurs in the terminal varicosities and is based on the rapid feedback inhibition of the synthesis of noradrenaline. As described earlier, tyrosine hydroxylase is the rate-limiting enzyme because its activity is regulated by the ultimate concentration of the end product of the synthetic processes — noradrenaline. In contrast, in the adrenergic cell body, an increase in sympathetic activity will only influence tyrosine hydroxylase activ-

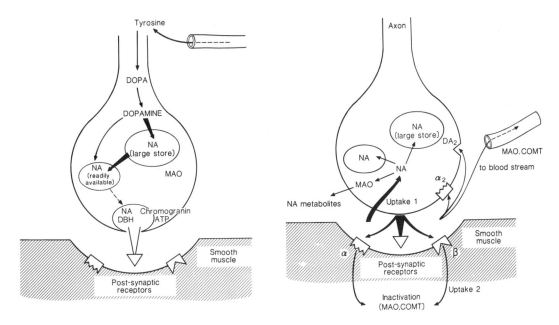

Fig. 26.6. *a*, The synthesis, storage and release of noradrenaline (NA). *b*, The uptake and inactivation of the released noradrenaline (NA). MAO, monoamine oxidase; DBH, dopamine β-hydroxylase; ATP, adenosine triphosphate; COMT, catechol-*O* methyl transferase; DA2, dopaminergic receptor.

ity after several hours and may not reach a peak for several days (slow regulatory mechanism). Thus, this latter mechanism appears to be associated with general overall alterations in physiological function whereas the former is a dynamic, rapidly accommodating process.

RELEASE OF NORADRENALINE

The physiological mechanisms which initiate, modulate and ultimately terminate the release of noradrenaline (and other adrenergic neurotransmitters) are of importance to the clinician. In particular, they are relevant to the practice of anaesthesia since it is these mechanisms which are, by and large, stimulated or inhibited as the clinician attempts to mimic or modify the actions of the physiological transmitter. However, although we will look at the various mechanisms in some detail, the discussion here will, of necessity, be somewhat didactic and the interested reader is referred to the reviews included in the Further Reading to this chapter for more in-depth analyses of the many pertinent investigations.

The presence of spontaneous excitatory junction potentials demonstrates that some noradrenaline is released spontaneously from the terminal varicosities. However, the amount released is small and its role uncertain. Thus, for the purposes of this chapter, we can accept that the release of noradrenaline from the terminal varicosities of a sympathetic neurone is initiated by depolarization of the terminal associated with the arrival of action potentials which originated in the cell body of the adrenergic neurone. It seems clear that the link between excitation and secretion depends on an influx of Ca^{2+} ions, although it also appears likely that the sites of action of Ca^{2+} ions are on the membrane of the varicosity and the membrane of the vesicle rather than on events occurring deep in the axoplasm. There is quite substantial evidence to indicate that nerve impulses release only the noradrenaline bound and held in the readily available stores in the vesicles: noradrenaline in extravesicular stores is unaffected. Noradrenaline is released in discrete packages. It seems that one quantum represents that part of the contents of a vesicle which can be released by exocytosis but that this is not identical for each vesicle.

To be effective, physiologically, the noradrenaline must reach the *synaptic cleft* and the actual mechanism or mechanisms by which this is achieved has stimulated considerable debate. Theoretically, at least, there are two principle ways by which noradrenaline, stored in the vesicles, could be 'transported' to the extracellular space. First, the noradrenaline could pass from the vesicle into the cytoplasm and then pass across the cell membrane into the synaptic cleft. In the second place, the individual vesicle(s), containing the noradrenaline, could move (or be moved) to fuse with the membrane of the varicosity and then release its contents directly into the extracellular space (exocytosis). Electron micrographs which show fusion of adrenergic vesicles with the membranes of axons support the latter hypothesis and, of the two, this is the preferred mechanism. Exocytosis is a *calcium-dependent mechanism* in which the vesicular membrane fuses with that of the varicosity, the phospholipids in the membrane are rearranged to form an opening through which the soluble contents of the vesicle (noradrenaline, chromogranin A, and dopamine β-hydroxylase) pass (*Fig. 26.6a*). These contents become relatively more soluble on exposure to the extracellular environment with its higher calcium concentration. The lipids associated with the vesicular membrane are retained, indicating that only the contents and not the whole vesicle are expelled.

However, although it is the preferred mechanism, exocytosis is not the only mechanism by which noradrenaline can be released from the nerve terminal. For example, the mechanism subserving the release of noradrenaline by indirectly acting sympathomimetic drugs such as tyramine is not dependent on an influx of Ca^{2+} ions and does not evoke the release of noradrenaline by exocytosis. It appears that, once inside the nerve terminal, tyramine either displaces noradrenaline from the vesicles into the cytosol, or increases the spontaneous loss of the noradrenaline which is present in the cytosol.

Although the next logical step in our discussion would be to consider those mechanisms (pre-junctional and post-junctional) which control the *release* of noradrenaline, there is merit in dealing first with the processes

by which the released noradrenaline is inactivated, and the neuronal stores of transmitter replenished.

Ultimately, the concentration of noradrenaline at the receptor and the termination of its activity depend on at least four factors (*Fig. 26.6b*): the re-uptake of noradrenaline into the nerve terminal, the uptake of noradrenaline into non-neuronal tissues, the metabolic breakdown of noradrenaline and the diffusion of noradrenaline from the synaptic cleft into the bloodstream.

NEURONAL UPTAKE OF NORADRENALINE (UPTAKE 1)

The effects of the released noradrenaline are terminated not by the direct enzymic breakdown of the catecholamine (no equivalent of the enzyme acetylcholinesterase exists in the adrenergic synapse), but by the transfer of the transmitter from its extracellular site of action back into the nerve terminal. This neuronal uptake of noradrenaline occurs over the entire surface of the adrenergic neurone and accounts for some 75 per cent of the released neurotransmitter. Once within the nerve terminal, most of the noradrenaline undergoes further redistribution into the intracellular storage vesicles (either newly formed or old). Noradrenaline not re-incorporated into the vesicles is subject to metabolic breakdown (by *monoamine oxidase*) followed by intra-neuronal reduction to 3,4-dihydroxyphenyl glycol — the principal intraneuronal metabolite of noradrenaline. The deaminated metabolite leaks passively out of the nerve ending into the extracellular space and, thence, to the bloodstream. The resultant low concentration of cytoplasmic noradrenaline increases the concentration gradient across the axonal membrane and facilitates the uptake of noradrenaline.

An appreciation of the existence of this uptake process is of value in understanding the various mechanisms by which drugs may interact with adrenergic mechanisms. For example, tyramine may obtain entry into the nerve terminal by this means and other indirectly acting sympathomimetic amines may not only release noradrenaline from the nerve terminal but also inhibit its re-uptake and hence potentiate its effects. Drugs such as cocaine and the tricyclic antidepressants inhibit the re-uptake of noradrenaline and their pharmacological effects are due, in large part, to this facility. Bretylium and guanethidine are drugs with 'local anaesthetic' properties (Chapter 1) which are structurally similar to noradrenaline. Thus, they can be concentrated selectively in the adrenergic nerve terminal and block the transmission of nerve impulses. Reserpine appears to act primarily by blocking another uptake process — the ATP/Mg^{2+}-dependent re-uptake and subsequent re-incorporation of noradrenaline into the granular vesicles. Since any noradrenaline accumulating in the cytoplasm will be deaminated by monoamine oxidase, the eventual outcome is a depletion of noradrenaline stores in the nerve terminal.

EXTRANEURONAL UPTAKE OF NORADRENALINE (UPTAKE 2)

Another route by which noradrenaline is removed from the synaptic cleft is uptake by certain non-neuronal tissues: in particular, vascular smooth muscle, cardiac muscle and certain glandular tissues. Uptake 2 differs from uptake 1 in its substrate specificity: it has a higher affinity for adrenaline than for noradrenaline and an even greater affinity for isoprenaline. Uptake by this process is followed rapidly by the *intracellular catabolism* of the catecholamine and it has been suggested that uptake 2 could 'constitute a mechanism for disposing of extracellular catecholamines by an "uptake-followed-by-metabolism" process, as opposed to the "uptake and retention" mechanism' described previously for uptake 1.

The physiological role of uptake 2 has been debated extensively without any definitive conclusions being reached. Its role is probably minor when compared with that of uptake 1, although its widespread distribution may be evidence of a physiological role, particularly in vascular smooth muscle. Certainly, in circumstances in which uptake 1 is blocked, uptake 2 may become the major uptake mechanism. Additionally, it may play a part in the rapid removal and inactivation of circulating adrenaline and noradrenaline.

Following uptake into extraneuronal tissue the noradrenaline is metabolized partly by *catechol-O methyl transferase* (and monoamine oxidase) into metabolites which have little biological activity. The metabolites are transported away by the bloodstream, conjugated in the liver and ultimately excreted.

This 'uptake and metabolic' inactivation system can be blocked either by substances that inhibit extraneuronal uptake (steroids, phenoxybenzamine) or by agents that inhibit the activity of monoamine oxidase or catechol-O methyl transferase. As a result, the effects of the catecholamines on vascular smooth muscle can be potentiated by certain of the corticosteroids (β-oestradiol corticosterone) and by drugs that inhibit catechol-O methyl transferase.

OTHER INACTIVATION MECHANISMS

The small amount of noradrenaline which escapes re-uptake enters the circulation where it is metabolized by both monoamine oxidase and catechol-O methyl transferase, primarily in the liver.

Less than 5 per cent of the released noradrenaline escapes uptake and/or breakdown to appear unchanged in the urine and this highlights the difficulty of judging the degree of sympathetic activity at the receptor by measuring the serum or urinary concentrations of noradrenaline — unless they are abnormally high, as in phaeochromocytoma. Measurement of the concentration of dopamine β-hydroxylase may be more useful in this respect.

MECHANISMS CONTROLLING RELEASE OF NORADRENALINE

The actual amount of noradrenaline released is related primarily to the frequency of stimulation (at least at physiological frequencies of between 2 and 16 Hz), and can be expressed as a fraction of the total available store of noradrenaline. In addition, however, it has become apparent that the release of noradrenaline is susceptible to modulation by drugs and by naturally occurring substances such as dopamine, angiotensin, prostaglandins, acetylcholine and even noradrenaline itself. The various factors thought to influence the release of noradrenaline are depicted diagramatically in *Fig. 26.6b* and summarized below (for reviews see Further Reading: Gillespie, 1980; Timmermans and Van Zwieten, 1982; McGrath, 1983).

INHIBITION OF THE RELEASE OF NORADRENALINE

The release of noradrenaline via the Ca^{2+}-dependent exocytotic mechanism can be inhibited by activation of *pre-junctional α-receptors* (α2-subtype) located on the terminal varicosity. Stimulation of these receptors, by noradrenaline, inhibits the further release of the neurotransmitter, due to a decrease in the amount of Ca^{2+} available to promote excitation coupling and exocytosis. The diagram depicts the presence of dopamine (DA2) receptors on the terminal varicosity, stimulation of which leads to inhibition of noradrenaline release as does an increase in the concentration of *prostaglandins of the E type* — an increase in the formation of which has been shown to follow stimulation of the sympathetic nervous system. The mechanisms involving pre-synaptic α-adrenoceptors and PGEs are independent and both are more effective when the rate of stimulation is low.

As alluded to earlier, the extraneuronal uptake of noradrenaline may be another method of inactivating the catecholamines and the potential of interaction between catecholamines and steroid hormones, for example, may have clinical implications (arterial hypertension in patients on hormone replacement therapy).

The terminal varicosities of the adrenergic neurones contain *cholinergic receptors* which respond to acetylcholine in two ways: activation of *muscarinic receptors* decreases the amount of noradrenaline released per impulse, whereas activation of the *nicotinic receptors* stimulates the release of noradrenaline. It has been suggested that the former mechanism may be of physiological significance in the heart, where vagal stimulation decreases the amount of noradrenaline released following stimulation of the sympathetic nervous system.

Basically these various mechanisms provide a type of 'autoregulation' such that as the synaptic concentration of transmitter increases, further release is inhibited.

FACILITATION OF THE RELEASE OF NORADRENALINE

In addition to frequency of stimulation a number of other mechanisms can facilitate the release of noradrenaline.

(*a*) *Angiotensin II* can increase the synaptic concentration of noradrenaline either by inhibiting uptake 1 or by facilitating the release of more noradrenaline per impulse — actions which can be counteracted by the administration of the angiotensin converting enzyme inhibitor, captopril.

(*b*) *Prostaglandins of the F type* are released during sympathetic stimulation and, in contrast to the PGEs described earlier, have been shown to enhance sympathetic neurotransmission in certain vascular beds.

(*c*) Recent studies have indicated that low concentrations of *adrenaline* augment the release of noradrenaline at many sympathetic terminals — an effect possibly mediated via pre-junctional β-receptors. The consensus of opinion favours a $β_2$-subtype and this effect of adrenaline may be of relevance in the aetiology of certain forms of arterial hypertension.

Unfortunately, although many of these fundamental mechanisms have been described individually, the exact means by which the various modalities act and/or interact to produce the facilitation (or, indeed, inhibition) of the release of noradrenaline are less clear.

MAINTENANCE OF NORADRENALINE STORES

The previous section considered factors that can influence the amount of noradrenaline released. The following section will discuss the physiological means by which this released noradrenaline induces a response at the post-junctional membrane. However, before addressing that question, it seems appropriate to consider briefly how the actual stores of noradrenaline (plus dopamine β-hydroxylase and chromogranin) are replenished so that an adequate amount of noradrenaline is always available. Having said that, however, it is worth noting that only a fraction of the total available store of noradrenaline is released by the action potential. Even continuous stimulation at high frequency does not appear to deplete the noradrenaline stores fully.

As described earlier, the available noradrenaline originates from the vesicular stores which are replenished by:

(i)   the axonal transport of noradrenaline from the cell body;

(ii) the local synthesis of noradrenaline;

(iii) the re-uptake of a considerable amount of the released noradrenaline.

Although the re-uptake of released noradrenaline would seem to be the most logical and efficient means of maintaining the noradrenaline stores, blockade of this mechanism does not interefere with transmission. As axonal flow supplies only a small percentage of the total daily storage of noradrenaline in the nerve terminals, it appears that local synthesis of noradrenaline is the most important means by which an adequate supply of noradrenaline is available. To this end, the rate of synthesis appears to follow not only the amount of noradrenaline released, but also the frequency of stimulation.

POST-JUNCTIONAL EFFECTS OF NORADRENALINE

Once released, noradrenaline diffuses across the synaptic cleft to interact with specialized components of the effector cell membrane — the adrenergic 'receptors' or *adrenoceptors*. Such adrenoceptive sites have been divided broadly into two main types designated α and β according to their responses to certain agonist and antagonist drugs. A detailed analysis of the precise locations and exact nature of these adrenoceptors is outwith the scope of this book, and the reader is referred to reviews by Gillespie (1980), Lees (1981) and McGrath (1983) listed in the Further Reading. Suffice to say that the two main types of adrenoceptor have quite different pharmacological properties (*Table* 26.1), and have been divided further into α_1 and α_2 and β_1 and β_2 sub-types. An effector organ may possess both α- and β-adrenoceptors which may either act synergistically or be antagonistic. If antagonist, the effects mediated by one of the receptors usually predominate.

Although the exact nature of the adrenoceptor is unknown, attempts have been made to determine the chemical processes involved. Thus, the interaction between neurotransmitter and receptor is thought to cause a change in the concentrations of certain compounds within the cell called second messengers. These modify the responses of the cell by controlling the activities of certain intracellular enzyme systems.

It has been suggested that the β-adrenoceptor is an integral part of the *adenylate*

Table 26.1. Catecholamine receptors: distribution and effects of stimulation

Receptor	Distribution	Response
α_1	Smooth muscle	Constriction: increase in systemic vascular resistance
α_2	Pre-synaptic Platelets Medulla	Inhibits release of noradrenaline
β_1	Heart	Increases heart rate Increases force of myocardial contraction
β_2	Smooth muscle	Relaxation of smooth muscle: uterus, airway, vascular dilatation
DA1	Smooth muscle: renal, mesenteric	Relaxation: increase in renal blood flow
DA2	Adrenergic nerve ending: pre-junctional	Decreases amount of noradrenaline released

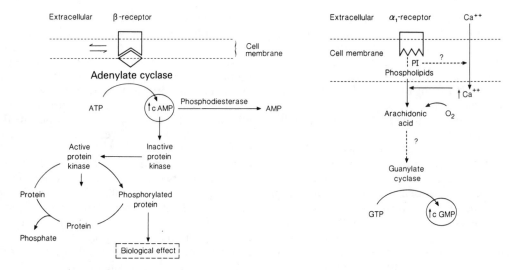

Fig. 26.7. Possible mechanisms involved in the mediation of adrenergic effects. *a*, Representation of β-adrenoceptor. *b*, Representation of α_1 receptor. ATP, adenosine triphosphate; AMP, adenosine monophosphate; cAMP, cyclic AMP; GTP, guanylate triphosphate; cGMP, cyclic GMP; PI, phosphatidylinositol.

cyclase (a membrane-bound enzyme) system. This enzyme has two components, one facing the exterior of the cell, the other facing the interior. The former recognizes the neurotransmitter and activates the latter. Activation of the internal component catalyses the conversion of adenosine triphosphate to cyclic 3′, 5′ adenosine monophosphate (cAMP) (*Fig. 26.7a*). This increase in intracellular cAMP appears to be responsible for those effects subserved by the β-adrenoceptor. The action of the cAMP is terminated by phosphodiesterase. The characterization of the *α-adrenoceptor* is less complete. However, it does seem likely that the chemical mechanisms subserving the two sub-types (α_1, α_2) differ. Activation of α_2-adrenoceptors appears to decrease the intracellular concentration of cAMP (via adenylate cyclase) whereas that of the α_1 sub-type is thought to induce a breakdown of phosphatidylinositol — a phospholipid confined mainly to the inner wall of the cell membrane (*Fig. 26.7b*).

The final step linking the catecholamine/receptor interaction and the mechanical event (constriction/relaxation) remains controversial but appears to involve the mobilization (immobilization) of *membrane Ca^{2+}* as the in-

itiator (inhibitor) of the actin–myosin system, a mechanism shared with skeletal muscle (Chapter 1).

THE ADRENAL MEDULLA

Although the adrenal medulla has been mentioned *en passant* earlier in this chapter, it has not been considered systematically. This seems an appropriate place to rectify this omission.

The *chromaffin cells* which make up the adrenal medulla arise embryologically from the same cells as those which give rise to the postganglionic noradrenergic neurones. However, the medullary cells do not develop long axons or threshold electrical characteristics. Instead, they acquire a considerable capacity to store, and release, catecholamines. Two types of chromaffin cell have been described: one which stores noradrenaline in large vesicles with a dense homogeneous core and the other which possesses larger vesicles with a larger less dense core and stores adrenaline. Although, on average, approximately 80 per cent of the secretion is adrenaline, the relative proportions of the two types of cell (and, hence, of the catecholamine secreted) varies under different physiological conditions, and may be dependent to some extent on hormones secreted by the adrenal cortex.

The adrenal chromaffin cells are innervated by cholinergic neurones originating in the spinal cord. The release of acetylcholine activates nicotinic receptors and causes a small, non-propagated depolarization of the cell. The subsequent release of the catecholamines into the bloodstream is due to a Ca^{2+}-dependent exocytotic mechanism.

Circulating adrenaline and noradrenaline have similar effects on the various organs as those brought about by direct stimulation of the adrenergic nerve ending, except that the effects last considerably longer (about ten times as long) because these hormones are inactivated much more slowly in the bloodstream. Usually, if the sympathetic nervous system is stimulated the entire system (or at least major portions of it) are activated. Thus, adrenaline and noradrenaline are released from the adrenal medulla in concert with direct stimulation of the adrenergic neurone. These two mechanisms support each other and may substitute for each other. For example, removal of the direct sympathetic nervous supply to an organ (transplantation) does not mean that the organ cannot respond to sympathetic 'activity': circulating adrenaline and noradrenaline can induce sympathomimetic responses indirectly. Similarly, removal of both adrenal glands has little significant effect on the physiological functioning of the sympathetic nervous system.

PARASYMPATHETIC NERVOUS SYSTEM

Compared with the sympathetic part of the autonomic nervous system, the parasympathetic innervation of the body is more limited in extent, and its response less diffuse. The basic lay-out of the parasympathetic component of the autonomic nervous system was presented in *Fig.* 26.1 and the description of the anatomical pathways detailed on page 260. Thus, this section will consider the physiological mechanisms by which the parasympathetic nervous system produces its effects.

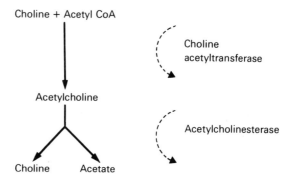

Fig. 26.8. Synthesis and inactivation of acetylcholine.

Synthesis and release of acetylcholine

In every instance, acetylcholine is the chemical transmitter between the postganglionic parasympathetic neurones and their effector cells. Acetylcholine is synthesized in the terminal endings of the cholinergic nerve fibre by the acetylation of choline in the presence of the enzyme *choline acetyl transferase* (*Fig.* 26.8). Most of the synthesis takes place in the axoplasm from where the acetylcholine is transported to the interior of the vesicles (agranular) where it is stored.

The mechanisms initiating and controlling the release of acetylcholine are similar at all cholinergic nerve terminals. These have been described in detail in Chapter 2.

CHOLINERGIC RECEPTORS (CHOLINOCEPTORS)

In the synaptic cleft acetylcholine forms reversible complexes with cholinoceptors on the post-synaptic membranes. Acetylcholine can activate two different types of cholinoceptor — muscarinic and nicotinic.

MUSCARINIC

This receptor was originally designated 'muscarinic' because muscarine, a poison from toadstools, could mimic the actions of acetylcholine at this site but would not activate the nicotinic receptor. Muscarinic receptors are found in all the organs innervated by postganglionic parasympathetic fibres (and those innervated by the postganglionic cholinergic neurones of the sympathetic nervous system: eccrine sweat glands). The responses to stimulation at muscarinic sites are characterized by decreases in heart rate, decreases in myocardial contractility, salivation, bronchoconstriction, increases in gastrointestinal tone etc., and so have been called (somewhat imprecisely) 'parasympathomimetic'. Atropine is the prototype blocking drug at the muscarinic receptor. However, the responsiveness to atropine appears to differ at different muscarinic sites (e.g. greater inhibition of the secretion of saliva than of the production of gastric acid) and indicates that muscarinic receptors may differ somewhat at different sites. Transmission in some ganglia is muscarinic but is not blocked by either atropine or hexamethonium.

NICOTINIC

Nicotinic receptors, so called because nicotine would mimic the actions of acetylcholine at this site, are found in the synapses between the pre- and postganglionic neurones of both sympathetic and parasympathetic systems, and at the neuromuscular junction. The prototype blocking drug is hexamethonium — although more familiar and more specific drugs are used now to block transmission at the ganglia, and at the neuromuscular junction.

INACTIVATION OF ACETYLCHOLINE

The action of acetylcholine is very brief — because of diffusion away from the receptor and hydrolysis to choline and acetic acid by *acetylcholinesterase* (true cholinesterase). Thus, one of the precursors of acetylcholine is also the product of its breakdown and in this way, the choline is available for re-incorporation into the nerve terminal and can be utilized for the synthesis of new transmitter. In this way, the parasympathetic system can compensate for the rapid hydrolysis and inactivation of acetylcholine and yet maintain adequate concentrations of active transmitter at the nerve ending.

True cholinesterase is present in high concentrations at cholinergic nerve endings and at the neuromuscular junction. Another enzyme, *pseudocholinesterase*, is present predominantly in plasma and is responsible for the hydrolysis of drugs with ester linkages — such as suxamethonium and certain local anaesthetic agents. Pseudocholinesterase does hydrolyse acetylcholine also but the rate of hydrolysis is too slow to be of any physiological significance. In contrast, the hydrolysis of acetylcholine by true cholinesterase is so rapid that the systemic administration of acetylcholine has no pharmacological value.

Drugs which inhibit true cholinesterase (and pseudocholinesterase) are termed anticholinesterases. Their pharmacological effects are due to the accumulation of endogenous acetyl choline and are most evident at the neuromuscular junction and at muscarinic receptors.

Table 26.2 presents the effects of stimulation of both the sympathetic and parasympathetic systems on different organs. It can be seen that although sympathetic stimulation produces excitation in some organs it has inhibitory effects in others. Likewise, stimulation of the parasympathetic system will cause excitation in some organs and inhibition in others. Moreover, the two systems may act reciprocally to each other: parasympathetic activity inhibiting and sympathetic activity stimulating a particular organ. Thus, although we have considered the autonomic nervous system as if it consisted of two functionally separate components, in practice the two parts of the autonomic nervous system appear to act frequently in concert, and the eventual physiological result is an amalgam of the various competing influences. This may be particularly noticeable if sympathomimetic influences (eg on the heart) are inhibited by drugs administered during anaesthesia such that parasympathetic effects (eg bradycardia) predominate. Nevertheless, under physiological conditions it is usual for one of the components to predominate and exert the major controlling influence on a particular organ, for example, parasympathetic on the gastrointestinal system, the sympathetic on blood vessels (*see below*).

AUTONOMIC CONTROL OF VISCERA

The previous section described the anatomical and physiological basis of the autonomic nervous system and, of necessity, focused primarily on the means by which information is

Table 26.2. Effects of sympathetic or parasympathetic stimulation on various organs

Organ	Sympathetic stimulation	Parasympathetic stimulation
Heart	Increased	Decreased
Rate	Increased	Decreased force of atrial contraction
Contractility		
Automaticity	Increased	—
Lung		
Bronchi	Relaxed	Constricted
Secretions	—	Increased
Intestines		
Motility	Decreased	Increased
Sphincter	Increased tone	Relaxed
Eye		
Pupil	Dilated	Constricted
Ciliary muscle	Relaxation (slight)	Contraction
Arterioles		
Coronary	Dilated (β_2) Constricted (α)	Dilated
Muscle	Dilated (β_2) Constricted (α) Dilated (cholinergic)	—
Skin	Constricted	—
Kidney	Constricted	—
Splanchnic	Constricted	—

passed from the centre *to* the periphery. However, since autonomic function depends substantially on the receipt of afferent information, we will now consider the means by which this is provided.

Although the autonomic nervous system innervates, to a greater or lesser extent, smooth muscle throughout the body, it does not itself control arterial pressure, or gastrointestinal function, or micturition, or other physiological homoeostatic processes. Autonomic function is but one of many interrelated factors which determine the level of activity in a particular organ or tissue. To emphasize this aspect we propose to consider certain examples which we believe highlight the integration of the autonomic nervous system with that of other control mechanisms. To this end we will discuss: (i) the autonomic regulation of cardiovascular function; (ii) the role of the autonomic nervous system in the regulation of gastrointestinal function; and (iii) the autonomic control of micturition. The first of these

is, obviously, of particular interest to the anaesthetist and will be described in some detail. Since the relevance of the other two examples is less immediate, although one must be mindful of the intensive care situation, they will be considered more briefly.

Autonomic regulation of cardiovascular function

The *raison d'être* of the circulation is the delivery of oxygen and other substrates to the tissues and the removal of the waste products of metabolism. Consequently, at 'grass-roots' level the regulation of cardiovascular function is dependent on those local mechanisms which ensure the optimal provision of nutrients to, and the adequate removal of waste products from, each individual tissue. Myogenic activity, or the contraction and relaxation of vascular smooth muscle, is the major mechanism controlling the blood flow to and within each tissue, and the distribution of blood flow between tissues. Since the contractility of vascular smooth muscle can be influenced by physical, chemical and autonomic factors, it is evident that the autonomic nervous system must have a role in the regulation of tissue blood flow. Undoubtedly, any change mediated via the autonomic nervous system would occur rapidly. However, since the effects produced would be widespread and involve many organs, it is not surprising that its role in the regulation of *local* tissue blood flow is comparatively minor, at least in the normal resting individual. Indeed, about 75 per cent of all the local blood flow in the body is controlled intrinsically by changes in the (perivascular) concentrations of locally produced vasoactive chemicals (*metabolic autoregulation*). The remaining 25 per cent of the total local blood flow — primarily that to the kidney and the skin — is independent of metabolic factors. As far as the kidney is concerned, the local blood flow to each nephron appears to depend on a mechanism intrinsic to the kidney which adjusts the blood supply to the rate (and, possibly, composition) of the excretion from that nephron. The principal factors modulating blood flow in the skin are impulses from the temperature regulating centres in the hypothalamus (Chapter 7), an example of one of the few situations in which there is a continuing role for the autonomic nervous system *per se* in the control of local blood flow.

If we now take this argument a step further, it will be obvious that, although local blood flow is dependent primarily on the factors described above, it must also depend, secondarily, on the maintenance of an adequate perfusion pressure (blood flow ∝ resistance and pressure). Let us suppose, for example, that activity in a particular tissue increases: the 'demand' for more oxygen will be met by a local metabolically induced increase in blood flow — as long as there is an adequate 'head' of pressure. Thus, it would be reasonable to assume that there must be certain specific mechanisms which can effect those changes in the heart and circulation necessary to maintain the stability of the arterial pressure and which could, if required, increase the volume of blood per unit time reaching the tissues should the former mechanism (maintenance of perfusion pressure) prove inadequate. Since these are adaptative mechanisms, one could reasonably assume that autonomic mechanisms would be involved. We will now consider to what extent this is so, highlighting in particular the integration of the autonomic with those other mechanisms that modulate cardiovascular function.

THE ROLE OF THE AUTONOMIC NERVOUS SYSTEM IN THE MAINTENANCE OF ARTERIAL PRESSURE

Two basic mechanisms underlie the physiological regulation of arterial pressure — neurogenic and non-neurogenic. The former is mediated through the autonomic nervous system, in particular, the sympathetic component of the autonomic nervous system, and is important in the acute modulation (seconds, minutes, hours) of arterial pressure. The latter is involved in the longer term control (many days, weeks) of arterial pressure and is related to the modification of blood volume by renal (excretion or retention of fluid) and/or humoral (angiotensin, aldosterone) mechanisms. Of the two mechanisms the former is the more pertinent here, and will be considered at this point. Although the non-neurogenic mechanism will be discussed later, consideration of it will be brief and will be used primarily to highlight the interplay between autonomic and other control mechanisms.

NERVOUS MECHANISMS IN THE CONTROL OF ARTERIAL PRESSURE

The neural control of arterial pressure can be understood readily if we use the analogy of a closed-loop, computer-controlled circuit (*Fig. 26.9*). Using this concept, the controlled variable (arterial pressure) is monitored continuously and any changes detected by the sensors (baroreceptors, chemoreceptors). The input from these sensors is integrated with other relevant information in the computer (central control system, vasomotor centre) and appropriate commands passed to the effector mechanism(s) (heart, blood vessels) via the efferent arm of the circuit (autonomic nervous system).

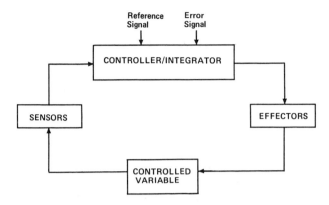

Fig. 26.9. Representation of computer-controlled, closed-loop, feedback system.

SENSOR MECHANISMS

High pressure baroreceptor mechanism

Reflexes in this system originate from mechanoreceptors which are located mainly in the adventitia and media of the carotid sinuses and in the wall of the ascending aorta. These receptors respond both to the degree of deformation (stretch) and to the speed of deformation. In this way, they sense both mean arterial pressure and the pulsatile variations in pressure, and respond to alterations in either. Afferent fibres from the *carotid sinuses* (a mixture of rapidly conducting myelinated fibres and slow-conducting unmyelinated fibres) join to form the carotid sinus nerve which then joins the glossopharyngeal nerve. Nerve fibres from the *aortic baroreceptors* form the depressor nerves and pass via the vagus nerve to the brain stem and the central control system. The receptors in the carotid sinuses are thought to be stimulated at lower values of arterial (transmural, more precisely) pressure than those in the aortic arch, and it has been suggested that the carotid baroreceptors respond to decreases in pressure below the normal range whereas receptors in the aorta respond mainly to increases in pressure. Whatever the nuances of their responses, an increase in pressure is accompanied by an increase in afferent discharge and vice versa.

The principal role of these baroreceptors is that of smoothing out those fluctuations in arterial pressure induced by everyday physiolo-gical 'stresses' such as changes in posture, alterations in environmental temperature, exercise etc. In addition, of course, they allow the individual to compensate in the face of more marked physiological trespass such as acute haemorrhage, increases in intrathoracic pressure and overtransfusion.

The sensitivity of the baroreceptors is increased during natural sleep, and can be decreased by increasing age, congestive cardiac failure, essential hypertension and the administration of a variety of anaesthetic agents. A measure of the gain (or sensitivity) of the baroreceptor reflex can be obtained clinically by noting the change in heart rate associated with an acute induced (usually with phenylephrine iv) increase in systolic arterial pressure. During prolonged hypertension the carotid and aortic baroreceptors 'reset' such that at the higher arterial pressure, afferent neural activity is similar to that observed in normotensive individuals. Whether this alteration in sensitivity has any part in the genesis of essential hypertension is debatable, although it has been postulated that the modest degree of sympathetic nervous system overactivity demonstrable in such patients could be secondary to such an alteration. Interestingly, it has been shown that the majority of the currently used anaesthetic agents — whether inhalation (halothane, enflurane, isoflurane) or intravenous (barbiturates, ketamine, alphaxalone-alphadalone acetate (Althesin)) — decrease the sensitivity of the baroreceptor reflex in a dose-dependent manner. Such an attenuation of physiological homoeostatic mechanisms could be of importance clinically when changes in posture, or the sudden loss of circulating blood volume, occur during (or immediately following) the administration of such drugs.

Low pressure baroreceptor mechanism

The low pressure baroreceptors or *cardiopulmonary mechanoreceptors*, are located in the endocardium at the junction of the superior and inferior venae cavae with the right atrium, in the left atrium, and at the junction of the pulmonary veins and the left atrium. Like the high pressure baroreceptors, they respond to stretch, and can, in this way, detect the degree of filling of the great veins, the atria and the pulmonary arterial system. When stimulated, impulses pass in myelinated nerve fibres to the central control system via the vagus nerve. The precise physiological significance of these sensors is unclear. However, the results of stimulation are an increase in heart rate (mediated by the efferent sympathetic supply to the sino-atrial node) and a water diuresis (mediated, possibly, by suppression of the release of antidiuretic hormone). In this way, they may act to maintain ventricular end-diastolic volume constant and so attenuate any effect of overfilling of the venous side of the heart on the Frank–Starling mechanism.

Chemoreceptor mechanism

The chemoreceptors situated in the *carotid bodies*, the aortic arch and the subclavian arteries, respond primarily to alterations in the chemical composition of the blood perfusing them: in particular, a decrease in oxygen content. In addition, however, they are activated by an increase in CO_2 content, acidaemia and significant arterial hypotension. Obviously, this means that their role in the overall control of arterial pressure in normal resting man is minimal. However, if arterial pressure decreases to less than 80 mmHg and, certainly, if it decreases to 50–60 mmHg, the central control system is activated and the integrated response involves a stimulation of respiration due to an interaction between the vasomotor and respiratory 'centres', increases in systemic vascular resistance and venous return pro-

duced by an increase in efferent sympathetic activity to the splanchnic venous reservoir and the resistance vessels in muscle and intestine, and a decrease in heart rate mediated by an increase in activity in the parasympathetic supply to the heart.

There are, in addition, *chemoreceptors situated centrally* within or adjacent to the central control system. Although their primary role is in the regulation of respiration they appear to be stimulated at very low values of arterial pressure (20–30 mmHg), possibly by the local tissue acidosis and increase in local carbon dioxide concentration which result from an inadequate blood flow. This has been termed a 'last-ditch' mechanism: certainly, there is an intensely powerful reflex activation of sympathetic efferent activity. There is maximum constriction of resistance and capacitance vessels with the result that mean arterial pressure can be increased dramatically (to more than 200 mmHg). However, the response is generally fairly short-lived (around 10 minutes) and its clinical relevance uncertain, although it has been suggested that it may have a role in patients in whom there has been acute severe blood loss.

Miscellaneous sensors

Afferent information can pass to the central control system from a number of other sensors. For example, there are *vagal receptors* scattered throughout the artria and ventricles which are stimulated by an increase in volume in the atria and/or ventricles. Reflex responses arise in the depressor neurones of the central control system (*see below*) and produce peripheral vasodilatation, bradycardia and a decrease in myocardial contractility. Sensors in the lung, the respiratory tract, the gastrointestinal tract and the skin can provide afferent information which may alter arterial pressure reflexly. It seems unlikely that any of this group of miscellaneous sensors has any role in the normal regulation of arterial pressure. However, they are included for completeness and because they are those stimulated frequently during surgery and anaesthesia — for example, on incision of the skin, manipulation of the intestines, intubation of the trachea and possibly overinflation of the lungs.

THE CENTRAL CONTROL SYSTEM

As its title suggests, this component of the overall system is situated centrally and, as such, provides a responsive rapidly-responding mechanism which can modulate a wide range of functions simultaneously. Primarily, the central control system is an integrator, or more precisely an integrator–comparator, which assimilates the information received from the peripheral sensors just described, from higher centres and from the environment and then, following its integration, compares that information with 'reference' information from the hypothalamus.

Conceptually, the central control system can be characterized as consisting of two discrete but functionally related groupings of cells which subserve 'pressor' or 'depressor' activity (*Fig. 26.10*). However, it seems likely that both these groupings of cells are under the influence of the *nucleus tractus solitarius* since this appears to act as a 'clearing house' for much of the afferent information from the various peripheral sensors (fibres from the baroreceptors and chemoreceptors terminate here). Certainly, it would appear from recent studies in which the nucleus tractus solitarius was either stimulated or ablated stereotactically, that it plays a major role in the regulation of arterial pressure.

Neural connections pass from the nucleus tractus solitarius to higher centres in the brain (*see Fig.* 25.1), and to the efferent pathways on the baroreflex arc (via the pressor and depressor areas and the vagal nucleus). As alluded to earlier, the *hypothalamus* is one of the higher centres thought to have a role in the regulation of arterial pressure: stimulation of certain specific sites in the anterior hypothalamus producing bradycardia, hypotension and inhibition of baroreceptor reflexes. That even higher centres influence arterial pressure can be deduced from the evidence that loud noises, emotional disturbances, mental arithmetic etc. can increase, and relaxation techniques decrease, arterial pressure.

The *pressor* (sympathetic) grouping of cells is located in the lateral (facilitatory) pathway of the *descending reticular formation* (*see Fig.* 3.1). Stimulation of this area will induce arteriolar vasoconstriction and increases in heart rate and myocardial contractility. Depressor (parasympathetic) cells lie in the *medial* (inhibitory) pathway and their primary role appears to be that of modifying activity in the tonically active pressor cells — an increase in depressor cell activity producing a reciprocal inhibition of activity in the pressor cells. As a result, parasympathetic activity will predominate peripherally and lead to arteriolar vasodilatation and decreases in heart rate and

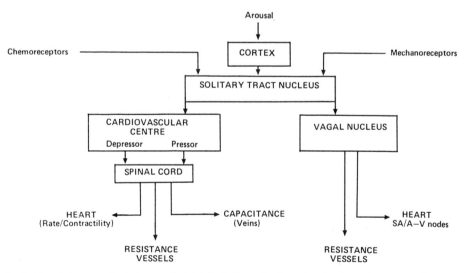

Fig. 26.10. Outline of anatomical sites and physiological mechanisms involved in the autonomic control of the cardiovascular system.

myocardial contractility. Conversely, any decrease in the activity of the depressor cells will allow pressor activity to predominate.

Earlier in the chapter we considered the place of the catecholamines in the peripheral autonomic nervous system and, obviously, they must have a cardinal role in the regulation of arterial pressure as the link between the efferent nerve and the effector mechanism. However, there seems little doubt that adrenaline and noradenaline, in particular, have also a substantial central role in the regulation of arterial pressure. Certainly, those areas of the brain which appear to subserve the regulation of arterial pressure contain many noradrenaline- and adrenaline-containing neurones. Pharmacological studies using drugs with selective adrenoceptor agonist or antagonist properties suggest that these central neurotransmitters exert their effects via α_2-adrenoceptors. More recent studies have reported that endogenous opioids, substance P and other peptides can be isolated from the nucleus tractus solitarius and the hypothalamus, and that the baroreceptor reflex can be attentuated by the central administration of enkephalin. Their precise role in the regulation of arterial pressure in man is unclear but there seems little doubt that they do have a place as witnessed by the selective effects of certain adrenoreceptor agonists and antagonists in patients with neurological disease.

From an anaesthetic point of view it has been suggested that certain of the available anaesthetic agents may inhibit selectively certain groups of cells. For example, cyclopropane, ketamine and di-ethyl ether have been thought to inhibit the depressor cells and this could underlie the evidence of sympathetic stimulation observed during their administration. In contrast, the barbiturates, halothane and enflurane, may inhibit selectively the pressor grouping of cells.

EFFERENT CONNECTIONS

The efferent pathways from the central control system to the effector organs have been detailed in the previous section. However, for completeness they are shown schematically in *Fig.* 26.10. From this diagram it is clear that the principle *effectors* are the heart, the resistance vessels, the capacitance vessels (and in a sense, the adrenal medulla).

EFFECTORS

Since arterial pressure is the mathematical product of the cardiac output and the systemic vascular resistance, it stands to reason that, if systemic vascular resistance remained constant, arterial pressure would be a direct function of the cardiac output. Obviously, of course, systemic vascular resistance (the sum of all the local resistances discussed earlier) must be changing continually. Nevertheless, it is the output of the pump which generates the 'head' of pressure considered so vital to the maintenance of local blood flow. Since this is so, we will consider first the role of the autonomic nervous system in the modulation of cardiac output and then the changes in systemic vascular resistance associated with autonomic activity.

REGULATION OF CARDIAC OUTPUT

Cardiac output is governed by three main mechanisms:

(i) the intrinsic adaptation of the myocardial muscle fibres to changes in ventricular end-diastolic volume;

(ii) the extrinsic, neurogenically mediated effects of changes in autonomic activity; and

(iii) the background control of blood volume.

At first glance it might seem as if, of the three mechanisms cited, only (ii) would be relevant to the present discussion. However, as we shall see, the autonomic nervous system plays some part in each, although that part is comparatively minor in relation to mechanisms (i) and (iii).

Cardiac output is the product of heart rate and stroke volume, both of which can be influenced by the autonomic nervous system.

Heart rate

Heart rate, at any one point in time, is determined by the balance between the activities of the sympathetic and parasympathetic components of the autonomic nervous system, as exerted primarily on the *sino-atrial node*. In the normal, healthy individual at rest, para-sympathetic activity predominates and the resting heart rate is around 60–70 beats/min. Heart rate increases to around 105 beats/min if both the sympathetic and parasympathetic neural connections to the heart are blocked or interrupted. Loss of sympathetic activity alone (spinal cord transection) results in a decrease in heart rate (to around 40 beats/min) on account of the loss of the sympathetically mediated suppression of parasympathetic activity. Heart rate decreases naturally during sleep, and can be decreased if parasympathetic activity is increased either physiologically (carotid sinus massage), iatrogenically (distension of a hollow viscus, tracheal suction, pressure on the eyeball) or pharmacologically (anticholinesterases). As discussed earlier, an increase in heart rate accompanies increases in sympathetic activity which, likewise, may be the physiological response to a change in posture, an increase in activity or emotional stress; or result from the administration of sympathomimetic drugs (or drugs that inhibit parasympathetic activity); or be due to iatrogenic stimuli (incision of the skin, skeletal pain, tracheal intubation).

Although heart rate can be a primary determinant of cardiac output, this is only really so when the heart rate decreases or increases substantially. Although cardiac output will decrease under both these situations, more minor fluctuations in rate are often accompanied by changes in stroke volume such that cardiac output changes little. However, during exercise a different situation pertains; cardiac output will increase in association with a substantial increase in heart rate because of the sympathetically mediated improvement in the diastolic filling and contractility of the heart which accompany the increase in venous return.

Stroke volume

The stroke volume is the volume of blood ejected from the heart with each contraction and represents the difference between ventricular end-diastolic and end-systolic volumes. As such, it can be influenced by a number of factors: those that affect end-diastolic volume (ventricular compliance, effective ventricular filling pressure and the time available for ventricular filling) and those that affect end-systolic volume (afterload, myocardial contractility). However, for the purposes of the present discussion, it is probably sufficient to indicate that the efficiency of the heart as a pump depends largely on intrinsic mechanisms (the Frank–Starling mechanism and the ability of the myocardium to develop tension from a given end-diastolic fibre length) and that these can be influenced by extrinsic factors such as alterations in the biochemical environment of the myocardial cells and by alterations in the activity of the autonomic nervous system, be this mediated neurogenically via the sympathetic nerves to the heart or by alterations in the concentrations of circulating catecholamines — whether endogenous (noradrenaline) or exogenous (isoprenaline). The Frank–Starling mechanism relates the force of contraction to the length of the myocardial muscle fibres at the start of systole. In this way the volume ejected during each cardiac cycle can be matched with the rate of filling (venous return). In addition, it provides an intrinsic mechanism which can maintain cardiac output in the face of alterations in arterial pressure. However, this relationship between stroke volume and ventricular filling is dependent on the inotropic state of the myocardium (myocardial contractility) — factors that increase contractility shift the Frank–Starling curve to the left: that is, stroke volume will increase for any given end-systolic fibre length.

The most important extrinsic factors affecting myocardial contractility are the level of neurogenic sympathetic activity and the circulating concentrations of catecholamines and other agents with inotropic (positive or negative) activity. Since ventricular muscle does not appear to receive any direct nerve supply from the vagus, changes in parasympathetic tone have no direct effect on myocardial contractility, although there may be a secondary effect mediated through changes in heart rate. Although it is difficult in man to determine the relative importance of the various mechanisms, it has been suggested that the intrinsic mechanisms alone can increase cardiac output by 2·5–3 fold. If an increase of greater magnitude is required, this is mediated through increases in autonomic activity.

Apart from the effects described above, the autonomic nervous system can influence stroke volume secondarily by the *mobilization* of blood from its store in the capacitance vessels. This is brought about, usually to compensate for a decrease in circulating blood volume, by sympathetically mediated venoconstriction (*see below*). In this way, the stroke volume (and hence, the cardiac output) can be augmented by a combination of the heart's own intrinsic mechanism and an extrinsic neurogenic mechanism.

VASCULAR RESISTANCE

The calibre of the resistance vessels, which comprise in the main the arterioles and pre-capillary sphincters, is under the control of local and general mechanisms. Once again, autonomic activity is integrated with other mechanisms in the overall regulation of vessel calibre.

Local mechanisms

Arteriolar smooth muscle has its own inherent tone which is quite independent of metabolic or extrinsic neurogenic mechanisms and which varies from organ to organ. For example, arteriolar tone is high in the myocardium, skeletal muscle and the brain (organs in which sympathetic innervation is sparse) and is virtually absent in cutaneous arteriovenous anastomoses.

From our previous considerations in this chapter it will be apparent that the degree of dilatation or constriction of an arteriole depends also on the activity of the local tissue (metabolic autoregulation, p. 273) and on the concentrations of various chemicals produced locally (histamine, 5-hydroxytryptamine). In most tissues alterations in vascular resistance can be mediated by changes in local tissue oxygen and/or carbon dioxide tensions: an increase in carbon dioxide tension and/or a decrease in oxygen tension producing vasodilatation.

General mechanisms

These are principally neurogenic or humoral. Under normal conditions the most important mechanism producing widespread vasoconstriction is an increase in activity in sympathetic vasoconstrictor nerves.

Most tissues receive a certain amount of resting sympathetic 'tone', changes in vascular calibre being brought about by changes in this tone. However, the degree of sympathetic 'tone' varies between organs — as does the importance of sympathetic activity in the control of vascular calibre. For example, the heart and the brain receive little sympathetic innervation yet the intrinsic vascular tone is high. The intestine and the kidney have a relatively greater sympathetic innervation but relatively less inherent vascular tone. As a result, any generalized increase in sympathetic activity will induce substantially more vasoconstriction in the splanchnic and renal vascular beds than in those of the heart and brain. In other words, such an increase in sympathetic activity can not only cause a *mobilization* of blood but also a *redistribution* of blood. In general terms, such a redistribution is considered to be of benefit to the organism in that in states of 'stress' the perfusion of the most vital organs is preserved. However, the vasoconstriction in the less vital organs can, if severe enough, cause a critical decrease in blood flow and the resultant release of toxic metabolites into the general circulation where they may affect adversely other organs which are not ischaemic of themselves.

Capacitance vessels

Veins have two physiological roles: they conduct blood back to the heart from the tissues and they act as low-pressure reservoirs in which a considerable volume of blood can be stored (65–70 per cent of the circulating blood volume) and from which it can be mobilized in an emergency. In general, adrenoceptors on the capacitance vessels appear to be α in type (receptors on resistance vessels are α and β) and, in contrast to the *selective* vasoconstriction of the resistance vessels which accompanies sympathetic stimulation, constriction of the capacitance vessels tends to occur uniformly throughout the body. Having said that, however, a large percentage of any blood so mobilized must come from the 'splanchnic venous reservoir' since this is probably the largest store of readily available blood in the body. In addition, it will be apparent that the effectiveness or otherwise of the selective redistribution of blood described earlier is dependent also on the transfer of blood volume from the intestinal vascular bed to other areas. Obviously, under conditions of physiological trespass the organism is markedly dependent on the ready availability of this store of blood within the splanchnic circulation. However, the sympathetic nervous system is not the only influence on this vascular bed: a number of humoral factors (eg 5-hydroxytryptamine) and certain circulating hormones (gastrin, secretin, etc.) can all affect directly the calibre of the splanchnic blood vessels.

Thus far we have considered the actions of sympathetic vasoconstrictor nerves on vascular resistance. Certainly, these are by far the most important from a physiological point of view, but we should remind ourselves that the autonomic nervous sytem also supplies *sympathetic vasodilator* (cholinergic) fibres and *parasympathetic vasodilator* (cholinergic) nerves. The parasympathetic fibres seem to have no role in the general control of the peripheral circulation. Sympathetic vasodilator fibres, on the other hand, are found in the arteries of skeletal muscle and perhaps also of the myocardium. These are the nerves that activate the vasodilatation in muscle vessels in preparation for exercise or muscular activity.

The last of the various mechanisms worthy of consideration is that related to the angiotensin-induced modulation of vascular calibre. *Angiotensin II* is the most active endogenous vasoconstrictor in the body. Its formation is dependent on the release of renin from the *juxtaglomerular cells* in the endothelium of the afferent renal arterioles, *renin* being released by (among other mechanisms) an increase in renal sympathetic activity.

While it is generally accepted that there is no basal sympathetic tone in the kidneys of man at rest, the sympathetic nervous system supplies richly the major arterial vessels in the renal cortex. Activation of the sympathetic nervous system results from stimuli received from the high- and low-pressure mechanoreceptors (arterial pressure) and the arterial chemoreceptors (hypoxaemia) mediated through the central control system. The vasoconstrictor response appears to be related to the degree of stress such that with severe stress, oliguria can result from the induced decreases in the renal blood flow and glomerular filtration.

In addition, and under specific circumstances, angiotensin II may induce an increase in the release of *antidiuretic hormone* (ADH). ADH is synthesized in the supra-optic and paraventricular nuclei of the hypothalamus (Chapter 25). It is stored in the posterior pituitary gland from whence it is released by several mechanisms: the low-pressure baroreceptors sense small decreases in blood volume; more marked decreases in blood volume are sensed by the high-pressure baroreceptors. In addition, changes in blood osmolarity stimulate *osmoreceptors* to modulate the release of vasopressin, as do high circulating concentrations of angiotensin II. Although the primary function of ADH is to maintain blood volume by increasing the reabsorption of water in the terminal part of the renal tubule, it can, if the plasma concentration is high, produce significant vasoconstriction in the muscle, splanchnic and coronary vascular beds. Originally ADH was called 'vasopressin' because it demonstrated these vasoconstrictor properties when administered in pharmacological doses. Vasoconstriction is not seen with physiological concentrations.

Regulation of gastrointestinal function

The basic design of the gastrointestinal system is that of a long tube surrounded by muscle and into which the secretions of various glands are passed. The muscular elements contract and relax to propel and churn the contents: the glandular secretions aid the breakdown of the food particles and facilitate the absorption of nutrients. Considered as a whole, the regulation of gastrointestinal function is a complex and confusing network of regulatory factors and feedback control mechanisms. However, in this section we will consider primarily the role played by the autonomic nervous system in these processes. The most relevant of the other control mechanisms will be introduced briefly so that the regulatory functions of the autonomic nervous system can be considered in context.

In the previous section we have touched upon the part played by the autonomic nervous system in the regulation of blood flow within the splanchnic circulation. In that discussion, it was noted that, in addition to neurogenic regulatory mechanisms, the arterioles in the gastrointestinal circulation could be influenced by hormonal factors. Likewise, it appears as if the gastrointestinal tract itself — its secretion, motility and possibly absorption — are regulated by the same two basic mechanisms: the autonomic nervous system, particularly the parasympathetic component, and by hormones released from the mucosal lining of the stomach and intestine during digestion.

NEUROGENIC CONTROL

The gastrointestinal tract is innervated extensively by sympathetic and parasympathetic efferent fibres, although, as will be evident from *Fig.* 26.1, the major portions of the autonomic (parasympathetic) supply are concentrated at the upper (down to the pylorus) and lower (from mid-colon to anus) ends. Although less important from a purely physiological point of view, the sympathetic component of the autonomic supply to the intestine is distributed more evenly and more widely throughout the length of the gastrointestinal tract. However, like most autonomically innervated organs, the gastrointestinal tract can act quite independently of any extrinsic neural mechanisms: it has its own *intrinsic nervous system.*

This consists of two layers of neurones and appropriate connecting fibres: the *myenteric plexus* (outer layer) lies between the longitudinal and circular layers of muscle, the *submucosal plexus* (inner layer) lying in the submucosa. This system provides the basic control mechanisms for almost all gastrointestinal functions — especially those subserving motility (myenteric plexus) and those subserving secretion (submucosal plexus). As far as both plexuses are concerned, the majority of the neurones occur in groups or ganglia which are joined together in mesh-like groupings of fibres. Many of the fibres contain *peptides* (substance P, enkephalin, somatostatin, vasoactive intestinal polypeptide (VIP)) and in some of the neurones there is evidence of the presence of two transmitter substances in a single neurone. In addition to the efferent activity described above, the submucosal plexus, in particular, may have a sensory role in that it receives information from receptors in the wall of the intestine which may respond to stretch (over-distension), and from the intestinal mucosa itself which may react to physical irritation, chemicals or other substances likely to be toxic to the organism.

In general, stimulation of the myenteric plexus increases the activity of the gut: the excitatory fibres are largely cholinergic — that is, they secrete acetylcholine. In addition, however, it has been suggested that some of the myenteric plexus fibres secrete other transmitters and that these are inhibitory to the intestine rather than excitatory (*see below*).

Rhythmic contractile activity is a characteristic of most types of smooth muscle and this is also true of the gastrointestinal tract. However, even although such activity is a basic characteristic of the gastrointestinal tract, it is depressed in portions of the intestine in which there is congenital absence of the myenteric plexus.

The neural connections and the distributions of the autonomic innervation to the gastrointestinal tract were described earlier and need not be considered further apart from reminding ourselves that the postganglionic parasympathetic neurones are integrated closely with the myenteric plexus: the preganglionic fibres terminate on the intrinsic enteric neurones and an increase in parasympathetic activity induces a general increase in those functions subserved by that plexus: for example, the intensity of peristalsis and its velocity of propagation. However, efferent preganglionic fibres from the vagus also innervate neurones which are neither cholinergic nor adrenergic and in which the transmitter may be VIP. Such neurones are inhibitory to the intestine and cause, for example, relaxation of the body of the stomach and vasodilatation in the colon.

In general, *parasympathetic* activation increases organized motor activity in the gastrointestinal tract, relaxes sphincters and, in this way, improves mixing and accelerates forward movement of the intestinal contents. In addition, parasympathetic activation stimulates the secretion of saliva, gastric and pancreatic juices and bile. Consequently, food is digested into simpler molecules which can then be absorbed by the small intestine. Vagal stimulation evokes directly the release of gastrin and indirectly the release of other *intestinal hormones*, through the stimulation of gastric secretion and emptying.

In general terms stimulation of the *sympathetic* nervous system has effects essentially opposite to those of the parasympathetic system: it inhibits activity in the gastrointestinal tract. This is achieved in two ways: first, by a direct effect of the noradrenaline released from the adrenergic nerve terminal on the smooth muscle of the gastrointestinal tract and, secondly, by an inhibitory effect of noradrenaline on the intrinsic nervous system. Although, in some ways, the sympathetic nervous system does not have a large part to play in normal gastrointestinal function, in certain stressful situations if the stimulation of the sympathetic system is strong enough, motility can be suppressed to such an extent that there is little, if any, movement of contents. In addition, the mucosal blood flow of the gastrointestinal tract can be reduced substantially under such conditions and this may result in ulceration or gangrene of the wall of the intestine.

Although the aforementioned are the main neurogenic components involved in the regulation of gastrointestinal function, it is obvious from everyday life that there is considerable modulation of these functions by higher structures in the brain. For example, at the highest cortical levels man must integrate his desire for food and his requirement for nutrition with his environment, the kind of food available and his state of health. It is obvious that anxiety can increase gastrointestinal motility and, indeed, the secretion of acid in the stomach. At a lower level, the modulation by higher autonomic integrated centres appears to involve an inhibition of incoming stimuli.

With this as a general introduction to the parts played by the major components of the autonomic nervous system in the regulation of gastrointestinal function, let us consider in a little more detail the mechanisms modulating function in those two areas of the intestinal tract which are of particular importance to the anaesthetist — the oesophagus and the stomach.

THE OESOPHAGUS: THE ROLE OF THE AUTONOMIC NERVOUS SYSTEM

In man, the muscular coat of the oesophagus can be divided into an upper (2–6 cm) striated section, a lower (lower third) smooth muscle section and an intermediate or middle section which contains a mixture of both types. The striated muscle of the oesophagus is innervated by special visceral efferent nerve fibres which terminate on motor endplates not too dissimilar from those found in skeletal muscle: action potentials are similar to those recorded in classic motor units. The smooth muscle in the oesophagus is innervated via the local nerve plexuses.

OESOPHAGEAL SPHINCTERS

The upper end of the oesophagus is closed by the so-called pharyngo-oesophageal sphincter: closure prevents the regurgitation of oesophageal contents into the pharynx and the aspiration of air into the oesophagus during inspiration. A zone of high pressure — some 2·5–4·5 cm in length — can be demonstrated and is thought to be due to the active contraction of motor units in the cricopharyngeus muscle. These are inhibited during swallowing, relaxation of the sphincter permitting the passage of food into the oesophagus. Likewise, at the lower end of the oesophagus, there is evidence of a high pressure zone (about 4 cm in length) which is situated partly within the abdomen and partly within the thoracic cavity. Intraluminal pressure measured in this zone is about 20 mmHg greater than that measured simultaneously in the fundus of the stomach and is considered to be one of the principal mechanisms preventing gastro-oesophageal reflux. The pressure developed depends on the degree of contraction, the 'tone', in the circular muscle of the oesophagus at this level plus that of the surrounding (extrinsic) muscle fibres and connective tissues of the diaphragm. This differentiation is of interest since the physiological (and possibly pharmacological) characteristics of the two types of muscle differ: the smooth muscle being influenced by intrinsic, the diaphragm by extrinsic factors.

Although the anatomical components of the lower oesophageal sphincter appear reasonably discrete, the physiological mechanisms involved are less clear. As alluded to above, the resting tone in the lower oesophageal sphincter appears to be an intrinsic property of the muscle(s) in that region. However, this tone may be influenced by a wide variety of neurogenic, hormonal and pharmacological factors. Obviously, relaxation of the lower oesophageal sphincter must be part of the normal process of swallowing and it may be that relaxation of the sphincter is associated with the stimulation of local mechanoreceptors which, acting via the local intramural plexuses, decrease sphincter tone. However, swallowing is an integrated coordinated physiological activity and it would seem only natural that there should be some role for neurogenic mechanisms extrinsic to the oesophagus itself. Certainly, there is evidence that the preganglionic (cholinergic) vagal fibres and the postganglionic (inhibitory) fibres described above are involved, although to what extent is unclear. However, it is thought that the former are under the control of the 'swallowing centre' (Chapter 20) and, since they pass distally in the wall of the oesophagus to synapse with inhibitory neurones in the smooth muscle of the sphincter, may have a role in the coordination of the movement of food through the oesophagus and into the stomach.

In addition to the neurogenic components, tone in the lower oesophageal sphincter can be modified by *humoral factors*. These can be inhibitory (GABA, adenine, prostaglandins E1 and E2) and cause relaxation of the sphincter, or stimulation (acetylcholine, histamine, 5-hydroxytryptamine) and induce an increase in tone. Likewise, drugs can be classified broadly into those, such as metoclopramide, domperidone, neostigmine and α-adrenoceptor agonists, that increase sphincter tone, those that decrease sphincter tone (for example, atropine, glycopyrrolate, volatile anaesthetic agents and β-adrenoceptor agonists), and those drugs that appear to have no direct effect on the degree of tone in the sphincter (cimetidine, ranitidine, propranolol, oxprenolol).

OESOPHAGEAL MOTILITY

In contrast to the other parts of the gastrointestinal tract, the oesophagus has little or no inherent spontaneous contractile activity. Certainly, this appears to be so as far as the upper and middle thirds of the oesophagus (the areas with striated muscle) are concerned. There is some evidence that there may be spontaneous contractile activity in the lower oesophagus, which is based on local neural circuits.

What is not in doubt is that contractile activity (peristalsis) can be induced in the oesophagus by neurogenic mechanisms and can be provoked by the presence of food (or foreign body). Swallowing induces a wave of contractile activity which commences in the posterior wall of the pharynx and progresses down the entire length of the oesophagus to the lower oesophageal sphincter: that is, it involves both the striated and smooth muscle components of the oesophagus.

In the striated muscle peristalsis is regulated neurogenically via a 'swallowing centre' in the medulla. This has neural connections with the cortex, with the substantia reticularis and with the motor nuclei of the Vth, VIIth, Xth and XIth cranial nerves. Peristalsis can be initiated voluntarily or as a result of local stimuli in the oropharynx, hypopharynx or in the oesophagus itself. Although there is some debate as to the precise mechanism for the progression of the peristaltic wave down the oesophagus, it must ensure the sequential firing of efferent impulses to progressively more distal segments in the oesophagus along with (probably) inhibition of contractile activity in those segments more distal to the advancing wave of contraction. It has been suggested that the circular muscle of the oesophagus receives not only postganglionic cholinergic (excitatory) impulses, but also impulses from the non-adrenergic, non-cholinergic (inhibitory) fibres described earlier. In this way, contraction at any level in the oesophagus is associated with inhibition in a more distal segment.

As far as the lower one-third of the oesophagus is concerned, three kinds of contractile waves have been described. The *primary peristaltic wave* (described above) is associated with the normal process of swallowing. A secondary wave, which is a reflex response to distension (provoked lower oesophageal contractions), may indicate the presence of a local myogenic mechanism in this part of the stomach. The third (tertiary) is a *non-peristaltic contraction* which is thought to result from various stimuli (for example, acoustic) induced some distance from the oesophagus. These are referred to as *spontaneous lower oesophageal contractions*. Interestingly, the amplitude of the secondary, and the frequency of the tertiary, contractions may be related to the depth of anaesthesia — variations in relevant amplitude or frequency being equated with variations in the depth of anaesthesia.

THE STOMACH: THE ROLE OF THE AUTONOMIC NERVOUS SYSTEM

The physiological importance of the stomach is clear: it receives and stores food and fluids temporarily, thus allowing us to eat meals at discrete times, it secretes a digestive juice which converts the ingested food into semiliquid chyme and it secretes intrinsic factor. However, of the many aspects of gastric physiology, two are of particular interest to the anaesthetist: the secretion and composition of gastric juice and the factors that influence the emptying of the stomach.

GASTRIC SECRETION

The juice actually secreted by the stomach is a mixture composed of the secretions from four different types of cells, three of which lie in the mucosal lining of the stomach: parietal cells, peptic cells, mucous cells and surface epithelial cells. The *parietal cells* elaborate a solution containing about 170 mmol/l hydrochloric acid (plus the intrinsic factor); the *peptic cells* secrete pepsinogen, the precursor of the proteolytic enzyme pepsin; the *mucous cells* produce a small volume of a complex organic gel (mucus) composed of various macromolecules.

The degree of activity in the various gastric glands is determined by an interplay between many stimulatory and inhibitory influences — as depicted diagrammatically in *Fig.* 26.11 from which it can be seen that gastric secretion is regulated by neurogenic and hormonal factors. Let us look at some of the more important influences and, in particular, at the role of the autonomic nervous system in their release.

Acetylcholine

Vagal efferent fibres release acetylcholine at three sites: at the serosal membrane of the parietal cell (influencing the secretion of acid); at the neurones of the intrinsic cholinergic nerves in the wall of the stomach (influencing gastric motility); and at the G cells in the antral mucosa (influencing the release of gastrin). The release of acetylcholine can be stimulated via influences from the hypothalamus, the medullary vagal centres or by local stimulation of the vagal nerves either directly (as by distension of the stomach) or indirectly via cholinergic reflexes. In addition, as might be expected, the release of acetylcholine can be induced by cortical influences: the anticipation or smell and taste of food, increasing the amount of acid secreted by the stomach (see Chapter 14).

Gastrin

As described above, parasympathetic activity plays a role in the secretion of gastrin — mainly during the 'cephalic' phase of gastric secretion and in association with distension of the stomach. However, the major secretion of gastrin is during the 'gastric' phase when food is actually in the stomach and the principal releasing agents are amino acids and peptides derived from the food, especially from protein.

Histamine

Although the gastric mucosa contains substantial amounts of histamine, the actual role played by histamine in the production of the gastric secretion(s) has been debated for decades. There is no doubt that the injection of histamine will increase the secretion of acid. Equally, it is clear that H_2-receptor antagonists inhibit the secretory response to gastrin, acetylcholine and other stimulators. It has been suggested that histamine is being released continuously in the gastric mucosa — in small amounts — and that, consequently, it is 'the

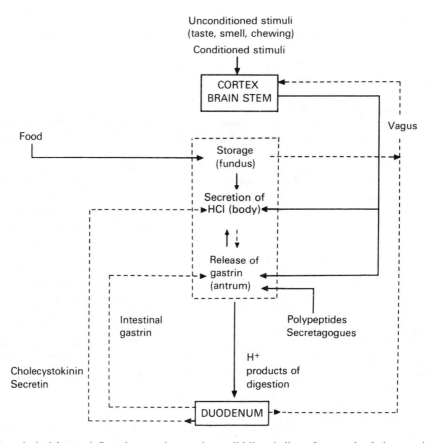

Fig. 26.11. The principal factors influencing gastric secretion: solid lines indicate factors stimulating gastric secretion, broken lines those inhibiting gastric secretion.

final common local chemostimulator of the parietal cells of the gastric mucosa'. In other words, it is possible that all the other stimulants of secretion such as acetylcholine and gastrin produce their stimulation of the parietal cells via histamine as a mediator.

Other substances

Corticosteroid hormones and increases in blood calcium concentration can influence the secretion of acid and pepsin. However, as the autonomic nervous system is not involved in these mechanisms, they will not be considered further.

Sympathetic nerves are distributed to the stomach, the stimulation of which inhibits the secretion of acid. Likewise, adrenoceptor agonists will suppress gastric secretion as does

the administration of antidiuretic hormone. In fact, gastrin itself — although a direct stimulant of the parietal cell — will decrease the secretion of acid indirectly via a decrease in blood calcium concentration. However, the most relevant negative feedback on the secretion of acid is the presence of acid itself on the antral mucosa and in the duodenum. In this instance a local inhibitory signal inhibits further secretion of gastrin: in the latter instance the release of *secretin, cholecystokinin and gastric inhibitory peptide* inhibit the further secretion of acid in the stomach.

GASTRIC EMPTYING

The importance of gastric emptying in the perioperative period is threefold: a delay in gastric emptying means that the volume of the gastric contents is increased and this may predispose to nausea and vomiting; the increase in the volume of acid gastric contents will increase the likelihood of pulmonary pneumonitis should these contents be inhaled into the lungs; and the absorption of orally administered drugs will be erratic.

Gastric motility is controlled by many factors: neurogenic, hormonal, chemical. The stomach is well supplied with nerve plexuses — the intrinsic (myenteric) plexus and extrinsic nerves from both parasympathetic and sympathetic components of the autonomic nervous system. In the upper (orad) half of the stomach stimulation of vagal (and sympathetic) efferent nerves induces relaxation. There is little contractile activity of this area, its main physiological role being to accommodate the ingested food, a function aided by the increase in distensibility induced by secretin and cholecystokinin. In the distal (caudad) half of the stomach, electrophysiological recordings show evidence of a basal intrinsic electrical rhythm (gastric slow wave), a partial depolarization of the muscle cell membrane which occurs every 20 seconds. This *basal electrical rhythm* does not initiate a mechanical contraction directly, although at a given point in the depolarization of the slow wave, a spike potential may be generated. This fast activity is associated with a mechanical contraction, the strength of the contraction depending on the muscle mass involved. However, the frequency of contraction is a function of the basal electrical rhythm. Although the basal electrical rhythm will persist if the vagus nerves are cut, it will lose its degree of coordination and the number of spike potentials will decrease. Conversely, stimulation of the *vagus nerves* will increase the number of spike potentials and, hence, the force and frequency of contractile activity in the distal half of the stomach. The frequency of the basal electrical rhythm is increased by *gastrin*: hence, the increase in gastric motility produced by gastrin.

Emptying of the stomach requires coordinated activity of these aforementioned factors: the intrinsic nerve plexuses, extrinsic neurogenic influences (particularly the autonomic nervous system), the inherent myogenic contractility of the stomach and various hormones. In addition, the nature and composition of the gastric contents influence emptying: fat and protein delaying emptying. Physiologically, the regulation of *gastric emptying* is under the control of a number of negative feedback mechanisms (*Fig. 26.12*): an increase in parasympathetic activity increases the rate of emptying, sensors in the duodenum respond to the presence of food in the duodenum and

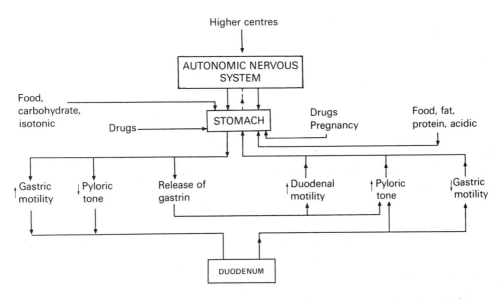

Fig. 26.12. Schematic representation of the major factors influencing the rate of gastric emptying.

Table 26.3. Some factors influencing the rate of gastric emptying

	Increase	*Decrease*
Physiological	Distension of the stomach Anxiety	Food Acid Posture High osmotic pressure
Pathological	Thyrotoxicosis	Pain/trauma/'shock' Pyloric stenosis Crohn's disease Coeliac disease Myocardial infarction
Pharmacological	Metoclopramide Neostigmine Propranolol Sodium bicarbonate Cigarette smoking	Anticholinergics Tricyclic antidepressants Aluminium hydroxide Alcohol Isoprenaline Opioid analgesics

decrease the rate of gastric emptying, and so on. Importantly, neural influences (pain, anxiety) can decrease gastric emptying, as can a variety of pharmacological agents (*Table* 26.3).

This is a fairly basic consideration of the role of the autonomic nervous system in the modulation of oesophageal and gastric function: certain aspects have been highlighted while other aspects have not been considered. However, we believe that those included are not only those which depict clearly the interrelations between autonomic control and other control systems, but are also those of most immediate relevance to anaesthesia.

The regulation of micturition

In its simplest terms, micturition can be considered as a local spinal reflex which is subject to regulation and modulation by higher centres in the brain itself. However, although micturition may appear simple in concept, in practice the actual mechanisms which subserve micturition are unique, and involve a coordinated series of reflexes which are integrated in a hierarchical fashion at many different levels within the central nervous system. Not surprisingly, therefore, we have chosen a consideration of these mechanisms as an appropriate

third example of the functional interrelationships which exist between the autonomic nervous system and other control mechanisms.

ANATOMICAL CONSIDERATIONS

The walls of the bladder are composed of thick layers of smooth muscle and it has been customary to consider this as consisting of two component parts: the *detrusor muscle*, which makes up the globular body of the bladder, and the funnel-shaped muscle at the outlet which comprises the *internal urethral sphincter*. More recent studies have challenged this view and shown that the intermingled network of the detrusor muscle extends down to the internal orifice of the bladder where it becomes organized into three layers: an external and an internal longitudinal layer and a middle circular layer. The muscle fibres of the internal longitudinal layer extend into the urethra. However, although there is no anatomical internal urethral sphincter, since the neck of the bladder and the proximal part of the urethra are made up of smooth muscle fibres and elastic fibres, they can be considered as comprising a physiological internal urethral sphincter. Some 2 cm distal to the base of the bladder the urethra passes through the *urogenital diaphragm*, the striated muscle of

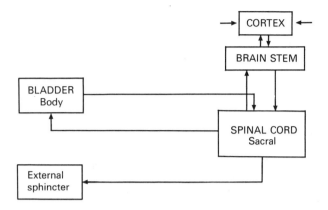

Fig. 26.13. Schematic representation of central and peripheral mechanisms subserving the control of micturition. The postganglionic sympathetic influence on parasympathetic ganglia has been omitted for clarity.

which constitutes the external urethral sphincter.

NEUROGENIC CONSIDERATIONS

Like other smooth muscle viscera the bladder has some inherent (non-neurogenic) contractile activity: if denervated the bladder will empty itself partially once a certain degree of filling has been achieved. However, when its nerve supply is intact, neurogenic control is superimposed on this autonomous activity. As far as neurogenic control is concerned, it is clear that in the normal healthy adult, this must involve central as well as peripheral mechanisms (*Fig.* 26.13): micturition can be initiated and/or terminated at will. However, it is just as clear that micturition can be mediated solely by peripheral reflex mechanisms as witnessed by the 'autonomic' bladder associated with transection of the spinal cord (above the sacral segments).

PERIPHERAL MECHANISMS

Stretch (mechano) receptors lie within the smooth muscle of the bladder and, possibly, in the submucosa. In the muscle these are arranged in series with the detrusor muscle fibres and are stimulated by increases in tension. There is, however, some debate as to whether these receptors are stimulated by the filling of the bladder *per se*, or whether they respond to an increase in the inherent rhythmic activity of the bladder — which has been produced secondarily as the smooth muscle is stretched during filling. Whatever the precise underlying mechanism, impulses generated in these sensory receptors are necessary prerequisites fo the initiation of micturition. Afferent information from these receptors reaches the spinal cord (S2–4) via the *pelvic nerves* and then travels to the brain stem primarily in the contralateral *spinothalamic tract*. It is believed that this 'supraspinal loop' involves the pontine micturition centre discussed below, and that this concept of a spino-bulbar-spinal reflex is fundamental to any consideration of the physiological control of micturition.

Bladder sensation may be preserved, however, after section of the spinothalamic tracts (which has produced sacral anaesthesia bilaterally), and the contribution of spinobulbar fibres (present in the superficial paramedian layer of the *dorsal column*) to the central transmission of information, relating in particular to passive distension of the bladder, has been recognized. Other sacrobulbar fibres ascend in the anterolateral part of the spinal cord having crossed in the lumbar segments. Afferent innervation of the urethra proximal to the prostate is by the *pelvic and hypogastric nerves*. Distal to the prostate sensory information is carried centrally in the *pudendal nerves*. The sensation that micturition is about to begin (urgency) is thought to originate in the urethra and be mediated centripetally via the pudendal nerves and the posterior columns.

The efferent arm of the reflex arc consists of parasympathetic fibres which originate in the spinal cord (S2–4) and travel via the *pelvic nerves* to ganglia on the surface of the bladder. *Postganglionic fibres* pass to the detrusor muscle and to the urethra, being distributed widely over the body and base of the bladder. Although acetylcholine is the most likely transmitter in man, at these postganglionic parasympathetic nerve endings there is some evidence that *adenosine triphosphate* may be the non-adrenergic, non-cholinergic transmitter in this pathway.

Many years ago it was suggested that the *parasympathetic* fibres had an inhibitory influence on the 'internal sphincter'. Recent studies have shown that parasympathetically mediated relaxation of the urethra can occur. Short *adrenergic* fibres which synapse in the pelvic ganglia and then pass directly to the urethra are thought to be involved.

In addition, the bladder is supplied by *sympathetic* fibres which travel via the *hypogastric nerves* and are distributed throughout the bladder and to the urethra. However, the relative number and type of adrenoreceptors vary in different locations. In the body of the bladder the adrenoreceptors are comparatively few in number and are predominantly β in nature. Contrariwise, sympathetic innervation is denser in the urethra and at the base of the bladder and α-adrenoceptors predominate. In general, the sympathetic nerves to the bladder play no direct part in micturition. However, it has been shown that sympathetic stimulation can induce a contraction of the bladder which is then followed by a relaxation. The contraction can be modified by phenoxybenzamine, the relaxation blocked with propranolol. In addition, sympathetic stimulation can facilitate or inhibit transmission through the pelvic (parasympathetic) ganglia — the actual effect being determined (possibly) by the amount of transmitter released. Sympathetic fibres do mediate the contraction of the bladder muscle that prevents semen from entering the bladder during ejaculation.

Voluntary contraction of the perineal muscles and the external urethral sphincter is mediated by the pudendal nerves in which continuous *somatic efferent* activity maintains the closure of the external urethral sphincter as the bladder fills.

CENTRAL MECHANISMS

Several areas within the brain stem have been characterized as having facilitatory or inhibitory influences on the sacral reflex arc. For example, a facilitatory area is said to exist in the pons and an inhibitory area in the mid-brain. Another facilitatory area has been identified in the posterior hypothalamus. However, most of this information has been obtained from investigations in animals and the position in man is much less clear. Nevertheless, it is likely that even in man, involuntary micturition is coordinated at this level. Indeed, an area within the brain stem reticular formation (*pontine detrusor nucleus*) has been identified as being responsible for the final integration and coordination of bladder (and sphincteric) function. The nucleus locus coeruleus has been suggested as a possible anatomical site.

Not surprisingly, there is a substantial cerebral representation as far as micturition is concerned, and numerous studies have attempted to localize the relevant areas. Clinical observations in patients with tumours or following leucotomy have indicated that, as far as man is concerned, the voluntary control of micturition is mediated by specific areas on the *medial surface of the superior frontal gyrus* and the adjacent part of the anterior cingulate gyrus. So precise is this localization that alterations in social awareness (in relation to bladder function) may be diagnostic of a lesion in this area of the brain. Inhibitory and excitatory pathways descend from these areas of cortex to influence the detrusor centre in the pons, the sacral preganglionic neurones and the motor neurones supplying the external urethral sphincter. Whatever the details of the central neural network this means that the autonomic control of the smooth muscle of the bladder is normally regulated via a central reflex arc which is 'subordinated to even higher, voluntary, neurogenic authority'.

FUNCTIONAL CONSIDERATIONS

As urine collects in the pelvis of the kidney the pressure increases, a peristaltic contraction is initiated and the urine is forced towards the bladder. Essentially, the bladder has two functions: the storage of urine and the voiding of urine. During storage the bladder can accommodate the increasing volume of urine by relaxation of the detrusor muscle. In addition, the stretch receptors in the wall of the bladder may be 're-set' — by activity from the brain stem centre — so that the reflex is not initiated when the volume of urine in the bladder is small. As the bladder fills, the resistance of the outlet increases as do neuronal impulses to the external urethral sphincter.

As alluded to earlier, the inherent rhythmic contractions of the smooth muscle of the bladder wall increase in frequency as the bladder enlarges. As a result afferent impulses pass to the spinal cord where they may or may not initiate neural activity in the efferent pathway depending on the balance between the inhibitory and facilitatory influences being transmitted from the higher centres. If the reflex is initiated the increase in parasympathetic activity will stimulate the detrusor muscle to contract more forcibly and the resistance at the outlet of the bladder will decrease due to relaxation of the external urethral sphincter, relaxation of the bladder neck being brought about by the contraction of the inner longitudinal layer of muscle described earlier. As the bladder contracts there is an increase in afferent activity which in turn produces more efferent activity — the cycle repeating itself until a strong and sustained contraction of the wall of the bladder has developed.

VOLUNTARY MICTURITION

The precise mechanism by which micturition is initiated voluntarily is unclear but may depend on relaxation of perineal muscles as a preliminary step. Certainly, it does appear as if the autonomous rhythmic activity can be initiated, at almost any degree of filling of the bladder, by relaxation of the perineal muscles, or there may be voluntary facilitation of (or removal of inhibition from) the sacral reflex arc. Obviously, voluntary contraction of the abdominal muscles can empty the bladder by increasing the intra-abdominal pressure. However, this mechanism is more normally invoked as an aid to micturition rather than as an initiator of micturition.

Micturition stops naturally once the bladder is empty or may be terminated deliberately by contracting the perineal muscles and the external urethral sphincter voluntarily. The ability to maintain the external urethral sphincter in a contracted state is the result of a learning process, and is one of the mechanisms that enables the adult to delay micturition until an appropriate opportunity presents itself.

From the foregoing discussion it will be apparent that neural disorders of bladder function could be classified as: (i) those due to the interruption of afferent fibres (polyneuritis, tabes dorsalis, neoplasm, herpes zoster); (ii) those affecting the efferent pathways from the spinal cord (polyneuritis, diabetes mellitus, surgical procedures, trauma, intrathecal or extradural blockade); (iii) those due to interruption of both afferent and efferent components of the reflex arc (cauda equina tumours, trauma, caudal anaesthesia); (iv) those which interfere with the facilitatory and/or inhibitory pathways in the spinal cord (spinal cord neoplasms, spinal cord transection, multiple sclerosis); (v) lesions of the medial frontal cortex which remove 'social' or learned inhibition of reflex emptying of the bladder.

Although this description of the factors involved in the physiological control of bladder function has strayed beyond the precise remit of this chapter, we believe this has been justified for two reasons: first, because it is a prime example of the interplay between the autonomic nervous system and a wide range of other control mechanisms; secondly, because it is an example *par excellence* of the hierarchical organization of such inter-relationships within the nervous system (receptor level, organ level, segmental level, brain stem level, cortical level, learning 'level').

DISORDERS OF AUTONOMIC FUNCTION

Our principal concern in this book is with normal (physiological) function. However, since by their very presence in a hospital environment, patients present evidence of alterations to, or impairment of, this normal function, we have felt it appropriate on occasions to relate the disorders of function to the normal pattern just described. We propose to do the same at this point since we believe that there is relevance in an understanding of certain of the clinical conditions associated with disorders of autonomic function. However, it must be understood that our consideration of this topic will not be exhaustive and the interested reader is referred to the more detailed descriptions suggested under Further Reading.

Assessment of autonomic integrity

If a substantial portion of the autonomic nervous system is diseased, many of its functions — including sweating, control of body temperature and sexual activity — can be affected. However, the most clinically important abnormality is a disturbance of the physiological mechanisms regulating cardio-vascular function such that arterial pressure cannot be maintained in the face of minor stresses, such as changes in posture (postural or orthostatic hypotension). Obviously, this must relate to some disruption of the sympathetic nervous system, at some point between the hypothalamus and the periphery, and a number of tests can be utilized in an attempt to localize the lesion and/or assess its clinical significance (*Table* 26.4).

MEASUREMENT OF ARTERIAL PRESSURE

Systemic arterial pressure may alter little or decrease by 10–15 mmHg in the normal individual on moving from the recumbent to the standing position. Diastolic arterial pressure will change little (±5 mmHg). Postural hypotension is said to be present when the systolic arterial pressure decreases by more than 20 mmHg with the same change in posture. Diastolic and pulse pressures will decrease also. In the patient with postural hypotension the rate of decrease in pressure may be rapid and the extent of the decrease uncertain: consciousness may be lost. Thus, conventional upper arm sphygmomanometry is too imprecise and intra-arterial pressure should be monitored so that the extent and rapidity of the decrease in pressure can be assessed readily. The change in posture (60 degrees head-up) should be brought about using a tilting table since the patient can not only be rapidly returned to the horizontal but, in addition, the effects of the change in posture are studied without the requirement for muscular activity.

Table 26.4. Measurements required, and evidence for, localization of a lesion on the cardiovascular reflex arc

1. Lesion in sympathetic efferent fibres to capacity and resistance vessels
   Postural hypotension.
   No overshoot in arterial pressure on release of increased intrathoracic pressure (Valsalva)
   No increase in arterial pressure with stress
   Low plasma noradrenaline concentration when resting
   No increase in plasma noradrenaline concentration on tilting

2. Lesion in sympathetic efferent fibres to the heart
   No increase in heart rate during Valsalva (Phase II)
   No increase in heart rate on tilting
   No increase in heart rate following arousal
   No increase in heart rate on isometric exercise

3. Lesion in parasympathetic efferent fibres to the heart
   No increase in sinus arrhythmia associated with increase in tidal volume
   No effect on heart rate associated with carotid massage
   No increase in heart rate following administration of atropine

Measurements required
   Arterial pressure: either indirect or direct
   Heart rate: beat-by-beat
   Pulse volume: finger photoplethysmography
   Respiration: rate, volume, ability to breath hold
   Sweating: response to generalized increase in body temperature

---

Theoretically, the lesion could be located in the sympathetic efferent fibres to the capacitance and resistance vessels, in the sympathetic efferent supply to the heart, in the parasympathetic efferent fibres to the heart, in the afferent pathways from the baroreceptors, or in a number of sites on the reflex arc. In addition, the instability of arterial pressure noted in association with autonomic failure may be due to supersensitivity of partially denervated vessels to noradrenaline. A number of mental and physical stimuli will increase arterial pressure acutely in the normal individual: a sudden loud noise, a startle, rapid mental arithmetic, the cold pressor test (hand immersed in water at 4°C for 90 seconds). An increase in arterial pressure demonstrates the integrity of the efferent supply to the capacitance and resistance vessels.

MEASUREMENT OF HEART RATE

In the context of the present discussion, heart rate is usually obtained from the ECG (three-lead): the signal is fed through a ratemeter which determines each R–R interval and plots continuously the heart rate for each beat. In this way, changes in absolute heart rate, to physiological or pharmacological manipulations, can be assessed. For example, bradycardia and a decrease in arterial pressure usually accompany carotid sinus massage in the normal individual: the response is absent in autonomic failure. Tachycardia is usually associated with the administration of atropine but does not occur if the parasympathetic efferent supply to the heart is damaged. Likewise, sinus arrhythmia depends on intact parasympathetic efferents to the heart, and is abolished by atropine and absent in autonomic failure. The integrity of the sympathetic efferent fibres to the heart can be assessed by noting the increase (if any) in heart rate associated with tilting, cortical arousal or isometric exercise.

ASSESSMENT OF PERIPHERAL PULSE VOLUME

Since the blood vessels in the pulp of the finger are innervated by sympathetic fibres, finger plethysmography with a photoelectric sensor can be utilized to demonstrate evidence for or against normal sympathetic function.

VALSALVA MANOEUVRE

In this test of circulatory integrity the three indices of cardiovascular function described previously (arterial pressure, heart rate, peripheral blood flow) can be monitored simultaneously during and following the application of an acute increase in intrathoracic pressure. Normally, this is brought about by asking the patient to take a deep breath and then expire forcibly through a tube connected to a mercury manometer. If possible, a pressure of 30 mmHg is maintained for 12 seconds.

The normal cardiovascular response to the increased intrathoracic pressure is divided classically into four phases (*Fig. 26.14*).

Phase I: A small increase in arterial pressure due to the pressure exerted on the aorta by the increase in intrathoracic pressure.

Phase II: Progressive decreases in systolic, diastolic and pulse pressures as a result of the decrease in venous return (and hence, in cardiac output). The decreases in the arterial pressures should cease after the first few seconds (increase in sympathetic efferent activity to the resistance vessels) and will be associated with an increase in heart rate (alteration in balance between parasympathetic and sympathetic influences on heart).

Phase III: Arterial pressure decreases suddenly and briefly. This phase follows immediately on the return of the intrathoracic pressure to its physiological value and is due to the sudden removal of the external pressure on the aorta.

Phase IV: Systolic and diastolic arterial pressures increase to above their baseline values. There is a compensatory reflex decrease in heart rate. Phase IV is complete once the arterial pressures have stabilized at or near their baseline values.

From the above description it will be evident that the normal response requires the integrity of the baroreceptor reflex, the central control system, the efferent pathways to the heart and peripheral vasculature and responsive effector organs. In an individual with sympathetic 'paralysis' the decreases in systolic and diasto-

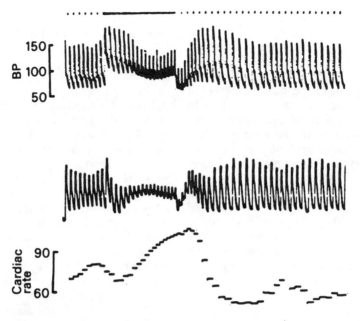

Fig. 26.14. Valsalva response in normal subject. *Upper trace*, arterial pressure; *middle trace*, finger plethysmograph; *lower trace*, beat-by-beat heart rate.

lic pressures (phase II) during the application of the increased intrathoracic pressure are more marked. There is no evidence of the pressures levelling off and there is no overshoot of the arterial pressure on removal of the positive intrathoracic pressure.

Impairment of parasympathetic activity is manifested by the lack of appropriate reflex changes in heart rate. Indeed, it has been suggested that measurement of the changes in heart rate provides the simplest and most reproducible assessment of autonomic function in association with the Valsalva manoeuvre.

$$\text{If } \frac{\text{Maximum heart rate in phase II}}{\text{Minimum heart rate in phase IV}} \times 100$$

is less than 100, the response is 'blocked': if greater than 125, the response is 'not blocked'.

Although there are a number of other tests available (responses to increases in body temperature, responses to hyperventilation, responses to the administration of insulin, or noradrenaline), should one wish to refine the diagnosis of an autonomic disorder further, we feel that those described are suitable for application in routine clinical practice should it be deemed helpful to evaluate autonomic

function in a patient prior to stressful procedures such as anaesthesia, surgery etc. However, it must be emphasized that autonomic lesions are rarely, if ever, single: generally they occur at more than one site. Moreover, they may be partial rather than complete and are usually progressive.

Clinical disorders of autonomic function

Disorders of autonomic function (dysautonomia) may be associated with a wide variety of systemic and neurological diseases (*Table 26.5*). Some are obvious (the ptosis, miosis, enophthalmos and facial anhidrosis which define Horner's syndrome), most are uncommon, a few are of some relevance to the anaesthetist and will be discussed briefly. Any reader interested in the wider spectrum of autonomic failure, or requiring more detail should consult the texts listed under Further Reading.

IATROGENIC CAUSES

The commonest cause of generalized impairment of autonomic, especially sympathetic,

Table 26.5. Examples of disorders which may be associated with autonomic failure

Iatrogenic
    Sympathectomy: surgical, phenol, drug-induced
    Cordotomy
    Drug-induced: systemic, extradural, intrathecal
Systemic
    Diabetes mellitus
    Chronic renal disease
    Amyloid
    Autoimmune disease: rheumatoid arthritis, Guillain-Barré syndrome
    Malnutrition: with or without alcoholism
Neurological
    Progressive autonomic failure
    Progessive autonomic failure with multiple system atrophy
    Progressive autonomic failure with Parkinson's disease
    Syringomyelia, haematomyelia
    Tabes dorsalis
    Acute transection of the spinal cord
    Tumours involving the hypothalamus or the mid-brain

function is the administration of those drugs used in the management of essential hypertension which act specifically on individual components in the sympathetic efferent pathways. As is well known, unfortunately, the desired pharmacological effect (decrease in arterial pressure) is often accompanied by undesirable side-effects such as postural hypotension, marked decreases in heart rate and impotence in the male which attest to the more widespread effects of such drugs on autonomic function.

Similarly, the extradural or intrathecal administration of local anaesthetic agents is accompanied (in the area of sensory/motor blockade) by vasodilatation, decreases in intestinal motility, and contraction of the intestine as evidence of the associated autonomic blockade. A number of other drugs have been implicated in the genesis of autonomic failure: antidepressants (monoamine oxidase inhibitors, tricyclic antidepressants), tranquillizers (phenothiazines, barbiturates), angiotensin converting enzyme inhibitors (captopril) and drugs like alcohol with selective neurotoxic capabilities (Wernicke's encephalopathy).

IDIOPATHIC ORTHOSTATIC HYPOTENSION

In the majority of patients with postural hypotension, the aetiology is clear, the postural hypotension is due to a recognizable disease process or is due to the administration of drugs. In some patients, however, there is no such association. Patients are usually middle-aged men in whom autonomic function has become impaired progressively over a number of years — or even decades. Symptoms progress steadily through loss of sweating, impotence, sphincter disturbances and postural hypotension. The hypotension results from the inability of the resistance and capacitance vessels to vasoconstrict in response to the change in posture: the response to the Valsalva manoeuvre is blocked. Physiologically it appears as if the lesion is located within the preganglionic sympathetic fibres: certainly at autopsy there is morphological evidence of cell loss in the intermediolateral columns of the spinal cord.

GUILLAIN-BARRÉ SYNDROME

In this condition an acute ascending polyneuritis produces motor weakness or paralysis, disturbances of sensation and the loss of tendon reflexes. In addition, there may be an associated imbalance in autonomic function which manifests itself in postural hypotension, profuse sweating, episodes of hypertension, etc. Although the severity of autonomic failure does not necessarily parallel the severity of the motor weakness, care is required on the institution of positive pressure ventilation in case the loss of circulatory reflexes — in the individual patient — is such that arterial pressure will decrease markedly. The Valsalva response is blocked and the capacitance vessels cannot react reflexly to neurogenic stimuli, although they will respond to stimulation by humoral agents.

TETANUS

Patients suffering from tetanus may demonstrate evidence of sympathetic overactivity which affects the peripheral blood vessels and the heart. Clinically, the patients may be tachycardic and hypertensive or there may be a marked increase in heart rate without any concomitant increase in arterial pressure. Perfusion of the skin and intestinal mucosa may be poor. Although treatment with a β-adrenoceptor blocking drug is helpful it must be given in markedly reduced dosage because of receptor supersensitivity: a normal pharmacological dose of, for example, propranolol often leading to severe bradycardia and/or systemic arterial hypotension.

DIABETIC NEUROPATHY

Diabetes is a relatively common cause of autonomic neuropathy: denervation of both parasympathetic and sympathetic components of the autonomic supply to the heart occurs. Vagal denervation occurs first with loss of sympathetic activity later in the progress of the disease. Loss of the normal beat-to-beat variation in heart rate with respiration or a persistent tachycardia are suggestive of parasympathetic involvement, the heart rate usually decreasing towards normal if sympathetic denervation is superimposed on an existing loss of vagal activity.

SPINAL CORD TRAUMA

Following a complete lesion of the spinal cord, the central control system can no longer modulate autonomic activity below the level of the lesion. This does not mean that there is no autonomic activity in this area: local vascular reflexes remain and function at a spinal level. However, the overall control of autonomic (particularly sympathetic) function is lacking and the integration of the various autonomic reflexes lost. If the lesion is above about T6 (the upper segmental level of the major parts of the splanchnic outflow), so much of the body is deprived of its normal control of vascular calibre that postural hypotension is the rule — and this may be severe enough to cause the loss of consciousness on movement or tilting of the patient, at least during the first few weeks following the injury. Other features of spinal cord trauma which result from the interruption of autonomic pathways are bradycardia, dilatation of the stomach, loss of normal bladder function, impairment of temperature regulation (poikilothermic below the lesion) and respiratory inadequacy. Obviously, the major component producing respiratory inadequacy (in patients in whom the phrenic outflow is intact) is the loss of motor power to the intercostal muscles. However, it has been suggested that, in addition, the unopposed action of the vagus (not transected) can increase bronchial secretions, induce bronchiolar constriction and, hence, increase the required work of breathing.

Autonomic hyper-reflexia is of particular concern to the anaesthetist. This occurs once the initial 'spinal shock' has worn off and is provoked commonly by the application of stimuli in areas of the body below the lesion: for example, distension of the bladder or in association with inadequate depth of anaesthesia. It is due to the loss of central control over local autonomic reflexes such that stimulation results in acute increases in arterial pressure and in cardiac arrhythmia. Fortunately, the condition does not arise if the lesion is below T7 but should be considered in any patient with spinal cord transection at a higher level.

As explained earlier, there has been no attempt to provide an exhaustive list of conditions associated with dysautonomia. The examples given may, however, highlight the need to consider the possibility that such problems may be of relevance in routine clinical practice.

Further reading

Appenzeller O. and Atkinson R. The autonomic nervous system. In: Swash M. and Kennard C. (ed.) *Scientific Basis of Clinical Neurology*. Edinburgh: Churchill Livingstone, 1985, pp. 463–88.

Bannister R. *Autonomic Failure: A textbook of clinical disorders of the autonomic nervous system*. London: Oxford University Press, 1983.

Berridge M.J. Inositol triphosphate and diacylglycerol as second messengers. *Biochem. J.* 1984; **220**, 345–60.

Burnstock G. Autonomic innervation and transmission. *Br. Med. Bull.*, 1979; **35**, 255–62.

Burnstock G. and Costa M. *Adrenergic Neurons: Their organisation, function and development in the peripheral nervous system*. London: Chapman and Hall, 1975.

Gillespie J.S. Presynaptic receptors in the autonomic nervous system. In: Szekeres L. (ed.) *Handbook of Experimental Pharmacology*, Vol. 54/1: *Adrenergic Activators and Inhibitors*. Berlin: Springer-Verlag, 1980, pp. 353–425.

Guyton A.C. An overall analysis of cardiovascular regulation. *Anesth. Analg.* 1977; **56**, 761–8.

Johnson R.H. and Spalding J.M. *Disorders of the Autonomic Nervous System* (Contemporary Neurology Series No. 11). Philadelphia: Davis, 1974.

Konturek S.J. Gastric secretion: physiological aspects. In: Duthie H.L. and Wormsley K.G. (ed.) *Scientific Basis of Gastroenterology*. Edinburgh: Churchill Livingstone, 1979, pp. 133–62.

Langer S.Z. and Hicks P.E. Physiology of the sympathetic nerve ending. *Br. J. Anaesth.* 1984; **56**, 689–700.

Lees G.M. A hitch-hiker's guide to the galaxy of adrenoceptors. *Br. Med. J.* 1981; **283**, 173–7.

McGrath J.C. The variety of vascular α-adrenoceptors. *Trends Pharmacol. Sci.* 1983; **4**, 14.

Maze M. Clinical implications of membrane receptor function. *Anesthesiology* 1981; **55**, 160–71.

Rand M.J., McCulloch M.W. and Story D.F. Catecholamine receptors on nerve terminals. In: Szekeres L. (ed.) *Handbook of Experimental Pharmacology*, Vol. 54/1: *Adrenergic Activators and Inhibitors*. Berlin: Springer-Verlag, 1980, pp. 223–66.

Reitan J.A. Control of the systemic circulation. In: Scurr C.F. and Feldman S.A. (ed.) *Scientific Foundations of Anaesthesia*. London: Heinemann, 1982, pp. 132–44.

Timmermans P.B.M.W.M. and van Zwieten P.A. α₂-Adrenoceptors: classification, localisation, mechanisms and targets for drugs. *J. Med. Chem.* 1982; **25**, 1389–401.

van Zwieten P.A., van Meel J.C.A., de Jonge A. et al. Central and peripheral α-adrenoceptors. *J. Cardiovasc. Pharmacol.* 1982; **4**, S19–S24.

Chapter 27

The cerebral circulation

Despite the small size of the brain (2–3 per cent of the total body weight), the central nervous system receives about 15 per cent of the resting cardiac output (750 ml/min), and consumes around 20 per cent of the oxygen (170 µmol $100 g^{-1} min^{-1}$) required by the body at rest. Moreover, a quarter of the glucose consumed by the entire body is utilized by the brain (31 µmol $100 g^{-1} min^{-1}$) and, since the brain, unlike muscle, does no mechanical work, the energy produced is required solely to sustain ionic pumps, maintain barriers (blood–brain barrier) and support the synthesis of transmitter substances. Thus, the normal functioning of the central nervous system is dependent upon the continuous provision of appropriate energy substrates and the adequate removal of the waste products of metabolism. As a result, mechanisms have been designed to ensure that, under physiological conditions, the flow of blood to the brain is protected. It is these mechanisms that we will principally consider in this chapter. However, it must be appreciated that, whereas physiological mechanisms can be expected to operate under physiological conditions, one should not be too surprised if they do not function normally in situations of disordered physiology — be this the result of intracranial pathology (traumatic injury, neoplastic disease, vascular insufficiency) or as a concomitant of extracranial problems (carotid arterial disease, profound systemic hypotension, systemic arterial hypertension, hypoglycaemia). Thus, we will consider, as appropriate, those alterations in physiological function produced by certain disease processes.

For obvious reasons, much of our present understanding of the mechanisms which modulate the cerebral circulation has been derived from investigations in experimental animals and, of necessity, results from such studies will be presented. However, there is no doubt that the available evidence from clinical studies appears to support strongly the understanding of the principles substantiated in animal models.

MEASUREMENT OF CEREBRAL BLOOD FLOW AND CEREBRAL METABOLISM

Any scientific appreciation of the physiology and, indeed, pharmacology of the cerebral circulation depends significantly on an awareness, and assessment, of the methods employed to measure cerebral blood flow. In all probability, methodology, more than any other factor, accounts for the major contradictions in interpretation. Thus, it is important that some consideration be given to the techniques by which cerebral blood flow and cerebral metabolism can be measured. Various possible methods by which cerebral blood flow can be measured in man are outlined in *Table* 27.1. However, since space does not permit of a discussion of each in detail, those aspects which are of clinical interest will be highlighted.

Techniques of measurement of cerebral blood flow and metabolism in man

The first quantitative estimations of cerebral blood flow and cerebral metabolism in man were made by Kety and Schmidt in 1945. The method, in which inhaled nitrous oxide is used as the tracer, is based on the Fick principle which asserts that 'the quantity of a substance taken up by an organ per unit time is equal to the product of the blood flow through that

Table 27.1. Techniques for the determination of cerebral blood flow in man*

Technique	Advantage(s)	Disadvantages
Direct measurement		
Electromagnetic flowmeter on carotid artery	Continuous assessment of flow Demonstrates any immediate change in flow	Requires surgical exposure Cannot assess changes in cerebral tissue perfusion Affected by changes in diameter of artery brought about by sympathetic stimulation
Non-diffusible indicators		
Estimation of mean transit time through brain following intracarotid injection of RISA	—	Requires puncture of carotid artery Qualitative assessment
Estimation of mode transit time following intravenous injection (technetium-99m)	Atraumatic Venepuncture only required	Measures velocity not actual tissue blood flow Difficult to detect regional variations in velocity
Diffusible indicators		
Kety–Schmidt technique (N_2O or ^{85}Kr)	Metabolic studies possible Used widely	Requires samples of arterial and jugular bulb blood Average hemisphere flow only
Intracarotid injection of ^{133}Xe or ^{85}Kr with external counting	Does not require blood sampling Measurements of regional flow possible Results available rapidly	Requires intracarotid injection of isotope Only limited metabolic information attainable
Inhalation/intravenous administration of ^{133}Xe with external counting	Atraumatic No blood samples required Tomography possible	Must correct for arterial recirculation of isotope and for clearance of isotope from scalp, skull, etc.
Inhalation/intravenous administration of positron-emitting radionuclides	Atraumatic Measurements of regional blood flow and metabolism possible Tomograms (usually)	Requires presence of on-site cyclotron Equipment expensive
Others		
Nuclear magnetic resonance	Atraumatic. Does not require radioisotopes	Low sensitivity

*The table is not comprehensive: techniques unlikely to be encountered in current clinical practice have been omitted.

organ and the arteriovenous concentration difference from that substance'.

$$Qt = Ft \times (Ca - Cv)$$

where Qt = quantity of substance taken up per unit time, Ft = blood flow per unit time, and Ca and Cv = the arterial and venous concentrations of the substance. By re-arrangement.

$$Ft = \frac{Qt}{(Ca - Cv)}$$

Unlike the kidney, the brain does not specifically and selectively remove foreign substances from the blood and excrete them — a process which would permit accurate measurement. What the brain can do, however, is absorb (in physical solution) an inert gas such as nitrous oxide when it is supplied to the brain via the lungs and the circulation. Thus, the amount of the inert tracer absorbed by the brain would be independent of the state of mental activity and, since the tracer is inert, it would not of itself alter the metabolic rate (and hence blood flow) of the brain.

The numerator of the Fick equation (Qt) is

the product of the concentration of the tracer in the brain, the weight of the brain and the blood–brain partition coefficient for nitrous oxide. The denominator has to be integrated with respect to time since the arterial and venous concentrations are changing continuously — whether blood flow is determined during the inhalation of nitrous oxide (the saturation technique) or on the cessation of inhalation (the desaturation technique). Metabolic rates are calculated by multiplying the arteriovenous difference for a substrate (for example, oxygen or glucose) by the cerebral blood flow

$$CMR_{O_2} = CBF \times (Ca_{O_2} - Cv_{O_2})$$

However, the basic Kety–Schmidt technique has a number of limitations. First, it is necessary to cannulate an artery (any artery), and the vein which drains the organ under study — in the case of the brain the appropriate sampling site is the jugular bulb. This requirement to obtain cerebral venous blood introduces the problem of what is, and what is not, true cerebral venous drainage. For example, in 10 per cent of the patients studied in one of the early investigations, the measured blood flow was abnormally low because the jugular bulb had not been entered at a high enough level, and a percentage of the venous blood sampled had drained from extracranial tissues (muscle, subcutaneous tissues, skin). Secondly, the actual technique is complex and time-consuming. Multiple accurately-timed arterial and venous samples are required together with skilled technical assistance to analyse the samples appropriately. Thirdly, the measurement of blood flow obtained is the mean flow through all the tissues draining into the vein from which the blood samples are obtained. In the case of the brain, in which samples are obtained from one jugular bulb, the measured flow is the mean flow from the area of brain (plus any extracranial tissues) draining into the jugular bulb from which the samples are drawn — that is, the ipsilateral cerebral hemisphere approximately. Furthermore, the value obtained is an average of all the rates of flow through different areas of grey and white matter: regional variations in flow are undetectable. Thus, the Kety–Schmidt technique has been utilized for studies of overall cerebral perfusion and metabolism and, as such, is of limited applicability when one wishes to delineate the alterations in local (regional) blood flow brought about by discrete pathological lesions.

In 1961, Lassen and Ingvar described the measurement of *local* blood flow through the exposed cerebral cortex of the dog by following, with a Geiger–Müller tube, the rate of clearance of the β-emissions of ^{85}Kr following the intracarotid injection of the isotope. Subsequently, the method was adapted to measure regional blood flow in man by recording the clearance of ^{133}Xe (γ-emissions) through the intact skull.

The introduction of the radioactive inert gases such as ^{85}Kr and ^{133}Xe obviated the necessity for arterial and venous cannulation as the rate at which the isotope left the brain could be determined by monitoring the decay in radioactivity (*Fig. 27.1*) with appropriate externally placed detectors. Like nitrous oxide, entry into and removal from the brain depends solely on physical properties (diffusion and solubility). Accordingly, if ^{85}Kr or ^{133}Xe (dissolved in saline) is injected into the internal carotid artery, the isotope will equilibrate rapidly between blood and brain tissue. When the injection of the isotope is stopped, the arterial concentration of isotope decreases to zero and the concentration gradient is reversed: isotope will leave the brain and the rate of 'washout' or clearance will depend on the blood flow. The more rapid the clearance, the more rapid the blood flow and vice versa. When introduced to the brain in this way there are no problems of arterial recirculation since both krypton and xenon have a much greater affinity for air than for blood and a high proportion (95 per cent) of the circulating isotope will be excreted into the alveoli on its first passage through the lungs.

The inert gas clearance method (as described above) has two distinct advantages over the classic Kety–Schmidt technique. First, no blood samples are required: the calculations of flow can be made from the clearance curves, and the result can be obtained rapidly. Flow can be calculated either by 'exponential stripping' or by 'height/area analysis'. In exponential stripping the slopes of the clearance curve are determined and, as these relate to the rates

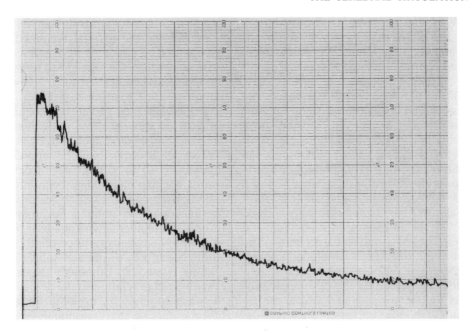

Fig. 27.1. Disintegrations of ^{133}Xe detected by external scintillation counting following the intracarotid injection of a bolus of isotope.

of clearance of radioactivity from the tissues, if there is more than one rate of blood flow in the tissue under study then more than one slope (exponential) can be 'stripped' from the clearance curve. Since blood flow in grey matter is four to five times as rapid as that through white matter, the two components of the clearance can be demonstrated and the appropriate flows calculated. Height/area analysis means that the peak height (the maximum radioactivity recorded after the injection of the isotope) is divided by the total area under the clearance curve. The value obtained is the mean blood flow through the area of tissue 'seen' by the detector (that is, the average of the flows in the grey and white matter into which the radioisotope has been introduced). Although this form of flow determination is less informative it can be calculated more rapidly, and is probably more reproducible. However, it is important to remember that this mean flow is not 'mean' in the usual sense, but is a mean value for the area of tissue 'seen' by the detector. This particular area may, or may not be, typical of the whole organ (*see below*).

The second advantage of the inert gas clearance method is that estimates of *regional* blood flow can be obtained. By using appropriately sized detectors and suitable collimation it is possible to focus down on small cones of tissue and, thus, localize variations in flow due to discrete pathological lesions such as tumours, or infarcts. Indeed, Scandinavian workers using a system with 254 individual detectors have demonstrated clearly that the technique is sensitive enough to detect changes in regional cerebral blood flow due to functional activity such as discrete motor activity or listening to music. If the radioisotope is injected only to the internal carotid artery it will pass exclusively to the brain and, therefore, the value obtained will refer solely to flow within brain tissue — despite the fact that the detector will be 'looking at' the core of tissue in front of it which includes skin, scalp, muscle and skull as well as brain.

The principle disadvantages of the inert gas clearance technique (as described above) are, first, the necessity for carotid artery puncture and, secondly, the technique provides no estimate of regional cerebral metabolism. In recent years, the necessity for carotid artery puncture has restricted severely the use of the basic technique in the United Kingdom except during procedures in which the artery is exposed surgically (carotid endarterectomy, carotid ligation). As a result, however, the development and evaluation of non-invasive inert gas clearance techniques have been stimulated, and their utilization increased substantially. Basically, the radioisotope can be administered either by inhalation, or by the intravenous administration of a bolus of ^{133}Xe dissolved in physiological saline solution. Both techniques use the same externally placed detectors as the intra-arterial technique and the same basic principles pertain. The miniaturization of the nucleonic equipment and the development of microprocessor-based computers have permitted the development of apparatus that is portable and which can be used readily in the operating theatre, the intensive care unit or the ward. Nevertheless, these non-invasive techniques suffer from certain theoretical disadvantages when compared with the intra-arterial technique.

INHALATION TECHNIQUE

The first theoretical disadvantage is that, during the period of inhalation, all the body tissues take up isotope. Consequently, the input function to the brain is influenced by the recirculation of isotope and is not a step function: consequently, the clearance curves will be distorted. To overcome this problem, the end-tidal concentration of ^{133}Xe gas is measured, and the clearance from the lung (as a measure of the clearance of xenon from the arterial blood) determined simultaneously with the clearance of the radioisotope from the brain. The cranial clearance is then subjected to a computerized correction to take account of the recirculation of xenon. The second disadvantage is the contamination of the clearance curves by the presence (and clearance) of radioactivity in the scalp and extracranial tissues. Over the years numerous refinements have been incorporated in an attempt to overcome this problem. For example, Obrist and colleagues decreased the period of inhalation of the isotope to two minutes and subjected the clearance curve to complex

computer analysis. Once the curves had been corrected for the arterial recirculation three exponential components were extracted — the slowest of which was thought to represent flow in the extracerebral tissues. However, to obtain accurate resolution of this third component the clearance had to be recorded for 30 minutes in the healthy individual — and probably for much longer under conditions of decreased flow. As will be appreciated 30 minutes or so is a long time over which to maintain stable physiological conditions (especially during anaesthesia) and is unsuitable in the uncooperative patient. Fortunately, more recent developments have made it possible to achieve a measurement of cerebral blood flow within 5 minutes (3 minutes inhalation and 2 minutes washout). Although the head must remain fixed in relation to the detectors during the washout phase the use of this brief interval of time means that reasonably steady-state conditions can be assured and the technique can be used, when necessary, on confused or uncooperative patients.

The main advantage of the inhalation technique is that it is atraumatic, and therefore may be used for studies in healthy subjects and outpatients, studies which may be repeated over hours or days or weeks, if required. The radiation dose to the lung (the critical organ) is 70 mrad (less than half that from a routine chest radiograph).

INTRAVENOUS TECHNIQUE

The inhalation technique described above was developed primarily for use in conscious patients and is less easily undertaken in patients undergoing artificial ventilation. In such patients ^{133}Xe gas under pressure must either be fed into a closed rebreathing system or into an open-loop breathing system — that is, mixed with the inspired gases. In the latter situation, in particular, decreases in inspired oxygen concentration are produced as is dilution of the anaesthetic gas mixture. To circumvent this problem, techniques based on the intravenous injection of ^{133}Xe have been developed and are of particular use in the operating theatre. Obviously, such a technique gives rise to the same two problems as the inhalation technique — recirculation of isotope from the rest of the body and contamination of the clearance curves by the presence of isotope in extracerebral tissue.

INTRA-ARTERIAL INJECTION OF RADIOACTIVE OXYGEN (^{15}O)

^{15}O-labelled water can be injected to the internal carotid artery and its clearance from the brain followed by externally placed scintillation detectors. Cerebral blood flow can be calculated using the equations developed for ^{133}Xe. However, with this technique it is also possible to obtain measurements of regional oxygen consumption. Thus, it is now possible to overcome the second major disadvantage of the regional ^{133}Xe clearance technique — the lack of any estimate of metabolic activity. The disadvantage of this particular technique is that the half-life of ^{15}O is 2·05 minutes and as a result, the technique can only be undertaken in close proximity to a cyclotron.

Although the rate of uptake and the clearance of ^{133}Xe has been recorded satisfactorily for many years using *stationary* detectors, the advent of the inhalation and intravenous techniques has prompted a re-appraisal of the degree of resolution obtained. Obviously, an atraumatic technique is obtained with the inhalation and intravenous techniques. However, the decrease in count rate obtained from the brain means that the field of view of each detector must be greater: consequently, the spatial resolution (the regionality) of individual measurements is less. In addition, the simultaneous labelling of both hemispheres and the extracerebral tissues with ^{133}Xe means that the resolution of depth is poorer than with the intra-arterial technique. As a result, equipment capable of producing tomographic images of the brain has been harnessed to provide (tomographic) measurements of regional blood flow.

Stable (non-radioactive) xenon can absorb X-rays and is used to enhance the images that can be obtained with standard X-ray transmission computed tomography (CT scanning). A sub-anaesthetic mixture of xenon gas in oxygen (35 per cent xenon: 65 per cent oxygen) is inhaled. The resultant changes in the absorption coefficients of the X-rays (Houndsfield numbers) depend on the solubility of the xenon and the perfusion of the tissue. These differences (with and without xenon enhancement), plus measurements of the end-expired xenon concentration (as indicative of the arterial concentration of xenon), can be used to calculate absolute values of local cerebral blood flow and of the local tissue/blood partition coefficients of xenon — the latter being of particular value if flow is to be determined in abnormal tissue. Unfortunately, the inhaled concentration has 'sedative' effects in certain individuals and this has limited the applicability of this technique.

In single-photon emission computed tomography *radioactive* xenon (^{133}Xe), or another suitable isotope (^{123}I-labelled *N*-isopropyl-*p*-iodoamphetamine), can be used to obtain tomographic images of cerebral blood flow (and cellular metabolism). A number of scintillation detectors are arranged in a movable gantry such that the three-dimensional distribution of the isotope can be reconstructed by the computer (as with conventional X-ray tomography), and maps of blood flow ('slices') demonstrated.

POSITRON-EMISSION TOMOGRAPHY

If a cyclotron is available it can be used also to generate other positron-emitting radionuclides (^{11}C, ^{13}N, ^{18}F). The local tissue concentrations following inhalation or intravenous administration can be used to measure, non-invasively, and to map (using the tomographic delineation of cerebral structures) functional processes in the human brain. This is a rapidly developing field at the present time. The interested reader is referred to the review by Phelps and colleagues (1982). Suffice to say that at the present time techniques have been developed which permit the determination of cerebral blood flow (intravenous (bolus) administration of ^{15}O, or the inhalation of $^{15}CO_2$), cerebral blood volume (inhalation of ^{11}C-labelled carbon monoxide), cerebral metabolic rates for oxygen (inhalation of ^{15}O-labelled oxygen) and glucose (^{18}F-labelled 2-fluoro-2-deoxy-D-glucose or ^{11}C-labelled glucose), selective blood–brain barrier and facilitated membrane transport for glucose (3-[^{11}C]methyl-D-glucose), and passive blood–brain barrier diffusion. Despite its relatively recent development, the technique has been applied to both fundamental studies of normal cerebral function and to those clinical problems posed by pathological alterations in function. Positron emission tomography offers the clinician the possibility of studying physiological function quantitatively as well as determining the anatomical distribution of that activity.

NON-DIFFUSIBLE ISOTOPES

Obviously, the measurement of cerebral blood flow (and cerebral metabolism) using freely diffusible tracers requires sophisticated apparatus, considerable technical support and relatively advanced data processing. Not surprisingly, therefore, there have been a number of attempts to find simpler alternatives. Measurement of the circulation time (mode transit time) of a non-diffusible isotope (the isotope remains in the circulation) is one such technique.

A bolus of a suitable non-diffusible isotope (for example technetium-99^m) is injected intravenously and the passage of the radioactivity through the brain monitored with an externally placed collimated scintillation detector (or a gamma camera). Unfortunately, the information obtained is limited. The method provides an index of the velocity of the blood flow within the cerebral vasculature and not a measure of cerebral tissue blood flow. It is qualitative rather than quantitative. In addition, the variability in values obtained between healthy subjects is considerable and makes it difficult to identify the individual with an abnormality.

NUCLEAR MAGNETIC RESONANCE

Previously, imaging of anatomical structures within the body has been achieved by measuring the differential absorption of X-rays. Nuclear magnetic resonance makes possible not only the display of morphology (normal and pathological) but, in addition, the recording of physiological and biochemical changes *in vivo*. The technique can demonstrate differences in cellular metabolism and display them as axial tomographic sections without the use of ionizing radiation. So far, all medical nuclear magnetic resonance images have been obtained with resonances from hydrogen nuclei (1H), largely because of the abundance of hydrogen in the body. In addition, however, hydrogen has a higher intrinsic nuclear magnetic resonance sensitivity than do other nuclei. Thus, hydrogen protons are ideal for imaging. ^{31}P is ideal for the spectroscopic examination of excised tissue because the spectra obtained from phosphorous compounds are relatively uncomplicated.

Although nuclear magnetic resonance is a comparatively new technique with which to study the brain, it appears promising and should be capable of providing information about, for example, regional blood flow, local alterations in metabolism, the evolution of strokes and the growth of tumours.

Obviously this description is brief and simple: it says nothing about the principles of the technique. For a more detailed description the reader is referred to the article by Smith (1983) (*see* Further Reading).

Physiological values of cerebral blood flow and metabolism

Physiological values for mean cerebral blood flow obtained by some of the techniques discussed above are summarized in *Table* 27.2. However, of particular interest is the demonstration in recent investigations of the marked heterogeneity of flow throughout the brain such that different, but physiological, values can be demonstrated not only between grey matter and white matter but also between different areas of the cortex, and between cortical grey matter and grey matter in the basal ganglia. The clinical relevance of these considerations relates to the changes in regional flow produced by functional activity, by discrete pathological lesions, and to the selective vulnerability of neuronal tissue to critical decreases in oxygen supply.

Most evidence indicates that, in conscious man under physiological conditions, the blood flow to the brain parallels the demand for energy by the brain and, consequently, the level of oxygen consumption and glucose utilization. When cerebral function is depressed, as in coma, and the requirement for energy decreased, total cerebral blood flow, oxygen consumption and glucose utilization are much

Table 27.2. Normal values for cerebral blood flow as determined using a selection of the techniques discussed in the text

Technique	Cerebral blood flow $(ml\ 100g\ min^{-1})$	Comments
Kety–Schmidt (arteriovenous difference)	45–50	Total hemisphere
[133]Xe: external scintillation counting	45–50	Mean: height/area calculation
	75–80	Fast compartment: probably grey matter
	20	Slow compartment: probably white matter
Positron-emission tomography: inhalation of ^{15}O-CO_2 (mean ± s.d.)	52 ± 10	Grey matter
	21 ± 3	White matter
	42 ± 6	Whole brain

lower than in the normal fully conscious state. In contrast, during seizures (the most severe form of functional activation of the brain), the demand for oxygen and glucose increases markedly and this must be met from a parallel increase in supply.

This coupling between the energy supplying processes (blood flow) and those processes that require energy (metabolism) (*Fig.* 27.2) has been demonstrated in all the functional subunits of the central nervous system. Thus, *under physiological conditions*, the heterogeneity of blood flow is mirrored by a heterogeneity of glucose utilization such that blood flow is greatest in areas of greatest glucose utilization (primary auditory cortex and neocortex) and least in those regions with the lowest demand for energy substrates (globus pallidus, white matter).

The hypothesis that the blood flow to the brain is determined primarily by cerebral metabolic activity was proposed initially by Roy and Sherrington in 1890, when they stated 'that chemical products of cerebral metabolism contained in the lymph which bathes the walls of the arterioles of the brain can cause variations of the calibre of the cerebral vessels ...; in this reaction the brain possesses an intrinsic mechanism by which its vascular supply can be varied locally in correspondence with local variations of functional activity'. However, despite the considerable volume of work undertaken since that date, it is still not

clear which products of metabolism mediate the alterations in cerebrovascular resistance.

Although evident under physiological conditions, this coupling between flow and metabolism can be modified by pharmacological and

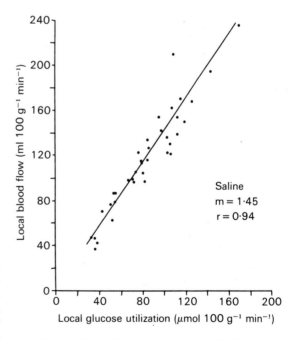

Fig. 27.2. Relationship between local cerebral glucose utilization and local cerebral blood flow in 37 anatomically discrete regions in the central nervous system: investigation in the conscious rat.

pathological factors. For example, the administration of drugs, such as the barbiturates, which suppress cerebral metabolism primarily, induces quantitatively similar decreases in blood flow and glucose utilization in various anatomically discrete regions. Thus, although the baseline indices of flow and metabolism are less than normal, the ratio between cerebral blood flow and glucose utilization is maintained. In other circumstances (prolonged metabolic acidosis, or following inhibition of prostaglandin synthesis), the ratio is altered but the alteration is of similar magnitude in each region of the central nervous system. In contrast, during many pathological processes the coupling between blood flow and glucose use is disturbed selectively and focally. This occurs in association with subarachnoid haemorrhage, following seizures and in the area around a brain tumour.

MAINTENANCE OF CEREBRAL BLOOD FLOW

Since the energy demands of the brain can only be met by the continuous supply of appropriate substrates, it will be obvious that the integrity of the central nervous system depends critically on the maintenance of its blood supply. Moreover, this supply must be such that it can respond adequately to any physiological trespass, such as a decrease in perfusion pressure or a decrease in inspired oxygen concentration which might otherwise impair the supply of oxygen and glucose. Since the anaesthetist can consciously or even unconsciously influence significantly such physiological variables as systemic arterial pressure (controlled, or inadvertent, arterial hypotension), cerebral venous pressure (increased intrathoracic pressure), intracranial pressure (increased carbon dioxide tension) and the inspired oxygen concentration, it behoves us to consider in some detail how the cerebral circulation reacts under such circumstances.

Influence of changes in perfusion pressure

For many years it was believed that the cerebral circulation responded passively to changes in systemic arterial pressure — that is, flow was thought to increase as the arterial

pressure increased and vice versa. This concept survived considerable scientific scrutiny until 1934, when it was shown conclusively that a decrease in systemic arterial pressure caused dilatation of the pial vessels and that, conversely, vasoconstriction of the pial vessels accompanied increases in arterial pressure. The introduction of quantitative measurements of blood flow permitted examination of the relationship between changes in arterial pressure and the blood flow through cerebral *tissue*. These investigations confirmed, in man as well as in animals, the remarkable stability of the blood flow to the *normal* brain despite quite wide fluctuations in cerebral perfusion pressure (the difference between the inlet pressure — arterial — and the pressure at the outlet — jugular bulb). Thus, the *normal* brain is said to have the ability to *autoregulate* (an *intrinsic* tendency of an organ to maintain constant flow despite variations in perfusion pressure). Although, at this point, we are considering primarily the responsiveness of the cerebral circulation to changes in systemic arterial pressure, autoregulation can be demonstrated also when the changes in perfusion pressure result from alterations in cerebral venous pressure or intracranial pressure (*see below*). Although this capability protects the brain from the effects of the physiological fluctuations in systemic arterial pressure that are part-and-parcel of normal daily living, the mechanism responsible for autoregulation requires a finite time (30–120 seconds) before it becomes established. Acute alterations in arterial pressure will be accompanied, initially at least, by concomitant alterations in blood flow.

The actual mechanism of autoregulation is debatable and, indeed, may vary from organ to organ. Classically, three possible hypotheses have been advanced to account for autoregulation in the cerebrovascular bed and, although each is supported by a body of evidence, no one theory is pre-eminent at the present time.

MYOGENIC HYPOTHESIS

This hypothesis states that the mechanism of autoregulation resides within the intrinsic ability of vascular smooth muscle (first noted in 1902) whereby a change in intraluminal pressure provokes contraction (or relaxation) of the smooth muscle in the vessel wall. Myogenic factors could theoretically operate to provide rapid compensation for alterations in perfusion pressure. However, it is likely that the capacity for such adjustments is limited to small fluctuations in pressure occurring for a brief period of time.

METABOLIC HYPOTHESIS

As discussed earlier in this chapter, the principal determinant of local levels of blood flow appears to be the local metabolic activity (oxygen consumption and glucose utilization) of cerebral tissue. According to the metabolic hypothesis, any decrease in perfusion pressure results initially in a transient decrease in blood flow and hence, oxygen delivery. As a result, an increase in the perivascular concentrations of certain vasoactive metabolites (the products of metabolic activity) occurs with a resultant decrease in cerebrovascular resistance and the restoration of blood flow. Alterations in the tissue hydrogen ion concentration or potassium concentrations are thought to be two of the major factors inducing vasodilatation of the cerebral vessels. However, other locally produced metabolites such as adenosine or adenosine di-phosphate may also produce the appropriate alterations in cerebral blood flow.

NEUROGENIC HYPOTHESIS

Extracranial and intracranial cerebral blood vessels are innervated by adrenergic and cholinergic nerves which originate principally in the extracranial autonomic nervous system. In addition, the intracranial vasculature may be supplied by adrenergic fibres arising in a brain stem nucleus. Thus, it has been proposed, on numerous occasions, that the alterations in the diameter of the cerebral resistance vessels which subserve autoregulation are mediated via this nervous supply. However, attractive as this hypothesis is, recent evidence would indicate that this is not the case. This does not mean that the cerebral blood vessels are completely unaffected by neurogenic factors — far from it — but it does appear that the mechanisms subserving autoregulation *per se* are not under nervous control.

A recent development which has attracted considerable interest is the observation that certain peptidergic and aminergic neurones are in direct contact with cerebral blood vessels, in addition to their conventional connections with other neurones. Such innervation could be evidence of a direct anatomical link between the energy-requiring processes in neurones and those that sustain the supply of energy (via the cerebral vasculature).

Factors modifying autoregulatory capability

1. UPPER AND LOWER LIMITS OF AUTO-REGULATION

Further studies on the relationship between changes in systemic arterial pressure and cerebral blood flow demonstrated that there

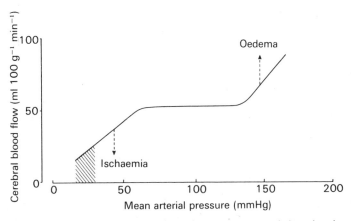

Fig. 27.3. Schematic representation of relationship between cerebral blood flow and alterations in mean arterial pressure.

are values of mean arterial pressure above which — and below which — the autoregulation of the cerebral circulation becomes ineffective (*Fig. 27.3*). Beyond these limits cerebral blood flow relates directly to perfusion pressure such that below the *lower limit of autoregulation* cerebral blood flow decreases in association with decreasing arterial pressure with the assumption that, if the mean arterial pressure decreases sufficiently, symptoms of cerebral ischaemia will appear. However, recent studies have demonstrated that the absolute value of the lower limit of autoregulation depends on the technique used to decrease the arterial pressure, the response to haemorrhagic hypotension being less perfect than that to similar decreases in arterial pressure produced pharmacologically. Presumably, this is one reason why the pharmacological induction of hypotension to relatively low values of mean arterial pressure can be undertaken without apparent hazard in healthy individuals.

It is important to realize, however, that what we have been considering — the lower limit of autoregulation — is the (lower) limit of mean arterial pressure *at* which blood flow remains similar to control. This is not the same as the lowest arterial pressure the brain can tolerate — the 'critical ischaemic threshold'. The lower limit of autoregulation is that value of mean arterial pressure at which the dilatation of the cerebral blood vessels becomes inadequate (rather than maximal). The smaller resistance vessels continue to dilate if pressure is decreased further. Once the blood flow has started to decrease, the brain can, at least initially, meet its oxygen requirements by increasing the amount of oxygen extracted from the blood. Symptoms of inadequate perfusion are not encountered until mean arterial pressure has decreased to around 35–40 mmHg and/or cerebral blood flow has decreased to approximately 70 per cent of its resting value.

At the other end of the pressure/flow plateau cerebral blood flow can be shown to increase markedly once mean arterial pressure has increased above a value of 130–140 mmHg in normotensive individuals. As a result, there is a forced dilatation of the arterioles at many discrete sites to produce a sausage string-like appearance. This is associated with disruption of the blood–brain barrier, reversal of hydrostatic gradients and the formation of cerebral oedema. Fortunately, it seems likely that brief periods of induced hypertension (as produced by anger, frustration, fright) to pressures above this *upper limit of autoregulation* can be tolerated without producing these adverse effects. However, should the increase in arterial pressure persist for some time, cerebral blood flow will not return to its resting or baseline value but will remain elevated even after the restoration of the arterial pressure to normal.

2. CHRONIC ARTERIAL HYPERTENSION

Not all patients presenting to the anaesthetist are normotensive: many are hypertensive and/or receiving some form of antihypertensive medication. Thus, it is of relevance to know what happens to the reactivity of the cerebral circulation under such conditions. The available evidence would suggest that, in chronic hypertension, although autoregulation is present the curve is displaced to the right (*Fig. 27.4*) that is, the upper and lower limits of autoregulation are observed at higher values of mean arterial pressure when compared with the values obtained in a normotensive individual. It seems likely that this shift of the curve is the result of the structural adaptation (medial hypertrophy) which has taken place in the walls of the cerebral blood vessels. However, this adaptation takes time. Thus, patients with *chronic* arterial hypertension will be protected against damaging vascular crises, whereas episodes of sub-acute hypertension, as seen in children with glomerulonephritis or in patients with toxaemia of pregnancy, will induce cerebral symptoms at values of arterial pressure tolerated readily by patients with chronic hypertension.

Of greater significance for the anaesthetist, however, is the displacement to the right of the *lower* limit of autoregulation since, for obvious reasons, such patients cannot tolerate the same degree of systemic hypotension as their normotensive peers. Fortunately, it has been demonstrated that adequate and effective treatment of chronic hypertension allows the

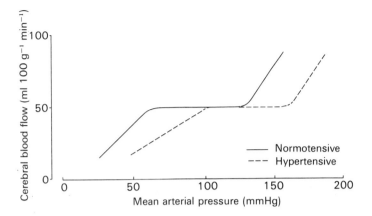

Fig. 27.4. Schematic representation of relationships between cerebral blood flow and changes in mean arterial pressure: comparison between normotensive and chronically hypertensive subjects.

curve to return to a more 'normotensive' position.

3. ALTERATIONS IN CARBON DIOXIDE TENSION

Although we will consider later the specific effects of variations in carbon dioxide tension on the cerebral circulation, it is relevant to point out here that the autoregulatory capability of the circulation can be modified by increases in carbon dioxide tension. Thus, during moderate hypercapnia, the degree of cerebral vasodilatation produced by the increased carbon dioxide tension limits the reserve available with which to maintain stable values of blood flow during concomitant decreases in systemic arterial pressure. In other words, the range of arterial pressure over which autoregulation pertains is reduced. Contrariwise, decreases in carbon dioxide tension not only decrease the absolute value of cerebral blood flow but also increase the range of autoregulation.

4. INCREASES IN VENOUS AND INTRACRANIAL PRESSURES

As cerebral venous pressure is comparatively low, it can be assumed to contribute little to the regulation of blood flow under physiological circumstances. However, just as the cerebral vessels can autoregulate to changes occurring in arterial pressure, so they can adapt to any significant alteration in cerebral venous pressure — whether produced by *extracranial* factors such as poor positioning of the head or neck, coughing and/or straining during anaesthesia or as a result of the application of a positive end-expiratory pressure or by *intracranial* factors such as an increase in intracranial pressure.

Likewise, the cerebral circulation can autoregulate to changes in intracranial pressure. As long ago as 1948 it was shown that the pial vessels would dilate in response to an increase in cerebrospinal fluid pressure and, more recently, it was demonstrated that cerebral blood flow remained stable until the cerebrospinal fluid pressure had been increased to over 35 mmHg. However, more detailed studies have indicated that this capacity for autoregulation depends not only on the absolute value of intracranial pressure but also on the rate of development and the aetiology of the intracranial hypertension. For example, autoregulation is demonstrable down to a perfusion pressure of 50 mmHg when intracranial pressure is increased by the infusion of fluid into the cisterna magna, presumably because the increase in intracranial pressure is distributed evenly among the various intracranial compartments. The situation is more complicated when the intracranial pressure is increased as the result of a space-occupying lesion. Under these circumstances, one has to consider not only the influence of the alterations in absolute pressure but, in addition, the effects of brain shift and the development of pressure gradients between the different intracranial compartments. In this context, a number of studies have demonstrated a pressure passive relationship in situations in which the increases in intracranial pressure were produced by the progressive inflation of an extradural balloon.

5. INFLUENCE OF INTRACRANIAL PATHOLOGY

Autoregulation is a physiological mechanism evident in the intact animal and in normal man. However, this ability of the cerebral circulation to compensate for variations in arterial, venous and intracranial pressures can be impaired markedly in the presence of intracranial pathology. We will discuss this particular aspect in more detail later. At this point it is sufficient to note that autoregulation may be defective following periods of hypoxia, in association with carotid artery occlusion, subarachnoid haemorrhage, space-occupying lesions and trauma, and in relation to seizure activity.

Influence of alterations in blood-gas tensions and acid-base balance

CARBON DIOXIDE

Alterations in arterial carbon dioxide tension have been recognized as having a potent influence on the cerebral circulation. Any increase in arterial carbon dioxide tension will cause an increase in flow and, conversely, a decrease in arterial carbon dioxide tension will induce cerebral vasoconstriction (*Fig.* 27.5). An increase in arterial carbon dioxide tension from its physiological value to 80 mmHg (10·6 kPa) will more than double blood flow. Decreasing the arterial carbon dioxide tension to 20 mmHg (2·7 kPa) approximately halves the flow — there appears to be little further decrease in flow at values of less than 20 mmHg — presumably because the cerebral blood vessels are incapable of constricting further. Although, in general terms, the magnitude of the response to carbon dioxide is approximately 5 per cent for each 1 mmHg change in

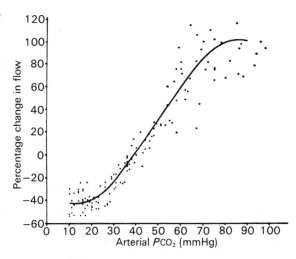

Fig. 27.5. Relationship between alterations in arterial carbon dioxide tension and cerebral blood flow: investigation in dogs.

arterial carbon dioxide tension, a recent observation suggests that the increase in flow due to hypercapnia is greater if the carbon dioxide tension is increased suddenly and acutely. For instance, the gradient of the Pa_{CO_2}/flow relationship is approximately 3–3·5 ml increase in blood flow for every mmHg increase in Pa_{CO_2} (22·5 ml/kPa) when the Pa_{CO_2} is increased acutely, whereas if the change is made more slowly — over several hours — the gradient is 1·5–2 ml/mmHg (15 ml/kPa).

OXYGEN

Cerebral blood flow responds in the reverse direction to changes in arterial oxygen tension — a decrease in Pa_{O_2} producing an increase in flow (*Fig.* 27.6). However, cerebral blood flow is comparatively insensitive to changes in arterial oxygen tension within the normal physiological range: only at Pa_{O_2} values of less than 50 mmHg (6·7 kPa) are marked increases in flow evident.

Increases in arterial oxygen tension cause only slight changes in cerebral blood flow. The administration of 100 per cent oxygen will decrease flow by approximately 10 per cent and the administration of oxygen at 2 ATA by just over 20 per cent.

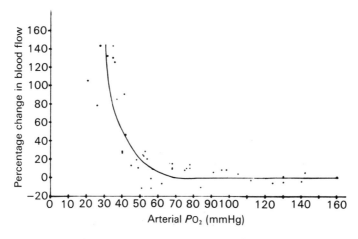

Fig. 27.6. Schematic representation of the changes in cerebral blood flow induced by progressive decreases in arterial oxygen tension.

ACID-BASE BALANCE

Systemic metabolic acidosis or alkalosis within the range pH 6·7–7·6 has no effect on the cerebral circulation as long as the arterial carbon dioxide tension remains constant. In contrast, changes of the pH in the cerebrospinal fluid (*see* Chapter 28) or, in particular, of the pH of the cortex (*see below*), can induce substantial alterations in blood flow.

MECHANISMS OF ACTION

The calibre of the cerebral arterioles is extremely sensitive to alterations in perivascular pH: acidosis provoking vasodilatation and alkalosis, vasoconstriction. The available evidence suggests that the effects of carbon dioxide on cerebral blood vessels are a consequence of such changes in perivascular pH, rather than being a direct effect of carbon dioxide on cerebrovascular smooth muscle.

Likewise, the underlying mechanisms through which hypoxic vasodilatation is achieved have been thought to involve alterations in perivascular pH, the decrease in oxygen supply leading to anaerobic glycolysis and the production of lactic acid. In recent years, a number of other putative mechanisms have been proposed — the two most favoured being changes in the concentration of potassium ions and in the concentration of adenosine. Certainly, each is a potent dilator of cerebral vessels and increases in the concentration of adenosine have been demonstrated in brain tissue during hypoxia. The alterations in vascular diameter produced by high arterial oxygen tensions are substantially less than those associated with critical decreases in oxygen tension (and, indeed, variations in arterial carbon dioxide tension). Consequently, the mechanism of this effect is, in all probability, quite different from that described above. A direct effect of the high oxygen tension on vascular smooth muscle (as noted also in alveolar capillaries) seems to be the most likely explanation.

But for the integrity of the blood–brain barrier — and its specific properties in relation to the passage of charged particles (*see* Chapter 28) — there is little doubt that variations in systemic acid-base balance would have a significant effect on brain extracellular pH and, *a priori*, produce quite substantial fluctuations in cerebral blood volume.

EFFECTS OF INTRACRANIAL PATHOLOGY ON NORMAL CEREBROVASCULAR FUNCTION

Obviously, a detailed consideration of those situations in which physiology is disordered is outwith the scope of this book. Nevertheless, we believe that it is important to discuss briefly those alterations to the normal dynamics of the cerebral circulation that are associated with a number of disease processes, since they form the basis for the appropriate clinical management of such patients.

Chronic brain diseases

The basic mechanisms controlling the cerebral circulation are unaffected by chronic diseases of the brain, such as senile dementia, which are associated with diffuse derangements of function and a decrease in metabolic rate. In such disease states there are parallel decreases in metabolism (oxygen demand) and perfusion (oxygen supply). As a result, the ratio between supply and demand is unaffected. These patients exhibit normal cerebrovascular reactivity to alterations in arterial carbon dioxide tension and possess also the normal physiological autoregulatory response to variations in systemic arterial pressure.

Acute brain injury

Such is not the case, however, in the presence of the acute *focal* brain damage that may follow head injury, subarachnoid haemorrhage or cerebral thrombosis. Neither is it the case following the *global* brain damage that may be associated with cardiorespiratory arrest, or profound decreases in systemic arterial pressure. The extreme sensitivity of neuronal tissue to low oxygen tensions and direct injury has been documented clearly and it seems likely that one of the consequences of such insults is an alteration in the normal physiological responses of the vascular system to variations in perfusion pressure, or alterations in blood-gas tensions. Since it would be inappropriate to dwell on this subject at any great length, only a few specific examples are given.

CAROTID ARTERY OCCLUSION

Following occlusion of one carotid artery there is a decrease in intravascular pressure in the circle of Willis. As a result, the vessels in the brain distal to the occlusion dilate to maximize the flow to the brain. However, once dilated, their ability to compensate for any additional 'stress', such as a decrease in arterial pressure or an increase in carbon dioxide tension, is limited and a pressure passive relationship develops.

SUBARACHNOID HAEMORRHAGE

It has been evident for some time that alterations to the normal reactivity of the cerebral blood vessels can follow subarachnoid haemorrhage. This may be associated with spasm of the larger vessels supplying the brain and/or a loss of responsiveness in the more distal arterioles to alterations in systemic arterial pressure and changes in blood-gas tensions. Thus, these patients may be susceptible to changes — even comparatively minor changes — in arterial pressure occurring in the perioperative period and, in particular, in the postoperative period.

INTRACRANIAL SPACE-OCCUPYING LESIONS

The influence of increases in intracranial pressure *per se* have been considered earlier in the chapter. Additionally, however, one must consider the effects of the space-occupying lesion itself on physiological function. As a tumour or haematoma increases in size, brain tissue is shifted in front of the advancing front of the lesion. Ultimately, this zone becomes compressed, its anatomical integrity threatened and its physiological function impaired. As you can imagine, the local blood flow in such an area is compromised by the increase in local tissue pressure, perivascular concentrations of the products of anaerobic metabolism increase, and the dilated blood vessels lose their physiological responsiveness. Indeed, not infrequently, such brain tissue will swell dramatically once the pressure has been relieved (by removal of tumour or evacuation of haematoma) since the perfusion of the dilated and unreactive vascular bed increases the cerebral blood volume (and probably the cerebral water content) substantially.

INTRACRANIAL TRAUMA

Clinical and experimental studies on the effects of concussional injury have demonstrated that, in and around areas of local brain contusion, there is evidence of a failure of the cerebral blood vessels to react to the normal stresses of changes in intravascular pressure. Although global loss of autoregulation is encountered infrequently following head injury, autoregulation is often impaired *focally*, and it seems likely that this suspension of autoregulation persists for several days following even relatively minor insults.

The inherent responsiveness of the cerebral circulation is an important physiological mechanism which 'protects' the brain from the efferents of those minor alterations in systemic arterial pressure and blood-gas tensions which occur normally during everyday living (for example during sleep, anger, isometric muscular work etc.). However, this normal regulatory mechanism can be modified, to a greater or lesser degree, by those factors considered briefly above. From an anaesthetic point of view it is important to appreciate that, in any patients in whom these physiological mechanisms are defective, the anaesthetist cannot rely on them to mitigate for the inadequate control of blood-gas tensions or the imperfect management of the systemic arterial pressure.

PHARMACOLOGY OF THE CEREBRAL CIRCULATION

Obviously, it would be quite inappropriate to consider the pharmacological aspects of the cerebral circulation systematically. It is a subject in its own right. Nevertheless, since the physiology, pathophysiology and pharmacology of the cerebral circulation are so closely interwoven in clinical practice, and, in particular, clinical anaesthetic practice, we believe that some consideration should be given to the ways in which drugs commonly used by the anaesthetist affect the cerebral circulation. However, our consideration will be brief, and we propose to present *principles* only, supported by a limited number of examples.

First, under physiological conditions the cerebral circulation is generally unresponsive to systemically administered monoamines (such as dopamine, noradrenaline and serotonin), prostaglandins or other drugs whose ability to cross the blood–brain barrier is limited (*see* Chapter 28), since, obviously, this restricts the access of these agents to cerebral tissue and cerebrovascular smooth muscle. Thus, before one can study the cerebrovascular effects of such drugs either their passage across the blood–brain barrier must be facilitated (by increasing the permeability of the barrier) or the drugs must be given in a manner which circumvents the blood–brain barrier (directly into the cerebral ventricles or by local perivascular microapplication around the pial vessels).

Obviously, if the blood–brain barrier has been damaged — by hypoxia or trauma — the cerebrovascular effects of drugs such as dopamine, adrenaline and noradrenaline will be substantially different from those described under more physiological conditions. For example, the systemic administration of noradrenaline, serotonin or angiotensin has minimal effects on cerebrovascular smooth muscle under normal conditions (intact blood–brain barrier, normal carbon dioxide tension). In contrast, each will induce vasoconstriction and decrease flow significantly if the blood–brain barrier is defective.

Secondly, in the *healthy* brain, the majority of the drugs which are of interest to the anaesthetist can be considered as affecting *primarily* either cerebral blood flow (by a direct action on cerebrovascular smooth muscle) or cerebral metabolism — usually in a dose-dependent fashion — and their pharmacological effects can be characterized from this information (*Table* 27.3).

Intravenous anaesthetic agents

A direct relationship can be observed between the level of consciousness and global oxygen consumption and glucose utilization by the brain. The administration of most of the intravenous anaesthetic agents, such as the barbiturates, alphaxalone and alphadalone acetate (Althesin) and etomidate, in anaesthetic concentrations, decreases cerebral oxygen consumption and cerebral glucose utilization by 20–50 per cent depending on the particular anaesthetic drug employed and the depth of anaesthesia achieved. Cerebral blood flow decreases secondarily to this decrease in metabolism since the demand by the brain for oxygen is less.

However, as can be seen from *Table* 27.3, those agents which produce dissociative anaesthesia, such as ketamine (and, possibly, nitrous oxide), increase glucose use and their adminis-

Table 27.3. Effects of a selection of pharmacological agents on cerebral blood flow and cerebral metabolism in healthy individuals

Drug	Effect on cerebral blood flow	Effect on cerebral metabolism
Intravenous anaesthetics		
Barbiturates	↓	↓
Etomidate	↓	↓
Althesin	↓	↓
Fentanyl	↓	↓
Ketamine	↑	↑
Volatile anaesthetics		
Halothane	↑	
Enflurane	↑↑	↓
Isoflurane (low conc.)	↓	↓
(high conc.)	↑	↓
Methoxyflurane	↑	↓
Direct-acting vasodilators		
Hydralazine	↑	—
Nitroprusside	↑	—
Nitroglycerine	↑	—

tration is accompanied by an increase in cerebral blood flow.

Inhalation anaesthetic agents

Likewise, the inhalation anaesthetic agents depress metabolism in a dose-dependent manner — and to a similar degree. However, as indicated, cerebral blood flow *increases* in spite of the significant suppression of metabolism and indicates that the precise coupling between flow and metabolism (described at the beginning of this chapter) has been impaired, possibly because these drugs (halothane, enflurane, isoflurane) affect vascular smooth muscle directly. This increase in cerebral blood flow and, hence, cerebral blood volume, is, of course, the means whereby these drugs produce increases in intracranial pressure (*see* Chapter 28).

For simplicity, *Table* 27.3 depicts the overall effects of the anaesthetic agent on global blood flow and metabolism. However, the advent of the autoradiographic techniques for assessing metabolism and flow, in anatomically discrete functional units in the brain, has demonstrated clearly that different anaesthetic agents can affect the various parts of the central nervous system differentially, the most pronounced decreases in metabolism being observed in the thalamocortical system, and the sensory relay nuclei in the brain stem.

Vasoactive agents

Numerous drugs which act directly on vascular smooth muscle (dopamine, dobutamine, nitroprusside, nitroglycerine) are used widely in anaesthetic practice. By their very nature, they influence the cerebral blood vessels as they do the systemic vascular bed, but have no effect on cerebral metabolism. *Fig.* 27.7 depicts the effects of the administration of sodium nitroprusside on cerebral blood flow; it is included at this point since the results bring together a number of the considerations discussed earlier in the chapter. Cerebral blood flow increased initially due to the vasodilatation produced by the nitroprusside. However, as the amount of nitroprusside administered was increased, the mean arterial pressure decreased progressively. The cerebrovascular resistance was now being 'attacked' on two fronts — the direct pharmacological effects of the drug, and the physiological mechanisms which decrease resistance as perfusion pressure decreases. The net result was that the vessels reached their critical vasodilatory threshold rapidly and once

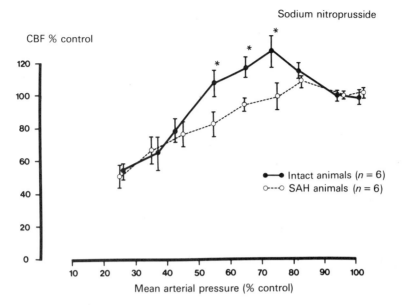

Fig. 27.7. Effects of nitroprusside-induced decreases in mean arterial pressure on cerebral blood flow. Investigations in intact baboons and in baboons 1 week after the induction of an artificial subarachnoid haemorrhage (SAH).

their reserve was exhausted flow decreased *pari passu* with any further decrease in systemic arterial pressure.

The *third* of the principles which ought to underly our understanding of cerebrovascular pharmacology is that — as for physiological mechanisms — the pharmacological effects of these drugs may be modified under pathological conditions. For example, the increase in intracranial pressure observed during the administration of halothane is augmented markedly in the presence of a space-occupying lesion (*see* Chapter 28): the characteristic relationship between cerebral blood flow and nitroprusside-induced decreases in arterial pressure (*Fig.* 27.7) is altered quite substantially 1 week after an experimentally induced subarachnoid haemorrhage. Thus, the clinician must be aware of these differences so that measures can be taken to use the relevant drug(s) appropriately in the individual patient.

Further reading

Edvinsson L. and MacKenzie E.T. Amine mechanisms in the cerebral circulation. *Pharmacol. Rev.* 1977; **28**: 275–347.

McDowall D.G. *Cerebral Circulation.* International Anesthesiology Clinics 7 (3). Boston: Little, Brown, 1969.

Phelps M.E., Mazziotta J.C. and Huang S.-C. Study of cerebral function with positron computed tomography. *J. Cereb. Blood Flow. Metabol.*, 1982; **2**: 113–62.

Roy C.S. and Sherrington C.S. On the regulation of the blood-supply of the brain. *J. Physiol. (Lond).* 1890; **11**: 85–109.

Smith F.W. Nuclear magnetic resonance in the investigation of cerebral disorder. *J. Cereb. Blood Flow Metabol.* 1983; **3**: 263–9.

Chapter 28

Cerebrospinal fluid: formation, composition and pressures

Once regarded as 'an uninteresting and fairly stagnant pool that passively fills the ventricles and cisterns of the central nervous sytem', the cerebrospinal fluid (CSF) is now thought to support and protect the brain and, along with the interstitial fluid of the brain, to provide that relative constancy of chemical environment which is necessary for optimal neuronal function.

Essentially, the brain is supported (within the arachnoid mater) by its blood vessels and nerve roots, and by the arachnoid trabeculae. The buoyancy provided by the CSF (in air the average brain weighs 1400–1500 g: buoyed by the CSF it weighs approximately 50 g) means the brain can be supported adequately by these relatively flimsy structures while, at the same time, being permitted a certain amount of movement within the confines of the skull.

The actual substance of the brain is densely packed with neurones and glial cells which, when examined by light microscopy, appear to abut each other 'like bricks laid without mortar'. However, the electron microscope has demonstrated convincingly that there is a narrow gap (average width 200 Å, 20 nm) between the cells as, indeed, between the cerebral capillaries and the cellular constituents of the brain. This space is filled with fluid (interstitial fluid) with a composition almost identical to that of the CSF (*see Table 28.1*). Two considerations of physiological interest ensue: first, there is no direct exchange of ions or molecules between neurones or between the neurones and the glial cells: any exchange takes place via this interstitial space. In the second place, the CSF is in free communication with the interstitial fluid such that the CSF plus the interstitial fluid make up the extracellular fluid of the brain. Not surprisingly, therefore, the CSF has been described as a 'major biological river' in that it can transport humoral messages from one region to another and provide a route for the

Table 28.1. Composition of cerebrospinal fluid: comparison with that of plasma

Constituent	CSF	Plasma
Sodium (mmol/l)	147	140
Potassium (mmol/l)	2·9	4·6
Chloride (mmol/l)	113	99
Calcium (mmol/l)	1·1	2·3
Bicarbonate (mmol/l)	23·1	24·8
Glucose (mmol/l)	<70% of simultaneously measured plasma concentration	4·0–5·5
Protein (g/l)	0·15–0·45	63–78
pH	7·28–7·33	7·38–7·72
P_{CO_2} (mmHg)	46–48	39–41

removal of the waste products of cellular metabolism (the brain does not possess a lymphatic system).

First in this chapter we will consider the formation, absorption and composition of CSF, and discuss briefly its physiological role. Secondly, we will describe the genesis and measurement of the pressure within the CSF and then consider, finally, why CSF pressure should increase and the effects of increases in CSF pressure.

Formation and absorption

FORMATION

In a relatively recent (1965) symposium concerned with the CSF, two consecutive papers opened with two contrasting statements. In the first, referring to the origin and fate of the CSF, the author stated that 'essentially the present viewpoint differs very little from that elaborated by Weed between 1914 and 1936'. In the second paper, the writer asserted that 'the results of recent investigations of CSF physiology have provided information which modifies substantially the old concept of the CSF circulation proposed by Weed in 1914'. Since both authors based their arguments on Weed's description, let us do likewise.

Weed's view was that the CSF was formed very largely in the *choroid plexuses* and moved thence into the *subarachnoid space* from which it was absorbed into the bloodstream through the *arachnoid villi*. This view has been modified, in the first place, by the likelihood that only about two-thirds of the CSF is actually formed by the choroid plexuses. By perfusing, on the one hand the ventricles and on the other the subarachnoid space with solutions of inulin, and then using the inulin clearance as a measure of the rate of absorption of CSF, it could be demonstrated (in the dog) that about 30 per cent of the CSF was produced outside the *ventricles*. The same appears to be true for the cat, while studies on hydrocephalic infants suggest that this concept may hold true in man as well.

The exact site (or sites) of CSF production *within* the ventricle is in itself somewhat unclear. What is not in doubt is that CSF *is* secreted by the choroid plexus, since it can be sampled directly from the surface of the plexus in an oil-filled ventricle. On the other hand, CSF can be formed in a lateral ventricle from which the choroid plexus has been removed surgically. The choroid plexuses consist of highly vascular tissue — each villous process being formed principally by a relatively large central (core) capillary surrounded by loose connective tissue. The epithelium of these capillaries is quite unlike that of other cerebral capillaries in that it is fenestrated and, being porous, permits the ready exchange of solutes. The choroidal epithelium consists of a single layer of modified *ependymal (columnar) cells*. These have apical brush borders and rest on a thin basement membrane. Adjacent cells are connected (near their apical or ventricular surfaces) by *tight junctions* which act as barriers to the passage of proteins and other large molecules from the blood to the CSF. This layer of ependymal cells is in continuity with those which line the walls of ventricles. Thus, although the bulk of the CSF is *secreted* (*see below*) via the choroid plexuses, it is also possible that some fluid can seep through the ependymal lining of the ventricles themselves and account for much of the extrachoroidal production of CSF.

Although the precise mechanisms underlying the secretory characteristics of the choroidal epithelium are incompletely understood, the primary process appears to be an *active secretion* (pumping) of sodium from blood to CSF. This is brought about by a cation pump (mediated by Na–K adenosine triphosphatase) located within the brush border of the epithelial cells. Potassium and hydrogen ions are pumped in the opposite direction, overall electrical neutrality being maintained by the associated movement of chloride and bicarbonate into the cell. The hydrogen ions and the bicarbonate ions are provided by the hydration of carbon dioxide under the influence of carbonic anhydrase. The movement of water into the CSF appears to result from the (extracellular) osmotic gradient which develops as the sodium is pumped out of the cells. Nerve endings (adrenergic and cholinergic) have been demonstrated in close proximity to the cells of the choroidal epithelium, and there is some evidence of the presence of α- and β-adrenoceptors in choroidal cell membranes. Thus, the autonomic nervous system may have some role in the regulation of the formation of CSF, although its precise role is not clear at the present time.

CIRCULATION

The CSF produced within the lateral ventricles circulates through the ventricular system before passing from the fourth ventricle via the foramina of Luschka and Magendie, into the *subarachnoid space*. CSF then passes either superiorly over the convexity of the brain or inferiorly into the subarachnoid space of the spinal canal. The 30 per cent or so of CSF which comes from extrachoroidal sources may contribute to the bulk movement of fluid within the brain parenchyma under physiological conditions. In grey matter, however, evidence is stronger for the existence of bulk flow under pathological conditions. Possible morphological conduits for such bulk flow may be the *Virchow–Robin spaces* which surround the intraparenchymal arteries and venules. These are bounded on one side by the basement membrane of the blood vessel and on the other by the basement of the glial cells, and are in continuity with the CSF in the subarachnoid space. Ultimately, the CSF reaches the arachnoid granulations or villi, and is absorbed into the venous circulation (principally into the *superior sagittal sinus*). As we shall consider in more detail later, the CSF pressure is not constant but fluctuates in concert with each heart beat and each respiratory cycle. At this point in our discussion it is sufficient to note that the amplitude of these pulsations is greatest in the lateral ventricles and that they decrease as one moves caudally in the cerebrospinal axis. It is thought that these cyclical and anatomical variations in CSF pressure help to agitate and circulate the CSF (and its constituents) around the subarachnoid space.

ABSORPTION

A second modification of the classical concept summarized by Weed resulted from the demonstration in 1961 of channels, lined with mesothelial cells, which were believed to penetrate the arachnoid villus. These channels had valve-like properties such that they were patent when the pressure in the subarachnoid space exceeded that in the superior sagittal sinus and, contrariwise, they closed when the pressure gradient was reversed. Thus, if the CSF pressure decreased to less than 70 mmH$_2$O (which approximates to the venous pressure in the sagittal sinus in the horizontal position), the reabsorption of CSF ceased. At CSF pressures above 70 mmH$_2$O (approximately) the rate of absorption of CSF was proportional to the CSF pressure. For example, the rate of absorption increased linearly from zero at 70 mmH$_2$O CSF pressure to around 1·5 ml/min when CSF pressure increased to 250 mmH$_2$O. Variations from the normal pattern of absorption have been described in patients with hydrocephalus (*see* p. 329).

The substitution of channels (of capillary diameter) for the semi-permeable membrane which was assumed previously to separate CSF and blood provided a ready explanation for the otherwise puzzling observations that labelled erythrocytes could pass from the CSF into the blood. Thus, it was no longer necessary to attribute the rapid disappearance of blood from the subarachnoid space to a peculiar faculty of the erythrocyte which enabled it to 'squeeze through' cellular membranes. However, this concept (of a microtubular system for the absorption of CSF) has been challenged recently following a series of detailed electron microscopic studies. These demonstrated, first, that the arachnoid villus was, in fact, covered with a complete 'cap' of mesothelial cells which were joined together by tight junctions. In the second place, it was noted that many of the mesothelial cells of the arachnoid villi contained vacuoles large enough to contain erythrocytes and the concept of a transcellular bulk flow of CSF was introduced. This postulates that the vacuoles are formed by an invagination of the basal (CSF) surface of the membrane and become an integral part of the cell. They then 'move across' the cell, fuse with the apical (blood) surface of the cell membrane and discharge their contents into the circulation.

Nevertheless, some doubt remains as to the *quantitative* importance of such mechanisms as far as the normal absorption of CSF is concerned. The time-honoured argument against the importance of the arachnoid villi as a drainage route, based on their absence in certain species of animal, and in many young animals, must carry some weight. To this must be added the demonstration that absorption of perfused artificial CSF can take place from ventricles which have been isolated from the subarachnoid space. Thus, although the arachnoid villi appear to be the main route for the reabsorption of CSF, there are almost certainly other possible pathways, perhaps through the ependymal lining of the ventricles or along the perineural sheaths of the spinal nerves. Thus, it would appear appropriate to think of the flow of CSF as taking place in a channel which, while it may begin at the choroid plexus and end at the arachnoid villi, is bounded by very leaky surfaces.

Before concluding this section on the general hydrodynamic aspects of CSF production and drainage, some reference should be made to the effects of variations in hydrostatic and osmotic pressures in the ventriculo-cisternal system on these processes. In the early 1960s Pappenheimer and his colleagues demonstrated elegantly that the rate of CSF *formation* (0·2–0·5 per cent of the total CSF volume per minute — or in adult man with a CSF volume of 150 ml the amount of CSF formed varies between 0·3 and 0·8 ml/min, average 0·35 ml/min or 500 ml per day) is virtually independent of the CSF pressure. This contrasts with the rate of *absorption* of CSF which, as has been mentioned previously, is sensitive to changes in pressure. The crystalloid osmotic pressure of the fluid perfusing the system affects predominantly the rate of formation of CSF. Perfusion with a fluid hypertonic with respect to plasma increases CSF production, although it should be noted that CSF continues to be formed even in the presence of a hypotonic perfusion fluid.

Composition

By virtue of the difference in composition between it and an ultrafiltrate of plasma, CSF must be regarded as a secretion, elaborated as a result of the selective activities of certain cells (p. 317). Moreover, the demonstration that substances such as diodrast and *para*-amino

hippuric acid can be transported actively out of the CSF into the systemic circulation against a concentration gradient means that the ultimate composition of the CSF may result from the combined contributions of secretory and reabsorptive processes in much the same way as the composition of urine is determined by the secretory and reabsorptive activities of the different parts of the nephron: in fact, CSF has been referred to as 'neural urine'.

Wherein does CSF actually differ from blood? *Table 28.1* includes a list of the normally accepted values for the constituents of CSF as obtained at lumbar puncture, and compares them with the concentrations present in plasma. CSF differs principally in having a very low protein concentration (0·20 g/l as against 60 g/l in plasma). Additionally, the concentrations of bicarbonate, glucose, urea, potassium, calcium and phosphate are lower in CSF than in blood, while those of sodium and chloride are higher.

The precise composition of the CSF is altered, under physiological conditions, as it passes along the cerebrospinal axis such that the composition of CSF sampled at lumbar puncture differs slightly from that obtained from the ventricles. Moreover, although the concentrations of the electrolytes (with the exception of phosphate) remain within narrow ranges under normal conditions, those of certain other constituents (for example, hydrogen ion) may vary substantially. However, the most marked alterations to the composition of the CSF are noted in association with pathological processes such as meningitis or cerebral neoplasia. Detailed consideration of the actual degree of change, and its diagnostic usefulness, is outwith the scope of this chapter. The interested reader is referred to the monograph by Fishman (1980) included in the list of Further Reading.

Blood–brain barrier

The initial concept that there was a barrier between the brain and the systemic circulation arose from studies carried out by Enrich in 1885 and Goldman in 1916. However, until the advent of electronmicroscopy the structural basis for this 'blood–brain barrier' was more a matter of conjecture than of demonstrated fact.

Twenty years ago Reese and Karnovsky injected horseradish peroxidase (an enzymic tracer which can be visualized under the electron microscope after a sequence of reactions) into mice. They noted that, although the tracer could pass freely from the systemic circulation into the extravascular space of tissues such as heart and skeletal muscle, it did not enter the brain: that is, there was a differential permeability of the brain to the tracer when compared with that in other organs. This difference in permeability is thought to be due primarily to the fact that the spaces between the endothelial cells which line the cerebral blood vessels (with the exception of those of the choroid plexuses) are true *tight junctions* and adhesions between the cerebral vascular endothelial cells 'could be said to form a morphological continuum'. Thus, unlike the situation in other organs, any substance passing from blood to brain must be taken up by the endothelial *cell* and then released on the contraluminal side of the capillary endothelium. In addition, unlike endothelial cells in peripheral vessels, those associated with the cerebral vasculature contain few, if any, vesicles. As a result, vesicular transport of substances is limited. We say 'limited' rather than non-existent because, although there is no evidence of vesicular transport as far as cerebral *capillaries* are concerned, parts of the arteriolar endothelium (vessels in the depths of sulci and those within the ventral diencephalon and adjacent brain stem), may be capable of the vesicular transport of substances from the lumen of the vessel to the extravascular space of the brain (or *from* the brain *to* the blood). Moreover, it has been suggested that the rate of such vesicular transport can be augmented by substances such as 5-hydroxytryptamine, noradrenaline and cyclic-3,5-adenosine monophosphate.

However, the morphological nature of the barrier means that not only does its permeability differ from that in other organs but also that the blood–brain barrier itself shows marked differences in permeability to substances of differing molecular weight, degree of ionization or lipoid solubility. Regardless of the actual nature of the barrier, the movement of a substance into the cells requires ultimately penetration of the plasma membrane — a bimolecular lipoid layer with an inner and outer adsorbed layer of protein. Penetration of such a membrane by any substance is facilitated by lipoid solubility: in general, the greater the lipoid solubility, the more rapid the penetration (for review see Pardridge, Connar and Crawford, 1975).

CSF–brain barrier

It is important to remember that as well as a blood–brain barrier there is also a CSF–brain barrier which consists of the *ependymal lining* of the ventricles plus the layer of neural tissue which lies immediately below the lining. The available evidence would suggest that the CSF–brain barrier does not possess the same structural features as the blood–brain barrier. If one injects horseradish peroxidase into the ventricular system there is evidence of diffusion into the parenchyma of the brain. In fact, quite large molecules (inulin, urea, creatinine, certain chemotherapeutic agents) can cross the CSF–brain barrier (possibly through the channels, p. 317, situated between the cells of the ependymal lining) and then diffuse readily through the interstitial space of the brain itself.

For the anaesthetist, the peculiar characteristics of the blood–brain and CSF–brain barriers are of interest and of practical importance — particularly in regard to the penetration of anaesthetic agents, physiological gases and acid-base components. The importance of lipoid solubility has been recognized for some time and is the basis of the Meyer–Overton law which relates anaesthetic potency to the lipoid solubility of various anaesthetic agents. Equally important is the failure of certain drugs to penetrate the barrier. Tubocurarine, given intrathecally, produces profound effects on the central nervous system which result in excitation and convulsions. That these do not occur after the intravenous administration of the drug is explained conveniently by a blood–brain barrier which prevents significant entry of this drug.

Carbon dioxide, oxygen, water and to a lesser degree, glucose, move freely between the systemic circulation and the brain. This is not unexpected since these molecules are necessary for the maintenance of the normal physiological and biochemical environment of the brain. Although glucose is the only metabolic substrate known to cross the blood–brain barrier in significant amounts, uptake is delayed to some extent. This, plus the unimpeded permeability of water, accounts for the initial decrease in brain mass that accompanies the intravenous infusion of a hypertonic solution of glucose — and the subsequent reversal of the osmotic gradient that then produces a rebound phenomenon and an increase in brain bulk. The rapid movement of carbon dioxide across the blood–brain barrier has profound and complex effects on the acid-base balance of the CSF, particularly since both hydrogen ions and bicarbonate ions penetrate much more slowly. This latter area is of considerable interest to the anaesthetist and will be discussed more fully later. Meantime, we should conclude our consideration of the blood–brain barrier by noting those circumstances under which the barrier may break down, and the consequences of such disruption.

Under physiological conditions, the blood–brain barrier is notable for its resistance to a wide variety of physical and pharmacological insults. However, 'opening' of the barrier can be produced experimentally (*see* Chapter 27) or may be associated with a number of disease processes: acute arterial hypertension, hypoxia, repeated seizure activity, neoplasia, lead intoxication, ionizing radiation, infection. A detailed description of all the situations in which there is disruption of the blood–brain barrier would be out of place in this book (*see* Further Reading). However, a brief consideration of the mechanism(s) of breakdown and of the clinical consequences of breakdown would seem relevant.

Disruption of the blood–brain barrier can be caused by insults which either increase the tension in the walls of small vessels (acute arterial hypertension, repeated seizures) or which damage the endothelial lining in other ways (radiation, direct trauma, heavy metal poisoning, inflammation). As far as brain tumours are concerned, it has been suggested that it might be more correct to talk of a complete absence of the blood–brain barrier rather than of a breakdown, since the morphological changes to the endothelial lining and basement membranes are substantial. As a result, there may be disruption of the tight junctions between the endothelial cells or there may be an activation of vesicular transport. Whatever the actual ultrastructural mechanism, vascular permeability is increased and leads to the accumulation of a protein-rich fluid in the extracellular space of the brain (vasogenic oedema). The fluid accumulates principally in the white matter producing, initially, a localized increase in tissue pressure which will compress adjacent veins and favour further exudation of fluid. Ultimately, the bulk of the brain increases and there will be a generalized increase in intracranial pressure.

The disruption of the blood–brain barrier may be reversible on removal of the insult (restoration of arterial pressure) or it may be possible to decrease the symptoms produced by the disruption with glucocorticoids, or osmotherapeutic agents. Glucocorticoids are probably the most effective agents in this context and may have a prophylactic role also in that they appear to make the cerebral vessels more resistant to those physical and chemical insults which induce disruption. Hypertonic solutions (urea, mannitol, glycerol) are used widely to decrease the bulk of the brain and, hence, reduce intracranial pressure. However, they act by reversing the osmotic gradient across an *intact* blood–brain barrier. Thus, although they can remove water from normal brain, they cannot do likewise from oedematous brain, since the vessels have lost their semi-permeable properties.

CSF acid-base balance

The hydrogen ion concentration of the cerebral extracellular fluid(s) plays a fundamental role in the regulation of ventilation (*see* Chapter 20), and may have a less fundamental but none the less important role in the physiological control of cerebrovascular resistance (*see* Chapter 27). Moreover, the acid-base status of the CSF may yield information about the adequacy, or otherwise, of cerebral oxygenation. In this section we will consider the basic mechanisms which regulate CSF pH, and highlight those aspects which are of particular clinical relevance.

The hydrogen ion concentration of CSF is maintained, under physiological conditions, at a value which is slightly less alkaline (7·28–7·33) than that of arterial blood (7·38–7·42). This difference is accounted for, in part, by a higher partial pressure of carbon dioxide (46–48 mmHg) in the CSF and, in part, by a lower bicarbonate concentration (approximately 23–24 mmol/l). As a result, there cannot be, even under steady-state conditions, complete equilibrium between the hydrogen ions in blood and those in the CSF. Thus, there is an *electrochemical gradient* (4 millivolts positive with respect to plasma) between the plasma and the CSF, the presence of which suggests that there must be a mechanism, or mechanisms, which act specifically to maintain the relative acidity of the CSF. What this mechanism is, is open to debate and need not concern us here, apart from indicating that the two most popular mechanisms are the 'active transport' of hydrogen ions (against the pH gradient and against the electrochemical gradient), and the 'passive diffusion' mechanism (the diffusion of the hydrogen ions along a concentration gradient from the intracellular fluid → extracellular fluid, including CSF, → blood).

In addition to the differences in acid-base components across the blood–brain barrier (or more correctly in relation to the present discussion the blood–CSF barrier), differences in the acid-base composition of CSF can be detected between cisternal CSF and lumbar CSF, even in normal individuals. Thus, at steady-state, lumbar CSF is more acid than cisternal CSF since the partial pressure of carbon dioxide is slightly higher in the lumbar fluid (the CSF bicarbonate concentration is the same at both sites). However, the differences are small in the normal individual and are unlikely to be of clinical significance. In contrast, in the acutely ill patient, or in unsteady states (as, for example, following an alteration in alveolar ventilation), the disparity in pH between the two sites is greater, since the changes in the acid-base balance of lumbar CSF lag behind those in cisternal CSF. Thus, there may be occasions when it would be inappropriate to depend on the results obtained from lumbar CSF.

At this point it may be relevant to digress slightly and point out that it is extremely difficult to measure CSF pH with any degree of accuracy. CSF contains negligible concentrations of buffer anions (other than bicarbonate) and, consequently, cannot buffer effectively those changes in pH produced by alterations in carbon dioxide tension. Thus, anaerobic conditions must be maintained during and after sampling, and the presence of air bubbles in the syringe will produce spurious results. Theoretically, valid measurements can only be obtained if ventilation is constant at the time of sampling. This is difficult to ensure under clinical conditions and it may be helpful to monitor the alevolar (end-tidal) carbon dioxide concentration to verify the stability of ventilation during sampling.

In addition to its acidity with respect to blood, there is another feature of CSF acid-base physiology which is worthy of note: the remarkable *constancy of CSF pH* in the face of changes in blood pH — other than those changes in blood pH due to alterations in blood carbon dioxide tension. For example, CSF pH remains virtually unaffected in experimental animals in which blood pH has been altered chemically by the infusion of acid or alkali. Likewise, most investigators agree that, in man, CSF pH changes little in association with chronic systemic non-respiratory acidosis (for example, renal insufficiency, diabetes) or alkalosis (hepatic disease, ingestion of bicarbonate). Although opinions differ as to the actual mechanism(s) of this regulation of CSF pH (and the role of respiratory compensation in the maintenance of CSF acid-base balance) this apparent dissociation between changes in blood and CSF must be due basically to the point made earlier, that hydrogen ions and bicarbonate ions penetrate the blood–CSF barrier with relative difficulty. In contrast, CSF pH will change rapidly in association with alterations in blood pH which are due to increases or decreases in blood carbon dioxide tension since, as we have noted earlier, carbon dioxide can diffuse rapidly across the blood–CSF barrier. As a result, hypocapnia (mechanical ventilation) and hypercapnia (respiratory inadequacy) can induce rapid, and substantial alterations in CSF pH. However, for reasons which should become clear later, the persistence of such alterations in CSF pH would be not only unphysiological but also inimical to neuronal function and to normal cerebrovascular reactivity. Thus, compensation (that is, a return of pH to its physiological value) must take place even if the stimulus to the change (hypocapnia, hypercapnia) persists.

Once again there appears to be disagreement as to the details of such compensatory mechanisms, but it is probably sufficient for our purposes to indicate that they involve the passage of hydrogen ions or bicarbonate ions across the blood–CSF barrier to balance the acid or alkaline shift in CSF pH. For the reasons given earlier, this normalization of CSF pH is a relatively slow procedure at the end of which, although CSF pH will be at or close to its physiological value, the bicarbonate concentration of the CSF will be greater than, or less than, its normal value. For example, in a group of patients with chronic obstructive airways disease and retention of carbon dioxide (Pa_{CO_2} = 62 mmHg, 8·2 kPa), CSF pH was at the lower limit of its physiological range (7·28): that is, compensation had occurred and was due to an increase in the CSF bicarbonate concentration from a normal value of 23 mmol/l to a value of 31 mmol/l. Conversely, prolonged hypocapnia due to passive hyperventilation will induce a compensatory shift of bicarbonate out of the CSF and a decrease in the bicarbonate concentration of the CSF.

The clinical relevance, at least as far as the anaesthetist is concerned, derives from the demonstrations by Leusen in the early 1950s and Pappenheimer and colleagues in the early 1960s of the cardinal role played by CSF pH in the control of respiration. The central chemoreceptors are situated just below the surface of the ventrolateral aspect of the medulla (Chapter 20) and are sensitive to changes in the hydrogen ion concentration of the CSF: an increase in hydrogen ion concentration stimulating respiration and, conversely, a decrease in hydrogen ion concentration depressing the central drive to respiration. Thus, if one attempts to wean a patient from mechanical hyperventilation following a prolonged period of deliberate hyperventilation he may continue to hyperventilate since any attempt to return his arterial carbon dioxide tension to normal will increase the partial pressure of carbon dioxide in the CSF and, hence, increase its

acidity — at least until the change in pH has been normalized by an increase in CSF bicarbonate concentration.

For many years anaesthetists have been concerned that the cerebral vasoconstriction induced by extreme hyperventilation (Pa_{CO_2} less than 20 mmHg, 2·7 kPa) might be detrimental on account of the substantial decrease in perfusion. Measurements of CSF acid-base status have been used to address this problem, and suggest that there is evidence of an acid shift in CSF pH (due, most probably, to an increase in the lactic acid concentration of the CSF) under these circumstances.

Cerebrospinal fluid pressure

If we insert a needle into the *cisterna magna* of an experimental animal, or into the *lumbar subarachnoid space* in a patient, CSF will usually flow out of the needle spontaneously, indicating that there is a pressure within the craniospinal axis which is greater than atmospheric. Since a variety of pathological processes (within the craniospinal axis) produce increases in the pressure(s) measured in the CSF, and since many only become symptomatic or life-threatening when they do so, it is important that we consider the genesis and measurement of the CSF pressure, the mechanisms inducing an increase in CSF pressure and the possible clinical sequelae of untreated high CSF pressure.

In clinical practice it is customary to use the terms 'CSF pressure' and 'intracranial pressure' as if they were synonymous. In this discussion we will use the term CSF pressure throughout to indicate that, in physiological terms, we are considering the pressure within the whole of the craniospinal axis and, indeed, will indicate those situations in which there may be differences in the measured value of CSF pressure in different anatomical sites. Intracranial pressure should, correctly, only be applied to CSF pressure (or brain tissue pressure, or extradural pressure) measured in the supratentorial compartment.

In the normal adult, the *volume* of CSF varies from 140 to 200 ml, with some 25–35 ml in the ventricular system, and the rest being distributed between the cerebral and spinal subarachnoid spaces. This compares with an

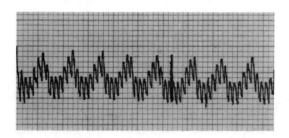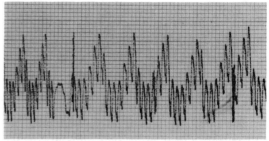

Fig. 28.1. Recordings of CSF pressure measured in the supratentorial compartment under conditions of normal (*a*) and increased (*b*) pressure. Each heavy horizontal line (vertical axis) represents 5 mmHg.

intracranial vascular volume of 100–150 ml, and a brain and spinal cord volume of 1200–1500 ml.

Under physiological conditions, the absolute value of the pressure within the craniospinal axis (measured with the subject in the horizontal position) varies between 7 and 12 mmHg, and is determined by the balance between the rate of formation of CSF and the rate of reabsorption — the latter being related to the pressure in the venous sinuses and the 'resistance' of the absorptive mechanism. As discussed earlier (p. 318) the absorption of CSF through the arachnoid granulations is related to the CSF pressure. Thus, if the CSF is to continue to circulate, the CSF pressure must be greater than the sum of the pressure in the dural sinus (at the point of entry of the arachnoid villi) *and* the pressure required to overcome the resistance of the villi, otherwise the CSF would cease to circulate.

In the horizontal position, and in the absence of any obstruction to the CSF pathways, the CSF pressure will be similar throughout the craniospinal axis. However, as one assumes the sitting position, the pressure measured supratentorially will decrease whereas that in the lumbar subarachnoid space will increase, due to the difference in hydrostatic pressure between the two sites. However, Davson has indicated that the CSF space can be considered to be a fluid-filled tube, closed at one end. Even if one turns such a tube into the vertical position, fluid will not run out of the bottom end since the pressure at the foot is no greater than atmospheric. In the context of the present discussion, this ought to indicate that CSF pressure in the lumbar area would not increase as one sat up. However, unlike the situation in a rigid tube, lumbar CSF pressure does increase (because the upper end — the intracranial dura — is not absolutely rigid) but the increase is only a proportion of that due, theoretically, to the hydrostatic difference.

Fig. 28.1 demonstrates clearly that CSF pressure is not constant but fluctuates in time with the heart beat, and with respiration. In the example illustrated, the variation in CSF pressure produced by each heart beat is approximately 4 mmHg, and that due to each respiratory cycle, around 9 mmHg. However, these values were obtained in the subarachnoid space over the convexity of the hemisphere and are representative of this site only. The amplitude of these pulsations is maximal in the lateral ventricles and decreases as one moves caudally, such that the amplitude of the pulsations in the lumbar subarachnoid space is only 40–50 per cent of that in the lateral ventricles. In addition to the difference in the absolute value of the pulsations (between ventricle and lumbar area), there will be a time delay as the pressure wave passes down the craniospinal axis, and it has been suggested that these cyclical changes in pressure help to mix the CSF, and to circulate it around the subarachnoid space. It is of interest to note that the amplitude of the pulsations produced by the heart beat is related also to the actual CSF pressure: if CSF pressure is high, the amplitude of the pulsations will be high also (*Fig.* 28.1*b*). Indeed, pulse amplitude has been used as an assessment of the compliance of the intracranial contents.

Classically, it was assumed that those pulsations synchronous with the heart beat arose from the pulsation of the choroid plexuses and, consequently, were greatest in the lateral ventricles. However, the argument that the pulsations originate as a result of the pulsatile changes in the volume of the large arteries around the base of the brain would be difficult to refute.

Fortunately, there is no divergence of opinion as far as the origin of the pulsations associated with respiration are concerned. The CSF spaces can be considered as a plethysmographic extension of the intrathoracic cavity. Consequently, changes in intrathoracic pressure will be reflected in changes in CSF pressure. The recordings depicted in *Fig.* 28.1 were obtained during positive pressure ventilation — the increases in CSF pressure being in accord with inspiration. In a patient breathing spontaneously the CSF pressure will decrease during inspiration as a result of the decrease in intrathoracic pressure. Although the CSF spaces can be considered as a plethysmographic extension of the thoracic cavity, one might well ask, How are the changes in pressure transmitted to the CSF spaces since there is no direct communication between the two? Any change in intrathoracic pressure is transmitted to the thin-walled veins in the thorax and then to the *jugular and vertebral veins*. If the pressure in these veins increases, for example, this is transmitted to the veins inside the skull — particularly the thin-walled veins which lie on the surface of the brain. The volume in these veins increases, total intracranial blood volume increases and the CSF pressure increases.

It will be obvious from this description that, should high inflation pressures or positive end-expiratory pressure be required in the management of an individual patient, or should the patient cough or 'fight the ventilator', CSF pressure will be increased acutely — at least in the short term. Likewise, CSF pressure will be increased if there is pressure on the jugular or vertebral veins due to poor positioning of the head. In the absence of intracranial pathology these changes are probably of little clinical importance in that they can be compensated for by a translocation of CSF from the cranial to the spinal CSF space; and by an increased reabsorption of CSF. However, for reasons which we will discuss

later, the clinical significance of such alterations in CSF pressure is much greater in the presence of intracranial space-occupying pathology.

At this point it would seem appropriate to consider in a little more detail the relationship between CSF pressure and the various pertinent venous pressures. First, there is the pressure in the veins on the surface of the brain itself: these are thin-walled and lack any significant muscle in their walls. Thus, they can dilate easily, and are subject to the pressure surrounding them — the CSF pressure. It will be evident that the pressure in these vessels must be greater than the CSF pressure: otherwise, the blood would stop circulating. Indeed, the pressure in these *surface veins* has been shown to be some 5–6 mmHg higher than the average CSF pressure. Secondly, there is the pressure in the *dural sinuses* within the skull. In contradistinction to the veins described above, these are 'protected' from changes in the CSF pressure by the rigid walls of the sinuses. Following the arguments adduced earlier in the chapter, it will be evident that the pressure in the dural sinuses must be less than the pressure in the CSF (to allow the reabsorption of CSF) and that, consequently, there must be a pressure drop at the point where the surface cerebral veins enter the sinus. Thirdly, there is the pressure in the *jugular vein*, a pressure that is influenced by the pressure in the dural sinuses, the *central venous pressure* and atmospheric pressure to which the jugular veins are exposed in the neck. However, whatever the various influences on this pressure, in absolute terms it must be less than that in the venous sinuses to permit the flow of venous blood to the heart.

In contrast to the significant influences of venous pressure on CSF pressure, arterial pressure has little effect *under physiological conditions*. As we have discovered already, there are systolic/diastolic fluctuations in CSF pressure which are due to the systolic/diastolic variations in arterial pressure. Otherwise, changes in arterial pressure do not affect CSF pressure as long as autoregulation is intact, and as long as the upper and lower limits of autoregulation are not exceeded (*see* Chapter 27). However, if these circumstances do not pertain, changes in arterial pressure will be mirrored by changes in CSF pressure, due to the transmission of a greater proportion of the arterial pressure to the venous side of the cerebral circulation.

The final point to consider in this discussion of the various physiological factors which influence the CSF pressure is the effect of alterations in the cerebral blood flow itself. Briefly, changes in cerebral blood flow parallel and induce immediate changes in CSF pressure. This is because any change in blood flow will alter the amount of blood in the thin-walled cerebral veins — the *cerebral blood volume* — and lead to an increase in CSF pressure, at least in the short term. However, in time, some compensation will occur and the CSF pressure will tend to return to its baseline values. Thus, if one induces hypocapnia, for example, with artificial ventilation, cerebral blood flow will decrease (*see* Chapter 27), less blood will reach the cerebral veins, the actual volume of blood inside the skull will decrease and, as a result, CSF pressure will decrease (at least temporarily).

MEASUREMENT OF CSF PRESSURE

METHODS

Traditionally, pressure has been measured following the insertion of a needle into the lumbar subarachnoid space or of a catheter into one or other lateral ventricle. Customarily, the needle is connected to a manometer held perpendicular to the patient's spine, and the catheter connected to an appropriate transducer via fluid-filled narrow-bore tubing. Of these two methods, the intraventricular is the more relevant clinically for a number of reasons. Using this system it is possible to obtain good quality recordings which show not only the physiological variations produced by the heart beat and respiration, but also those that occur as a result of alterations in intracranial compliance (*see below*); the pressure can be measured continuously without movement of the patient creating a problem and, very importantly, pressure measured in the lumbar subarachnoid space will not be representative of supratentorial pressure once obstruction of the CSF pathways has occurred.

CSF pressure can be measured in the subarachnoid space over the convexity of the hemisphere either by placing a catheter in the subarachnoid space, or by inserting a bolt in the skull using a specially manufactured drill. As with the catheter systems, the bolt is connected to a transducer via a fluid-filled system. If the dura mater has been opened, the bolt will measure subarachnoid (subdural) CSF pressure: if the dura mater is left intact, it will measure extradural pressure.

VALUE

With the advent of CT scanning, the monitoring of intracranial pressure (ICP) has become virtually obsolete as a diagnostic tool. Nevertheless, this does not mean that it is no longer of value as a guide to appropriate management in an individual patient as, for example, in those head injured patients in an intensive care unit who are in receipt of neuromuscular blockade and artificial ventilation.

There are three sources of information available from the ICP record: first, the mean intracranial pressure and its trends; secondly, information derived from the size of the fluctuations in mean intracranial pressure as a response to nursing procedures, physiotherapy and tests of intracranial compliance; and thirdly, the actual amplitude of the variations in intracranial pressure associated with heart rate and respiration. The normal physiological intracranial pressure is around 10 mmHg with, as we have seen, superimposed pulsations corresponding to heart rate and ventilation. There is general agreement that a sustained value greater than 15 mmHg is abnormal but, for clinical purposes, it has been suggested that values greater than 20 mmHg should be considered moderately increased and those above 40 mmHg markedly increased.

From what we have discussed previously about the relationship between intrathoracic pressure and CSF pressure, it will be evident that the pressure inside the skull can be altered quite substantially, by many so-called routine clinical manoeuvres such as movement of the patient, tracheal suction, chest physiotherapy and so on. For reasons which will become apparent later, the changes in CSF pressure induced by such manoeuvres are substantially greater in the patient with intracranial pathology and, indeed, may be of sufficient magnitude to decrease the perfusion pressure to the brain significantly.

Of the other information available from the recording of intracranial pressure, it is worth noting that the amplitude of the circulatory and ventilatory oscillations is also increased in the presence of intracranial pathology (*Fig. 28.1b*) and may be used to provide a continuous and useful monitor of the degree of intracranial compression — the greater the oscillations, the 'tighter' the intracranial contents.

Having now alluded to the influence of intracranial pathology on CSF pressure it is appropriate to note at this point that, in addition to the normal physiological fluctuations in CSF pressure, three distinct waves are recognized in association with increases in mean intracranial pressure.

'A' waves or plateau waves

These are defined as periods of intracranial pressure above 50 mmHg (*Fig. 28.2a*) which persist for at least 5 minutes and which increase and decrease rapidly, generally to their original value. These occur against a background of an increase in intracranial pressure and are usually precipitated by some stimulus — physiotherapy, hypercarbia, pain, the administration of a volatile anaesthetic.

'B' waves

'B' waves are smaller than 'A' waves (10–15 mmHg in amplitude) and occur at intervals of 30 seconds to 2 minutes (*Fig. 28.2b*). Like 'A' waves they are an important sign of intracranial compression: *Fig. 28.2c* depicts a series of 'B' waves preceding and leading eventually to a series of 'A' waves.

'C' waves

'C' waves occur at a rate of around five per minute, are of low amplitude and are thought to correspond to certain variations in arterial pressure.

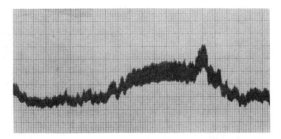

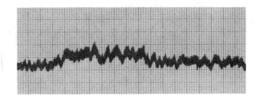

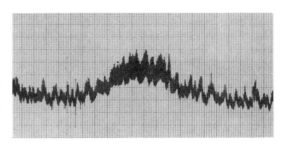

Fig. 28.2. Recordings of CSF pressure measured in the lateral ventricle of one patient with intracranial hypertension. *a*, Plateau waves, *b*, 'B' waves, *c*, a series of 'B' waves proceeding to 'A' waves. Vertical axis, pressure: each heavy line = 10 mmHg; horizontal axis, time.

Mechanism of the increase in intracranial pressure

The adult skull is a rigid and virtually closed container, containing four tissue/fluid compartments (*Table* 28.2): cells (neurones and glia), cerebrospinal fluid, interstitial fluid, and blood, the blood being present in both arteries and veins. An increase in the volume of any one of these compartments leads to a decrease in the space available for the other three. For example, an increase in the cellular component by a tumour leads initially to distortion of the normal anatomical architecture of the brain

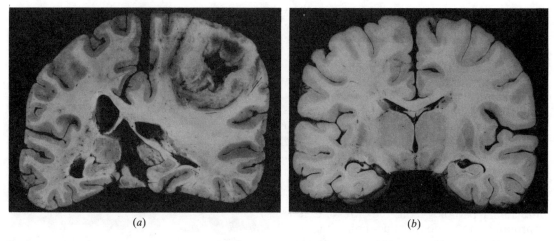

(a)   (b)

Fig. 28.3. Coronal sections of the brain showing alterations to the normal anatomical architecture produced by neoplastic disease (a) and by cerebral oedema (b). Kindly supplied by Professor D. I. Graham.

Table 28.2. Intracranial tissue and fluid compartments (with average volume)

Compartment	Approx. volume (ml)
Cellular compartments	
Glia	700–900
Neurones	500–700
Fluid compartments	
CSF	100–150
Interstitial	75
Blood	100–150

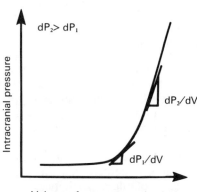

Fig. 28.4. Changes in CSF pressure resulting from a progressive increase in intracranial volume.

(*Fig.* 28.3a) and eventually to movement of the brain within the skull — this being a form of spatial compensation for the increase in the *cellular compartment*. Ultimately, however, if the movement is sufficiently great, coning will occur and lead to obstruction to the cerebrospinal fluid pathways. *Fig.* 28.3b shows a brain in which there is evidence of considerable cerebral oedema (an increase in water content). This increase in *interstitial fluid volume* has been offset to some extent by a decrease in another of the compartments — the *cerebrospinal fluid compartment*. As alluded to above, this also is referred to as 'compensation', and explains the commonly depicted pressure/volume compliance curve (*Fig.* 28.4) in which the pressure generated within a closed or virtually closed container, is related to changes in the volume of that container. The essential point of this graph is that, initially, the intracranial space can compensate for changes in intracranial volume, but that as the relationship moves towards the right-hand side of the graph, compensation becomes exhausted and any further increases in volume are accompanied by more marked increases in CSF pressure: the 'tighter' the brain the more marked the induced alterations in CSF pressure (*Fig.* 28.5).

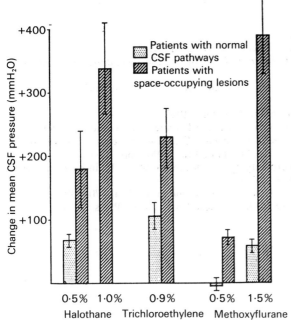

Fig. 28.5. Changes in CSF pressure (mean ± s.e. mean) produced by the administration of certain volatile anaesthetic agents to patients with and without intracranial space-occupying lesions.

Although we do not wish to dwell too long on the abnormal, it is pertinent to consider certain points since they provide evidence of the limits of physiological control, and are of clinical importance. First, the major compensatory mechanisms are the translocation of cerebrospinal fluid from the intracranial space to the intraspinal space, and the extrusion of blood from the thin-walled veins on the surface of the brain. As a result, there is a limit to the degree of compensation possible. Secondly, compensation takes some time to develop. Thus, any sudden alterations in the volume of another compartment, regardless of the position of the patient on the curve, will increase intracranial pressure acutely. In this context we refer back to those changes that can be induced by the administration of a volatile anaesthetic agent, physiotherapy, straining, 'fighting the ventilator' and so on. Thirdly, of the four compartments depicted in *Table* 28.2, the anaesthetist cannot influence the cellular compartment at all, can influence the interstitial fluid compartment only slowly as, for example,

with mannitol, and can do little with the volume of the cerebrospinal fluid compartment *per se*, unless he inserts a ventricular or spinal drain. The anaesthetist can, however, alter *cerebral blood volume* and this has obvious clinical relevance.

Of the four compartments we have been discussing, the cerebral blood volume is the only compartment which is capable of increasing or decreasing its volume quickly. Thus, manipulation of this compartment can produce rapidly effective changes in the clinical condition of a patient. For example, the application of hyperventilation and the associated decrease in carbon dioxide tension may decrease rapidly cerebral blood volume and hence, CSF pressure. Contrariwise, of course, the administration of pharmacological agents which decrease cerebral vascular resistance (*see Table* 27.3) and, consequently, increase cerebral blood volume, will increase CSF pressure acutely.

Fourthly, as far as the CSF compartment itself is concerned, increases in the volume of CSF within the craniospinal axis are rarely due to an increase in the amount of CSF produced: usually, they result from some defect in absorption. In non-communicating hydrocephalus due, for example, to a stenosis of the aqueduct there is impaired access to the absorptive mechanism. Two types of communicating hydrocephalus are described (at least in children). In one (Type I) the pressure at which the absorption of CSF occurs first is greater than normal (by around 13 mmHg) but the relationship between the rate of change in CSF pressure and the rate of absorption remains physiological. In the other (Type II) the critical 'opening' pressure is normal but the relationship is altered: the conductance to the outflow of CSF is decreased.

The cerebral circulation is unique in that the variations in the diameter of the cerebral blood vessels and the alterations in cerebral blood volume take place within an almost completely closed 'container'. Although specific physiological mechanisms mitigate the potential disadvantages of this arrangement, it is important, for the clinician, to appreciate the limits of such physiological compensation as well as the situations in which it is inoperative.

Further reading

Bradbury M. *The Concept of a Blood–Brain Barrier*. Chichester: Wiley, 1979.

Brooks C. McC., Kao F.F. and Lloyd B.B. (ed.) *Cerebrospinal Fluid and the Regulation of Ventilation*. Oxford: Blackwell, 1965.

Cutler R.W.P., Page L., Galicich J. et al. Formation and absorption of cerebrospinal fluid in man. *Brain* 1968; **91**: 707–20.

Davson H. *Physiology of the Cerebrospinal Fluid*. London: Churchill, 1967.

Fishman R.A. *Cerebrospinal Fluid in Diseases of the Nervous System* Philadelphia: Saunders, 1980.

Pappenheimer J.R. *The ionic composition of cerebral extracellular fluid and its relation to control of breathing. The Harvey Lectures 1965–1966*. New York: Academic Press, 1967, pp. 71–94.

Pardridge W.M., Connor J.D. and Crawford I.L. Permeability changes in the blood–brain barrier: causes and consequences. *CRC Crit. Rev. Toxicol.* 1975; **3**: 159–99.

Plum F. and Siesjo B.K. Recent advances in CSF physiology. *Anesthesiology* 1975; **42**: 708–30.

Rapoport S.I. *Blood–Brain Barrier in Physiology and Medicine*. New York: Raven Press, 1976.

Index